Student Workbook

Outdoor Emergency Care

**Comprehensive Prehospital Care
for Nonurban Settings**

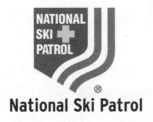

National Ski Patrol

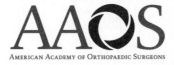

American Academy of Orthopaedic Surgeons

JONES AND BARTLETT PUBLISHERS

Sudbury, Massachusetts

BOSTON   TORONTO   LONDON   SINGAPORE

Outdoor Emergency Care: Comprehensive Prehospital Care for Nonurban Settings, Fourth Edition

Student Workbook

World Headquarters
40 Tall Pine Drive
Sudbury, MA 01776
978-443-5000
info@jbpub.com
www.jbpub.com

Jones and Bartlett Publishers Canada
6339 Ormindale Way
Mississauga, ON L5V 1J2
CANADA

Jones and Bartlett Publishers
International
Barb House, Barb Mews
London W6 7PA
UK

ISBN-10: 0-7637-1194-2, ISBN-13: 978-0-7637-1194-8

This Student Workbook is intended solely as a guide to the appropriate procedures to be employed when rendering emergency care to the sick and injured. It is not intended as a statement of the standards of care required in any particular situation, because circumstances and the patient's physical condition can vary widely from one emergency to another. Nor is it intended that this Student Workbook shall in any way advise emergency personnel concerning legal authority to perform the activities or procedures discussed. Such local determinations should be made only with the aid of legal counsel.

Note: The patients depicted in *Calls to the Scene* are fictitious.

Editorial Credits

Author: Rhonda J. Beck, NREMT-P

National Ski Patrol

Editors: Judy Over, Leif Borgeson

Contributors:

Karen Anderson-Hadden, RN
Anthony N. Brown
Michael J. Costa
Marcia Ellis, PA-C
Steve Francisco
Daniel Goldberger, MD
Dayle Hadden
Bryant F. Hall, BS (MT), MBA
Erica Krol, PA-C

Charles L. Lentz, MA
Robert T. Maybury, RN, CFRN, EMT-P
Robert Offerle
Frank Saylor
Suzanne Wise
Ann T. Wood, EMT
David Worfel
Kathleen A. Young

American Academy of Orthopaedic Surgeons

Vice President, Educational Programs: Mark W. Wieting
Director, Department of Publications: Marilyn L. Fox, PhD
Managing Editor: Lynne Roby Shindoll
Senior Editor: Barbara A. Scotese
Associate Senior Editor: Susan Morritz Baim

Production Credits

Publisher, Emergency Care: Kimberly Brophy
Emergency Care Associate Editor: Carol Brewer
Manufacturing Buyer: Therese Bräuer
Senior Production Editor: Linda S. DeBruyn

Interior Design: Anne Spencer
Cover Design: Studio Montage, Philip Regan
Composition: AnnMarie Lemoine, Laura Wiegleb
Printing and Binding: Courier Company

Printed in the United States of America

11 10   10 9 8 7 6 5

Table of Contents

Technology Resources

An important part of learning to become a great outdoor rescuer is doing. You will find numerous types of interactivities and simulations at our website: **www.OECzone.com**.

www.OECzone.com

Anatomy Review–
interactive anatomic figure labeling

Web Links–
present current information including trends in health care, the outdoor rescue community, and new equipment.

Online Outlook–
activities further reinforce and expand on topics covered in each chapter.

Online Chapter Pretests–
prepare students for training with instant results, feedback on incorrect answers, and page references to the Fourth Edition.

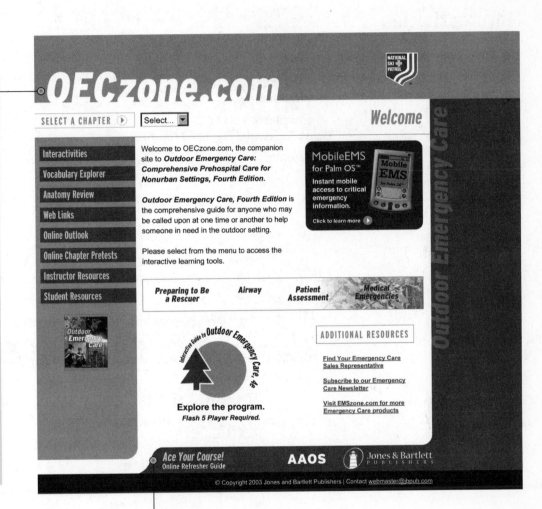

Online Refresher Guide–
prepare for annual refreshers and continuing education sessions with this handy guide providing instant results, feedback, and page references.

Interactivities

Videos: Skills in Action–

watch an experienced provider perform critical skills.

Interactive Simulations–

practice rescuer skills in the safety of a virtual environment.

Assessment in Action–

scenarios challenge your problem-solving abilities and give feedback.

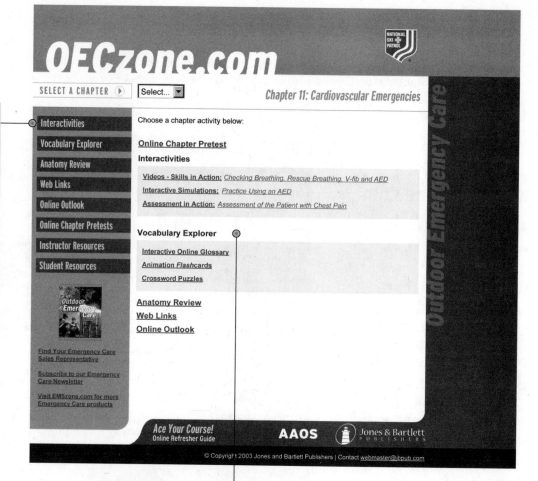

Vocabulary Explorer

Interactive Online Glossary–

expand your medical vocabulary, complete with sound and images.

Animated FlashCards–

review vital vocabulary and key concepts.

Workbook Activities

The following activities have been designed to help you. Your instructor may require you to complete some or all of these activities as a regular part of your OEC training program. You are encouraged to complete any activity that your instructor does not assign as a way to enhance your learning in the classroom.

Chapter Review

The following exercises provide an opportunity to refresh your knowledge of this chapter.

■ NOTES ■

Matching

Match each of the items in the left column to the appropriate definition in the right column.

_____ 1. BLS

_____ 2. EMT-B

_____ 3. OEC

_____ 4. OEC technician

_____ 5. EMS

_____ 6. Medical Director (advisor)

_____ 7. Americans with Disabilities Act

_____ 8. Abandonment

_____ 9. Certification

_____ 10. Consent

_____ 11. Duty to act

_____ 12. Expressed consent

_____ 13. Implied consent

_____ 14. Negligence

_____ 15. Standard of care

_____ 16. Refresher

A. OEC professional trained in BLS

B. unilateral termination of care

C. a system to provide prehospital care to the sick and injured

D. the physician who helps/oversees rescue groups develop protocols and perform in the field

E. process that recognizes that a person has met set standards

F. basic lifesaving interventions, such as CPR

G. a system to provide comprehensive prehospital care for nonurban settings

H. granted permission

I. protects disabled individuals from discrimination

J. legal responsibility to provide care

K. specific authorization to provide care expressed by the patient

L. failure to provide standard of care

M. accepted level of care consistent with training

N. legal assumption that treatment was desired

O. continuing education process to maintain skills and OEC certification

P. EMS professional trained in BLS

Introduction to Outdoor Emergency Care

Multiple Choice

Read each item carefully, then select the best response.

_____ 1. The major goal of quality improvement is to ensure that:

    A. quarterly reviews of the patrol protocols are done.

    B. OEC technicians have received BLS/CPR training.

    C. the public receives the highest standard of care.

    D. the proper information is received in the national office.

_____ 2. Your main concern while responding to a call should be the:

    A. safety of the other rescuers and yourself.

    B. number of potential patients.

    C. request for mutual assistance.

    D. type of call.

_____ 3. The first phase of the emergency care continuum consists of:

    A. recognition of the emergency by the public.

    B. patient assessment, stabilization, packaging, and transport.

    C. safe delivery of the patient to definitive care.

    D. accurate relay of information by the dispatcher.

_____ 4. Care for burns, splinting, and management of patients with behavioral problems are conditions covered in which category of OEC training?

    A. care of life-threatening problems

    B. care of problems that are not life-threatening

    C. important nonmedical problems

    D. These are outside the OEC standard of training.

_____ 5. Understanding legal and ethical issues, learning difficult transport techniques, and using special equipment are covered in which category of OEC training?

    A. care of life-threatening problems

    B. care of problems that are not life-threatening

    C. important nonmedical problems

    D. These are not the concern of OEC technicians.

_____ 6. Which of the following groups is responsible for the national standard training curriculum for EMT-Bs?

  A. American Academy of Orthopaedic Surgeons (AAOS)

  B. Department of Transportation (U.S. DOT)

  C. American Heart Association (AHA)

  D. National Ski Patrol (NSP)

_____ 7. Negligence is based on the OEC technician's duty to act, cause, breach of duty, and:

  A. expressed consent.

  B. termination of care.

  C. mode of transport.

  D. real or perceived damages.

_____ 8. While treating a patient with a suspected brain injury, he becomes verbally abusive and tells you to "leave him alone." If you stop treating him you may be guilty of:

  A. neglect.

  B. battery.

  C. abandonment.

  D. slander.

_____ 9. Good Samaritan laws generally are designed to offer protection to persons who render care in good faith. They do not offer protection from:

  A. properly performed CPR.

  B. acts of negligence.

  C. improvising splinting materials.

  D. providing supportive BLS to a DNR patient.

_____ 10. Which of the following is generally NOT considered confidential?

  A. assessment findings

  B. patient's mental condition

  C. patient's medical history

  D. the location of the emergency

_____ 11. An important safeguard against legal implication is:

  A. responding to every call within a specific amount of time.

  B. checking equipment once a month.

  C. transporting every patient to an emergency department.

  D. a complete and accurate incident report.

Vocabulary www.OECzone.com vocab explorer

Define the following terms using the space provided.

  1. Outdoor Emergency Care (OEC):

  _____

  _____

  _____

2. First responder:

_____

_____

_____

3. OEC technician:

_____

_____

_____

4. Expressed consent:

_____

_____

_____

5. Good Samaritan laws:

_____

_____

_____

6. Implied consent:

_____

_____

_____

7. Negligence:

_____

_____

_____

Fill-in

Read each item carefully, then complete the statement by filling in the missing word(s).

1. OEC training should meet or exceed the guidelines of _____.

2. In some areas, OEC rescuers may provide selected ALS care such as

   _____, use of airway adjuncts, and assisting patients in taking

   prescription _____.

3. The appropriate care for injury or illness as described by the local medical

   director through written form is _____.

4. The determination of _____ is based on duty, breach of duty,
   damages, and cause.

5. Abandonment is the _____ of care without transfer to someone
   of equal or higher training.

6. _____ consent is given directly by an informed patient, whereas

   _____ consent is assumed in the unconscious patient.

7. Mentally competent patients have the right to _____.

True/False

If you believe the statement to be more true than false, write the letter "T" in the space
provided. If you believe the statement to be more false than true, write the letter "F."

1. _____ The OEC scope of training is identical to EMT-B training for "like"
   topics.

2. _____ A professional appearance and manner by the rescuer will help a
   patient build confidence.

3. _____ Failure to provide care to a patient once you have been called to the
   scene is considered negligence.

4. _____ For expressed consent to be valid, the patient must be a minor.

5. _____ If a patient is unconscious and a true emergency exists, the doctrine
   of implied consent applies.

Short Answer

Complete this section with short written answers using the space provided.

1. Describe the OEC technician's role in the EMS system.

   _____

   _____

   _____

2. List five roles and/or responsibilities of being an OEC technician.

_____

_____

_____

_____

_____

3. When does your responsibility for patient care end?

_____

_____

_____

■ ■ ■ CLUES ■ ■ ■

Across

1. Ability to make rational decisions
6. Advanced lifesaving procedures, ie, defibrillation
8. BLS intervention in cardiac arrest
9. A serious situation, such as an injury or illness
10. Designed to protect individuals with disabilities
11. Developed outdoor emergency care training
12. Characteristic of the outdoor and wilderness environment
13. Assumed permission to provide care

Down

1. Recognition of meeting standards
2. Direct permission to provide care
3. Responsibility to provide care
4. Touching another person without their expressed consent
5. Unilateral termination of care
7. Failure to provide standard of care

Word Fun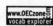

The following crossword puzzle is an activity provided to reinforce correct spelling and understanding of medical terminology associated with emergency care. Use the clues in the column to complete the puzzle.

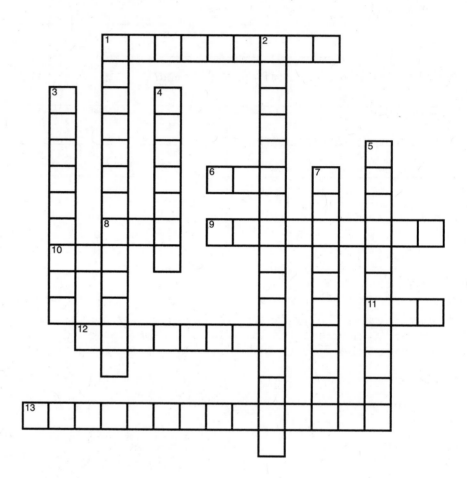

Calls to the Scene

The following case scenarios provide an opportunity to explore the concerns associated with patient management. Read each scenario, then answer each question in detail.

1. There is only one patroller on duty in the aid room when two people walk in. One person is complaining of pain and pressure in the chest; the other has a laceration on the palm of the hand from trying to fix a binding.

How would you best manage this situation?

_____

_____

_____

_____

_____

_____

_____

_____

2. You are "flagged down" by a teenager at a local playground. She tells you there is a small boy injured on one of the baseball diamonds. You arrive to find a 10-year-old boy complaining of a "twisted ankle." There is obvious deformity to his right ankle with a noted loss of function. He says he came to the park to play with his friends while his mother went shopping. There are no adults immediately available.

What actions are necessary in the management of this situation?

_____

_____

_____

_____

_____

_____

_____

_____

3. It is late in the night when you stop at an auto crash. After identifying yourself, a police officer directs you to the back of his patrol car. Sitting on the seat is your patient, snoring loudly with blood covering his face. The officer states that the patient was involved in a drunk driving accident in which he hit his head on the rear-view mirror. The patient initially refused care at the scene. The patient's wound continues to bleed. Assessment reveals a sleeping 56-year-old man with a deep, gaping wound over the right eye with moderate venous bleeding. During assessment, the patient wakes suddenly and pushes you away. He tells you to "leave him alone."

What actions are necessary in the management of this situation?

_____

_____

_____

_____

_____

_____

_____

_____

Notes

Workbook Activities

The following activities have been designed to help you. Your instructor may require you to complete some or all of these activities as a regular part of your OEC training program. You are encouraged to complete any activity that your instructor does not assign as a way to enhance your learning in the classroom.

Chapter Review

The following exercises provide an opportunity to refresh your knowledge of this chapter.

NOTES

Matching

Match each of the terms in the left column to the appropriate definition in the right column.

_____ 1. Acclimatization

_____ 2. Aerobic capacity

_____ 3. Occupational Safety and Health Administration

_____ 4. Posttraumatic stress disorder

_____ 5. Body substance isolation

_____ 6. Pathogen

_____ 7. Transmission

_____ 8. Cardiovascular fitness

_____ 9. Evaporation

_____ 10. Hepatitis

_____ 11. Exposure

_____ 12. Infection control

_____ 13. Hypoxia

_____ 14. Shell

_____ 15. Contamination

A. body's ability to take, transport, and use oxygen

B. assuming all body fluids are potentially infected

C. regulatory compliance agency

D. body adjusts to new environment

E. capable of causing disease in a susceptible host

F. delayed stress reaction

G. skin, muscles, and extremities of the body

H. conditioning the heart and circulatory system to meet an active body's need for blood

I. insufficient oxygen reaching the body tissues

J. an infection of the liver

K. contact with blood, body fluids, tissues, or airborne particles

L. the presence of infectious organisms in or on objects, or a patient's body

M. conversion of a liquid into a vapor

N. the way in which an infectious agent is spread

O. procedures to reduce transmission of infection among patients and health care personnel

The Well-Being of the Rescuer

Multiple Choice

Read each item carefully, then select the best response.

_____ 1. Wool garments are effective as cold weather clothing because they:
  A. dry quickly.
  B. are warm even if wet.
  C. are tough and durable.
  D. are windproof.

_____ 2. The condition that denotes a lack of oxygen is called:
  A. hyperventilation.
  B. hypoventilation.
  C. hypoxia.
  D. apnea.

_____ 3. Presumptive signs of death would not be adequate in cases of sudden death due to which of the following causes?
  A. hypothermia
  B. acute poisoning
  C. cardiac arrest
  D. all of the above

_____ 4. Definitive or conclusive signs of death that are obvious and clear to even nonmedical persons include all of the following except:
  A. profound cyanosis.
  B. dependent lividity.
  C. rigor mortis.
  D. putrefaction.

_____ 5. Heat is lost from the body in five ways. What are they?
  A. external, internal, conduction, respiration, radiation
  B. radiation, external, respiration, conduction, evaporation
  C. conduction, radiation, respiration, internal, evaporation
  D. evaporation, conduction, respiration, convection, radiation

_____ **6.** When exposed to the cold, the body attempts to overcome the heat loss by increasing the production of heat from within the body and reducing the:

A. blood flow to the heart, lungs, and brain.

B. basal metabolic rate.

C. circulation of blood to the skin.

D. shivering rate.

_____ **7.** If exposed to extremely cold conditions without shelter, a person should:

A. run in place to build up body heat.

B. avoid eating and drinking.

C. keep moving, slowly but constantly.

D. stay quiet and still to retain heat.

_____ **8.** To reduce heat loss from infrared radiation, winter snowsports enthusiasts should:

A. calculate the current windchill factor.

B. apply sunscreen lotion.

C. wear protective sunglasses or goggles.

D. wear a hat.

_____ **9.** Shivering is the body's method of:

A. warning of an impending infection.

B. maintaining or increasing its core temperature.

C. maintaining or reducing its core temperature.

D. maintaining fluid consistency of the tissues.

_____ **10.** When providing support for a grieving person, it is okay to say:

A. "I'm sorry."

B. "Give it time."

C. "I know how you feel."

D. "You have to keep on going."

_____ **11.** When grieving, family members may express:

A. rage.

B. anger.

C. despair.

D. all of the above

_____ **12.** To prevent problems from excessive environmental heat, maximize heat loss and:

A. wear vapor-barrier garments.

B. minimize heat gain.

C. minimize cooling.

D. increase muscular activity.

_____ **13.** Signs of anxiety include all of the following except:

A. diaphoresis.

B. fear.

C. hyperventilation.

D. tachycardia.

_____ **14.** Layering involves:

A. coverings for the hands and feet.

B. garments for the core body.

C. accessories for the head and face.

D. all of the above

_____ **15.** If you find that you are the target of the patient's anger, make sure that you:

   A. are safe.

   B. do not take the anger or insults personally.

   C. are tolerant, and do not become defensive.

   D. all of the above

_____ **16.** When acknowledging the death of a child, reactions vary, but _____ is common.

   A. shock

   B. disbelief

   C. denial

   D. all of the above

_____ **17.** Factors influencing how a patient reacts to the stress of an incident involving injury include all of the following except:

   A. family history.

   B. age.

   C. fear of medical personnel.

   D. socioeconomic background.

_____ **18.** Physical symptoms of stress include all of the following except:

   A. fatigue.

   B. changes in appetite.

   C. increased blood pressure.

   D. headaches.

_____ **19.** Events that can trigger critical incident stress include:

   A. mass-casualty incidents.

   B. serious injury or traumatic death of a child.

   C. death or serious injury of a coworker in the line of duty.

   D. all of the above

_____ **20.** The quickest source of energy is _____; however, this supply will last less than a day and is consumed in greater quantities during stress.

   A. glucose

   B. carbohydrate

   C. protein

   D. fat

_____ **21.** The safest, most reliable sources for long-term energy production are:

   A. sugars.

   B. carbohydrates.

   C. fats.

   D. proteins.

_____ **22.** A _____ is any event that causes anxiety and mental stress to emergency workers.

   A. disaster

   B. mass-casualty incident

   C. critical incident

   D. stressor

_____ **23.** A CISD meeting is an opportunity to discuss your:

    A. feelings.

    B. fears.

    C. reactions to the event.

    D. all of the above

_____ **24.** You should begin protecting yourself:

    A. as soon as you arrive on the scene.

    B. before you leave the scene.

    C. as soon as you are dispatched.

    D. before any patient contact.

_____ **25.** _____ is the way an infectious agent is spread.

    A. The route

    B. The mechanism

    C. Transmission

    D. Exposure

_____ **26.** _____ is contact with blood, body fluids, tissues, or airborne droplets by direct or indirect contact.

    A. Transmission

    B. Exposure

    C. Handling

    D. all of the above

_____ **27.** Modes of transmission for infectious diseases include:

    A. blood or fluid splash.

    B. surface contamination.

    C. needlestick exposure.

    D. all of the above

_____ **28.** _____ is the presence of an infectious organism on or in an object.

    A. Virulence

    B. Contamination

    C. Immunity

    D. Transmission

_____ **29.** To protect against accidental exposure to bloodborne infections, rescuers should at least:

    A. wash their hands before touching an open wound.

    B. irrigate the wound with clean, warm water.

    C. wear rubber gloves.

    D. irrigate the wound with isopropyl alcohol or iodine.

_____ **30.** After removing rubber or latex gloves and other items contaminated with blood, they should be temporarily stored in a:

    A. wastebasket.

    B. cardboard box.

    C. plastic bag.

    D. sink.

_____ **31.** The proper method for removing rubber or latex gloves is to:

    A. wipe your gloves with alcohol and then remove.

    B. remove the gloves so they are inside out and the contaminated side is not exposed.

    C. have your rescue partner remove your gloves while wearing face shield, gown, and gloves.

    D. remove the gloves so the contaminated side is exposed.

Vocabulary www.OECzone.com vocab explorer

Define the following terms using the space provided.

1. Critical incident stress management (CISM):

_____

_____

_____

2. Posttraumatic stress disorder (PTSD):

_____

_____

_____

3. Critical incident stress debriefing (CISD):

_____

_____

_____

4. Conduction:

_____

_____

_____

1

5. Convection:

_____

_____

_____

6. Evaporation:

_____

_____

_____

7. Radiation:

_____

_____

_____

8. Windchill:

_____

_____

_____

9. Layering principle:

_____

_____

_____

Fill-in

Read each item carefully, then complete the statement by filling in the missing word.

1. The personal health, safety, and _____ of all rescuers are vital to outdoor prehospital care.

2. The struggle to remain calm in the face of horrible circumstances contributes to the _____ of the job.

3. Determination of the cause of death is the medical responsibility of a _____ .

4. In cases of hypothermia, the patient should not be considered dead until the patient is _____ and dead.

5. Almost all dying patients feel some degree of _____ because of internalized anger and other factors.

6. The best way to develop effective pulmonary function is to incorporate aerobic activity that uses the _____ and _____ at the same time.

7. Most HIV and HBV infections are acquired by transmission through body fluids such as _____ , _____ , and _____ .

8. After removing and disposing of personal protective equipment, the rescuer should immediately _____ his or her hands.

9. Blood-stained clothing should be treated with _____ before washing with soap and hot water.

True/False

If you believe the statement to be more true than false, write the letter "T" in the space provided. If you believe the statement to be more false than true, write the letter "F."

1. _____ Developing self-control is aided by proper training.
2. _____ A low or decreased body temperature is sufficient evidence of death.
3. _____ Rigor mortis is a softening of body muscles shortly after death.
4. _____ The exchange of oxygen and carbon dioxide occurs in the alveoli.
5. _____ Denial is generally the first step in the grieving process.
6. _____ Body fluids are generally not considered infectious substances.
7. _____ Illnesses and injuries that interfere with the proper delivery of oxygen to the tissues are rare in the wilderness and at alpine ski areas.
8. _____ Physical conditioning and nutrition are two factors the rescuer can control in helping reduce stress.
9. _____ As the wind velocity rises, the "effective" temperature drops.
10. _____ An effective vaccine for hepatitis B is available for health care workers.

Short Answer

Complete this section with short written answers using the space provided.

1. Describe the basic concept of body substance isolation (BSI).

_____

_____

_____

2. List six survival requirements.

_____

_____

_____

_____

_____

_____

3. How does the body adjust to high altitude?

_____

_____

_____

_____

4. Identify voluntary methods of increasing heat gain.

_____

_____

_____

_____

_____

5. Identify involuntary methods of increasing heat gain.

_____

_____

_____

_____

6. Identify voluntary methods of decreasing heat loss.

_____

_____

_____

7. Identify involuntary methods of decreasing heat loss.

_____

_____

_____

8. What are some ways to prevent problems from excessive heat?

_____

_____

_____

9. Describe the adage "if your feet are cold, put on your hat."

_____

_____

_____

10. Emergency food taken on rescues should have what four characteristics?

_____

_____

_____

_____

11. List six groups of nutrients.

_____

_____

_____

_____

_____

_____

12. The physical training program should include four phases. What are they?

_____

_____

_____

_____

13. List three important items used to protect the rescuer from HBV and HIV infections.

_____

_____

_____

14. Describe the process for proper handwashing.

_____

_____

_____

15. List the three layers of clothing recommended for cold weather.

_____

_____

_____

Word Fun www.OECzone.com vocab explorer

The following crossword puzzle is an activity provided to reinforce correct spelling and understanding of medical terminology associated with emergency care. Use the clues in the column to complete the puzzle.

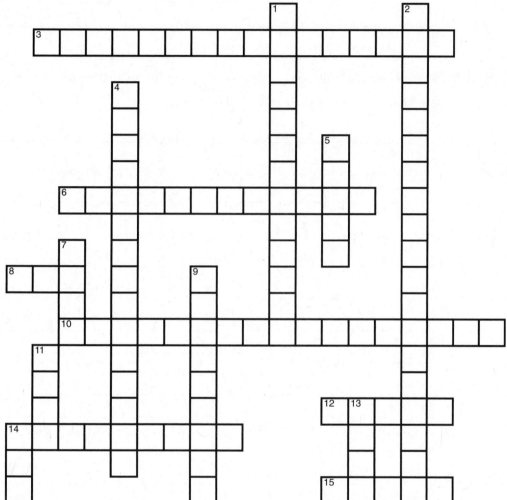

Across

3. Increase in rate and depth of breathing
6. Disease of the lungs
8. Infection control process
10. Blood settling to the lowest point of the body
12. Impenetrable barrier for tactical use
14. Infection of the liver
15. A single thickness covering a surface

Down

1. Exposed by physical touching
2. Disease spread from person to person
4. Index of cardiovascular fitness
5. Emotional response to the loss of a loved one
7. Confidential group discussion of severe incident
9. Emitting energy in the form of waves or particles
11. Central nervous system, heart, lungs, and other internal organs
13. Federal workplace safety agency
14. May progress to AIDS

Calls to the Scene

The following case scenarios provide an opportunity to explore the concerns associated with patient management. Read each scenario, then answer each question in detail.

1. You and a friend are planning a 2-day winter camping/ski-touring trip for the weekend. Your local weather forecast says there is a 20% chance of precipitation and strong winds, with temperatures ranging from 30° to 40°F.

   What preparations do you make, including equipment and clothing? Why?

   _____

   _____

   _____

   _____

   _____

_____

_____

_____

_____

_____

2. You find a patient with hypothermia who is unresponsive and has no reflexes. How would you best manage this situation?

_____

_____

_____

_____

_____

_____

_____

_____

_____

_____

3. In the following table the left column lists ways that the oxygen supply can be interrupted. In the right column, list mechanisms of injury that could lead to the problems identified in the left column.

Oxygen supply obstructed via:	Mechanisms:
Insufficient oxygen in the outside air	• High altitude • • • Near drowning •
Obstruction of the upper airway	• • •
Obstruction of the lower airway	• Inhaled foreign body •

Interference with lung function
 	
   Acute
 	
   Chronic
	Acute
	•
	
	•
	
	•
	
	Chronic
	•
	
	•
	
	•

Interference with chest integrity or function	• • •
Interference with the brain's control of breathing	• Head Injury • • Stroke •

Abnormal function of the circulatory system
 	
   Illness
 	
   Injury
	Illness
	•
	
	•
	
	•
	
	Injury
	•
	
	•

Interference with the blood's oxygen-carrying capacity	• •

Skill Drills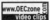

Skill Drill 2-1: Proper Glove Removal Technique

Test your knowledge of skill drills by placing the photos below in the correct order. Number the first step with a "1," the second step with a "2," etc.

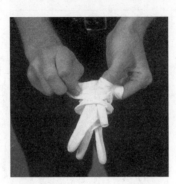

Grasp both gloves with your free hand, touching only the clean, interior surfaces.

_____

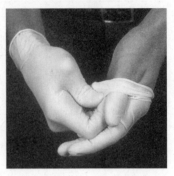

Partially remove the first glove by pinching at the wrist. Be careful to touch only the outside of the glove.

_____

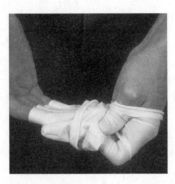

Pull the second glove inside out toward the fingertips.

_____

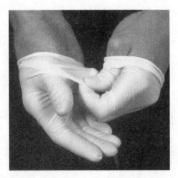

Remove the second glove by pinching the exterior with the partially gloved hand.

_____

Notes

Workbook Activities

The following activities have been designed to help you. Your instructor may require you to complete some or all of these activities as a regular part of your OEC training program. You are encouraged to complete any activity that your instructor does not assign as a way to enhance your learning in the classroom.

Chapter Review

The following exercises provide an opportunity to refresh your knowledge of this chapter.

■ NOTES ■

Matching

Match each of the items in the left column to the appropriate definition in the right column.

_____ 1. EMS	A. Physician's instructions
_____ 2. EMT-Basic	B. Multidisciplinary system that provides prehospital emergency care and transport
_____ 3. Medical control	C. A transfer of a patient by the treating rescuer to the receiving ambulance crew
_____ 4. Local procedures	D. Point to which an initial incident report or injury is sent
_____ 5. AED	E. Protocols established with medical resources
_____ 6. Dispatch	F. EMT trained in basic emergency care skills
_____ 7. Documentation	G. Automated external defibrillator
_____ 8. Turnover	H. Completing detailed reports supporting all major events involved with an incident

Multiple Choice

Read each item carefully, then select the best response.

_____ 1. In addition to focusing on initial emergency care and stabilization, OEC-trained rescuers must focus on:

    A. providing definitive medical care.

    B. getting patients to and into the EMS system.

    C. driving the patients to the hospital.

    D. none of the above

Interfacing with EMS and Other Medical Personnel

_____ **2.** Before a physician can participate as a medical director at a ski area, who must be informed?

  A. area management

  B. patrol director

  C. physician's hospital

  D. local clinic

_____ **3.** BLS excludes:

  A. cardiac monitoring.

  B. advanced airway skills.

  C. IV medication skills.

  D. all of the above

_____ **4.** The National Ski Patrol's Outdoor Emergency Care program is:

  A. regulated by state EMS statutes.

  B. regulated by the American Academy of Orthopaedic Surgeons.

  C. not regulated by state EMS statutes.

  D. not a credentialed program.

_____ **5.** The standard prehospital emergency care procedures are expanding in scope to include:

  A. treatment of cardiac arrests.

  B. helicopter medical evacuation services.

  C. general pharmacology.

  D. all of the above

Vocabulary www.OECzone.com vocab explorer

Define the following terms using the space provided.

  1. Advanced life support (ALS):

  _____

  _____

  _____

2. Basic life support (BLS):

_____

_____

_____

3. Standard of training:

_____

_____

_____

4. Standard of care:

_____

_____

_____

5. First responder:

_____

_____

_____

Fill-in

Read each item carefully, then complete the statement by filling in the missing word(s).

1. _____ is a cornerstone of quality management.

2. _____ _____ have responsibilities defined by state statutes, local protocols, and/or on-line medical control.

3. When an initial incident or injury report needs to be sent from a ski area, it

   should go to _____ .

4. Outdoor rescuers must make important _____ decisions in the field.

5. An important interface between the _____ and EMS is the preparation of the patient prior to EMS transport.

True/False

If you believe the statement to be more true than false, write the letter "T" in the space provided. If you believe the statement to be more false than true, write the letter "F."

1. _____ OEC technicians are not licensed by any state regulatory agencies.

2. _____ Physicians generally cannot actively patrol for a ski area.

3. _____ NHTSA is the lead agency that provides national curricula guidelines for the OEC program.

4. _____ Cross training between local EMS personnel and OEC-trained patrollers is not advised.

5. _____ The initial emergency care solutions in the outdoor setting can be substantially different from urban EMS.

Short Answer

Complete this section with short written answers using the space provided.

1. Identify three ways to involve physicians at ski areas.

_____

_____

_____

2. Differentiate the roles and responsibilities of the OEC technician and the EMT-B.

_____

_____

_____

3. Characterize the various methods used to access the following systems in your patrol or community.

   A. Incident Command System

_____

_____

_____

   B. Local law enforcement

_____

_____

   C. Search and rescue interface

_____

_____

   D. Ambulance interface

_____

_____

_____

E. EMS system

_____

_____

_____

■ CLUES ■

Across

2. Point or center for notification and report

6. Common transportation equipment used by EMTs

8. The first medically trained individual to arrive at an emergency scene

11. Official or legal permission to do a specific thing

Down

1. Invasive emergency lifesaving care

3. Guideline for handling specific procedures

4. Common transportation equipment used by winter rescuers

5. An essential component of emergency care

7. Noninvasive emergency lifesaving care

9. Nonurban prehospital emergency care

10. Urban prehospital emergency care

Word Fun www.OECzone.com vocab explorer

The following crossword puzzle is an activity provided to reinforce correct spelling and understanding of medical terminology associated with emergency care. Use the clues in the column to complete the puzzle.

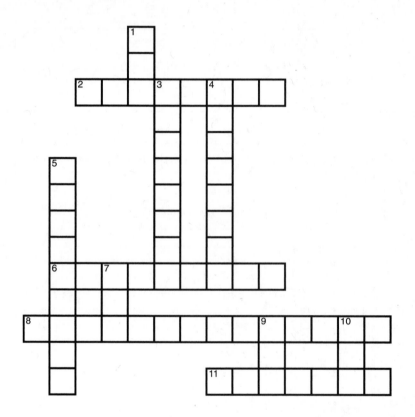

Calls to the Scene

The following case scenarios provide an opportunity to explore the concerns associated with patient management. Read each scenario, then answer each question in detail.

1. You have been dispatched to an intermediate slope to attend a patient with a reported leg injury. Upon arrival, you cross your skis above the incident to better protect the scene and to guide the patroller who will be bringing the toboggan to the right location. As you are doing your initial assessment, a gentleman stops and identifies himself as a doctor. He says he will take over. You have never seen this individual before, nor are you familiar with his name.

   How would you manage this situation?

   _____

   _____

   _____

   _____

   _____

   _____

   _____

   _____

   _____

2. Your rescue group has had some difficulties with the local ambulance service involving misunderstandings and acceptance of techniques. You are responsible for planning your annual preseason refresher and would like to work on improving this relationship.

   What steps could you take?

   _____

   _____

   _____

   _____

   _____

   _____

   _____

   _____

Workbook Activities

The following activities have been designed to help you. Your instructor may require you to complete some or all of these activities as a regular part of your OEC training program. You are encouraged to complete any activity that your instructor does not assign as a way to enhance your learning in the classroom.

Chapter Review

The following exercises provide an opportunity to refresh your knowledge of this chapter.

NOTES

Matching

Match each of the terms in the left column to the appropriate definition in the right column.

_____ 1. Anterior

_____ 2. Capillary

_____ 3. Anatomic position

_____ 4. Superior

_____ 5. Midline

_____ 6. Carotid

_____ 7. Medial

_____ 8. Inferior

_____ 9. Femoral

_____ 10. Proximal

_____ 11. Brachial

_____ 12. Distal

_____ 13. Midaxillary

_____ 14. Radial

_____ 15. Posterior

A. closer to the midline

B. farther from the midline

C. farther from the head; lower

D. standing, facing forward, palms facing forward

E. imaginary vertical line descending from the middle of the forehead to the floor

F. front surface of the body

G. closer to the head; higher

H. imaginary vertical line descending from the middle of the armpit to the ankle

I. back or dorsal surface of the body

J. closer to the midline

K. connects arterioles to venules

L. major artery that supplies blood to the head and brain

M. major artery that supplies blood to the lower extremities

N. major artery of the lower arm

O. major artery of the upper arm

For each of the bones listed in the left column, indicate whether it is an upper extremity bone (A) or a lower extremity bone (B).

_____ 16. Acetabulum

_____ 17. Patella

_____ 18. Clavicle

_____ 19. Fibula

A. upper extremity bone

B. lower extremity bone

Human Anatomy and Physiology

_____**20.** Calcaneus

_____ **21.** Ulna

_____**22.** Acromion

For each of the muscle characteristics described in the left column, select the type of muscle from the right column.

_____**23.** Attaches to the bone

_____**24.** Found in the walls of the gastrointestinal tract

_____**25.** Carries out much of the automatic work of the body

_____**26.** Forms the major muscle mass of the body

_____**27.** Under the direct control of the brain

_____**28.** Found only in the heart

_____**29.** Responds only to primitive stimulus, such as heat

_____**30.** Can tolerate blood supply interruption for only a very short period

_____ **31.** Responsible for all bodily movement

_____**32.** Has its own blood supply and electrical system

A. skeletal

B. smooth

C. cardiac

For each of the parts of the nervous system in the left column, select the phrase in the right column with which it is associated.

_____**33.** Spinal cord

_____**34.** Central nervous system

_____**35.** Sensory nerves

_____**36.** Motor nerves

_____ **37.** Brain

_____**38.** Peripheral nervous system

A. exits the brain through an opening at the base of the skull

B. transmits electrical impulses to the muscles, causing them to contract

C. brain and spinal cord

D. links the central nervous system to various organs in the body

E. carries sensations of taste and touch to the brain

F. controlling organ of the body

Multiple Choice

Read each item carefully, then select the best response.

_____ **1.** The topographic term used to describe the location of an injury that is toward the midline of the body is:

  A. lateral.

  B. medial.

  C. midaxillary.

  D. midclavicular.

_____ **2.** Topographically, the term distal means:

  A. near the trunk.

  B. near a point of reference.

  C. farther from a point of reference.

  D. toward the center of the body.

_____ **3.** The firm cartilaginous ring that forms the inferior portion of the larynx is called the:

  A. costal cartilage.

  B. cricoid cartilage.

  C. thyroid cartilage.

  D. laryngo cartilage.

_____ **4.** Which of the following types of muscle carries out the automatic work of the body?

  A. striated

  B. skeletal

  C. smooth

  D. sensory

_____ **5.** Which of the following is the main supporting structure of the skeleton?

  A. thorax

  B. upper extremities

  C. lower extremities

  D. spinal column

_____ **6.** The ilium, ischium, and pubis are fused together, forming the:

  A. clavicle.

  B. sternum.

  C. pelvis.

  D. olecranon.

_____ **7.** The leaf-shaped flap of tissue that prevents food and liquid from entering the trachea is called the:

  A. uvula.

  B. epiglottis.

  C. laryngopharynx.

  D. cricothyroid membrane.

_____ **8.** Which of the following systems is responsible for releasing chemicals that regulate body activities?

  A. nervous

  B. endocrine

  C. cardiovascular

  D. skeletal

_____ **9.** Which of the following vessels does NOT carry blood to the heart?

    A. inferior venae cavae

    B. superior venae cavae

    C. pulmonary vein

    D. pulmonary artery

_____ **10.** The peripheral nervous system is composed of the:

    A. brain, spinal cord, and motor nerves.

    B. brain, and sensory and connecting nerves.

    C. motor, sensory, and connecting nerves.

    D. spinal cord, and sensory and motor nerves.

N O T E S

Labeling

Label the following diagrams with the correct terms.

1. Directional Terms

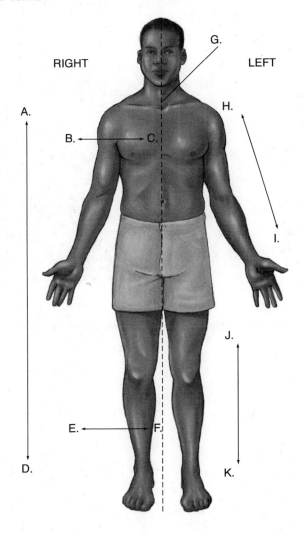

RIGHT   LEFT

A. _____

B. _____

C. _____

D. _____

E. _____

F. _____

G. _____

H. _____

I. _____

J. _____

K. _____

2. Anatomic Positions

Fill in the names of the anatomic positions shown.

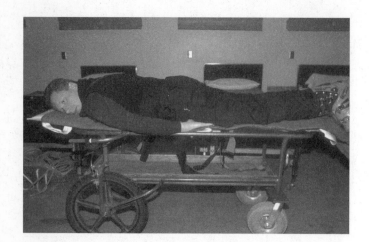

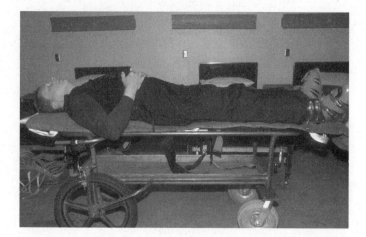

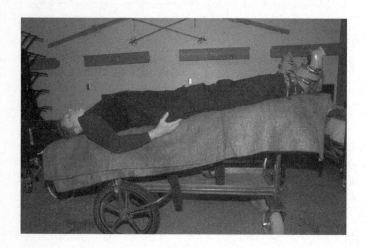

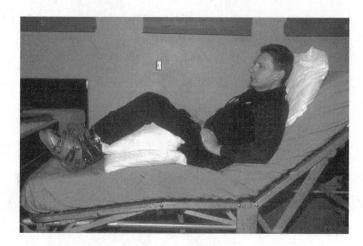

3. The Skeletal System

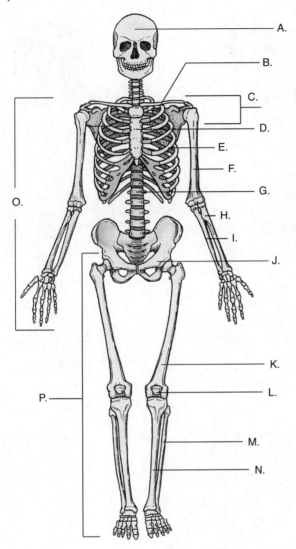

A. _____

B. _____

C. _____

D. _____

E. _____

F. _____

G. _____

H. _____

I. _____

J. _____

K. _____

L. _____

M. _____

N. _____

O. _____

P. _____

4. The Skull

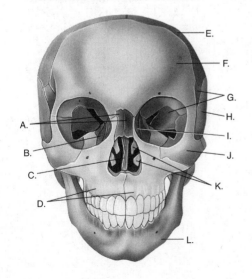

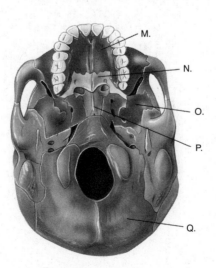

A. _____

B. _____

C. _____

D. _____

E. _____

F. _____

G. _____

H. _____

I. _____

J. _____

K. _____

L. _____

M. _____

N. _____

O. _____

P. _____

Q. _____

5. The Spinal Column

A. _____

B. _____

C. _____

D. _____

E. _____

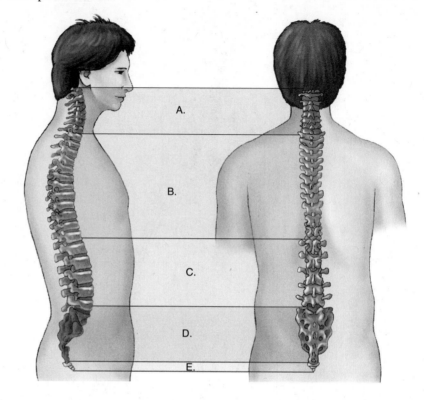

6. The Thorax

A. _____

B. _____

C. _____

D. _____

E. _____

F. _____

G. _____

H. _____

I. _____

J. _____

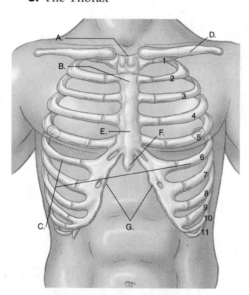
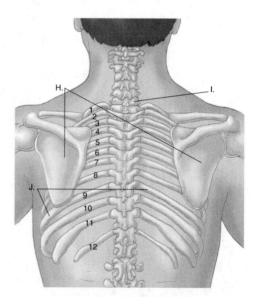

7. The Pelvis

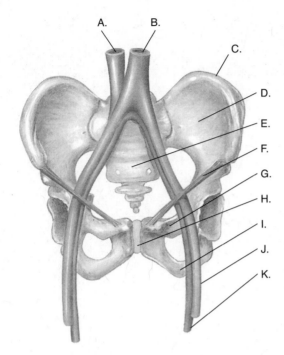

A. _____

B. _____

C. _____

D. _____

E. _____

F. _____

G. _____

H. _____

I. _____

J. _____

K. _____

8. The Lower Extremity

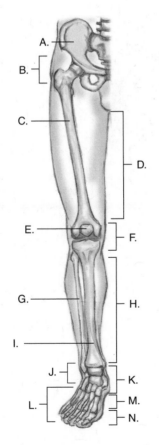

A. _____

B. _____

C. _____

D. _____

E. _____

F. _____

G. _____

H. _____

I. _____

J. _____

K. _____

L. _____

M. _____

N. _____

9. The Shoulder Girdle

A. _____

B. _____

C. _____

D. _____

E. _____

F. _____

G. _____

H. _____

I. _____

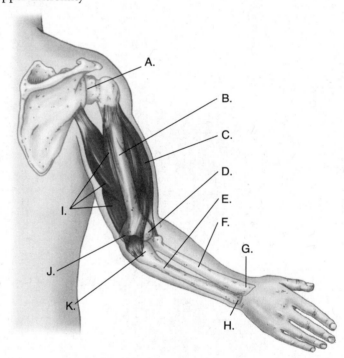

10. The Upper Extremity

A. _____

B. _____

C. _____

D. _____

E. _____

F. _____

G. _____

H. _____

I. _____

J. _____

K. _____

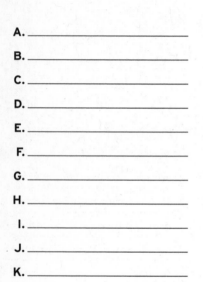

11. Wrist and Hand

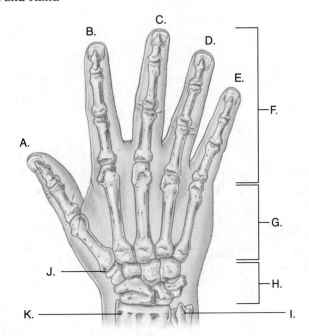

A. _____

B. _____

C. _____

D. _____

E. _____

F. _____

G. _____

H. _____

I. _____

J. _____

K. _____

12. The Respiratory System

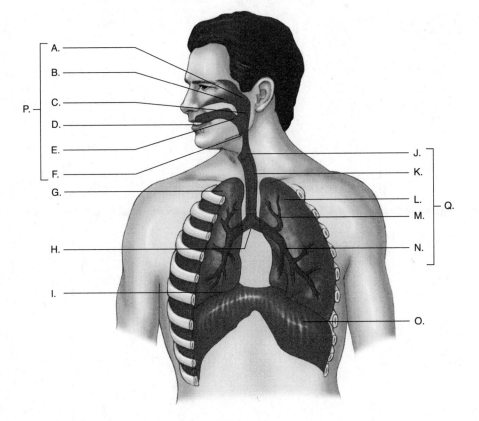

A. _____

B. _____

C. _____

D. _____

E. _____

F. _____

G. _____

H. _____

I. _____

J. _____

K. _____

L. _____

M. _____

N. _____

O. _____

P. _____

Q. _____

13. The Circulatory System

A. _____

B. _____

C. _____

D. _____

E. _____

F. _____

G. _____

H. _____

I. _____

J. _____

K. _____

L. _____

M. _____

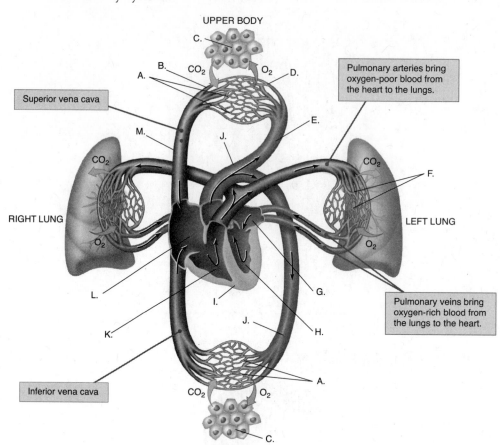

14. Electrical Conduction

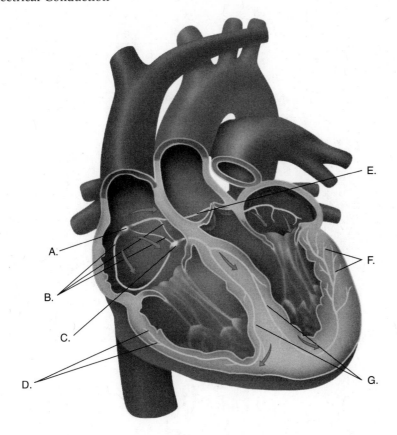

A. _____

B. _____

C. _____

D. _____

E. _____

F. _____

G. _____

1

NOTES

15. Central and Peripheral Pulses

A. _____

B. _____

C. _____

D. _____

E. _____

F. _____

G. _____

H. _____

I. _____

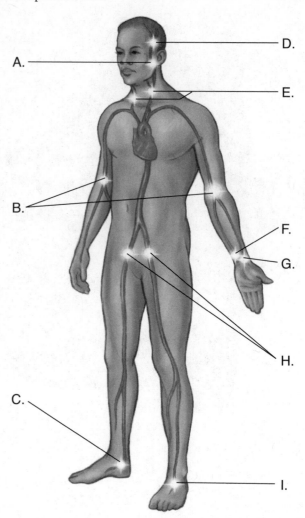

16. The Brain

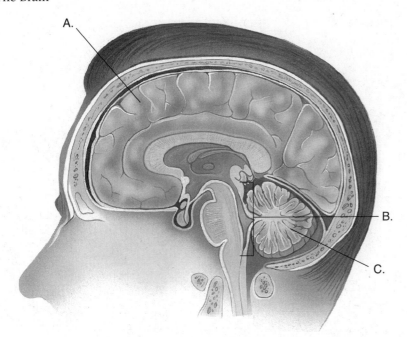

A. _____

B. _____

C. _____

17. Anatomy of the Skin

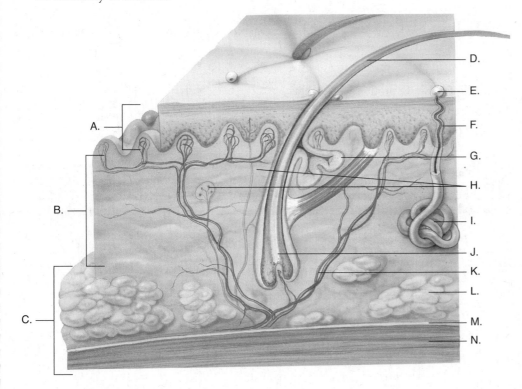

A. _____

B. _____

C. _____

D. _____

E. _____

F. _____

G. _____

H. _____

I. _____

J. _____

K. _____

L. _____

M. _____

N. _____

18. The Male Reproductive System

A. _____

B. _____

C. _____

D. _____

E. _____

F. _____

G. _____

H. _____

I. _____

J. _____

K. _____

L. _____

M. _____

N. _____

O. _____

P. _____

Q. _____

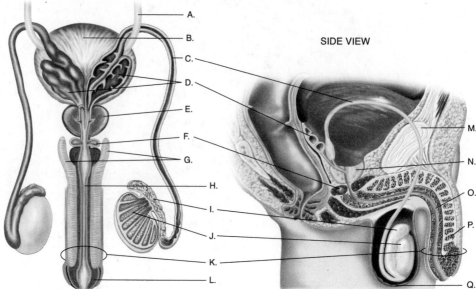

FRONT VIEW

SIDE VIEW

19. The Female Reproductive System

A. _____

B. _____

C. _____

D. _____

E. _____

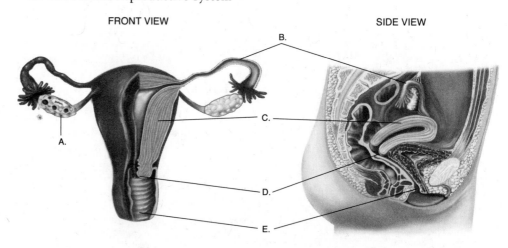

FRONT VIEW

SIDE VIEW

Vocabulary [www.OECzone.com vocab explorer]

Define the following terms using the space provided.

1. Perfusion:

_____

_____

_____

2. Agonal respirations:

_____

_____

_____

3. Autonomic nervous system:

_____

_____

_____

4. Pleural space:

_____

_____

_____

5. Trendelenburg's position:

_____

_____

_____

6. Fowler's position:

_____

_____

_____

7. Somatic nervous system:

_____

_____

_____

8. Endocrine system:

_____

_____

_____

9. Peripheral nervous system:

_____

_____

_____

10. Epiglottis:

_____

_____

_____

11. Metabolism:

_____

_____

_____

12. Brain stem:

_____

_____

_____

Fill-in

Read each item carefully, then complete the statement by filling in the missing word.

1. There are _____ cervical vertebrae.

2. The movable bone in the skull is the _____.

3. There is a total of _____ lobes in the right and left lungs.

4. There are _____ pairs of ribs that attach posteriorly to the thoracic vertebrae.

5. The spinal column has _____ vertebrae.

6. The vocal cords are located in the _____.

7. The ankle bone is known as the _____.

8. The 11th and 12th ribs are called _____.

True/False

If you believe the statement to be more true than false, write the letter "T" in the space provided. If you believe the statement to be more false than true, write the letter "F."

1. _____ The aorta is the major artery that supplies the groin and lower extremities with blood.

2. _____ The largest joint in the body is the knee.

3. _____ The phalanges are the bones of the fingers and toes.

4. _____ The right atrium receives blood from the pulmonary veins.

5. _____ There are 12 ribs that attach to the sternum.

Short Answer

Complete this section with short written answers using the space provided.

1. List the four components of blood and each of their functions.

_____

_____

_____

_____

2. List the five sections of the spinal column and indicate the number of vertebrae in each.

_____

_____

_____

_____

_____

3. What organs are in each of the quadrants of the abdomen?

RUQ_____

_____

LUQ_____

_____

RLQ_____

_____

LLQ _____

_____

4. List in the proper order the parts of the heart that blood flows through.

1. _____   6. _____

2. _____   7. _____

3. _____   8. _____

4. _____   9. _____

5. _____

Word Fun

www.OECzone.com
vocab explorer

The following crossword puzzle is an activity provided to reinforce correct spelling and understanding of medical terminology associated with emergency care. Use the clues in the column to complete the puzzle.

Across

1. Inner layer of skin
8. Nearer to the feet
10. Lower chamber of the heart
13. Front surface of the body
14. Away from the midline, sides
15. Slow, dying respirations or pulse
16. Bone on thumb side of forearm

Down

1. Nearer the end
2. Behind the abdomen
3. Lower jawbone
4. Adequate circulation of blood
5. Upper chamber of the heart
6. Back surface of the body
7. Appears on both sides
9. Windpipe
11. Large solid organ in RUQ
12. Sitting up with knees bent

Calls to the Scene

The following case scenarios provide an opportunity to explore the concerns associated with patient management. Read each scenario, then answer each question in detail.

1. A skier coming down a most difficult run loses it and takes a windmill-type fall. In one of the tumbles, the ski comes off and the person rolls over a pole, which jabs him hard in the right upper quadrant of the abdomen.

   Using medical terminology, indicate which organ(s) might be affected. How would you describe this patient's injuries?

   _____

   _____

_____

_____

_____

_____

_____

_____

2. An 8-year-old boy flew out of the alpine slide track and is complaining of pain to his left forearm just above his wrist. You see that the wrist bone is sticking out at an odd angle.

Using medical terminology, how would you describe this patient's injuries?

_____

_____

_____

_____

_____

_____

_____

_____

3. A 14-year-old skier was accidentally hit by a passing snowboarder. Upon arrival, you find the patient's left lower leg to be deformed and swollen.

Using medical terminology, how would you describe this patient's injuries?

_____

_____

_____

_____

_____

_____

_____

_____

Workbook Activities

The following activities have been designed to help you. Your instructor may require you to complete some or all of these activities as a regular part of your OEC training program. You are encouraged to complete any activity that your instructor does not assign as a way to enhance your learning in the classroom.

Chapter Review

The following exercises provide an opportunity to refresh your knowledge of this chapter.

NOTES

Matching

Match each of the terms in the left column to the appropriate definition in the right column.

_____ 1. Pulse

_____ 2. Auscultation

_____ 3. Palpation

_____ 4. Perfusion

_____ 5. Blood pressure

_____ 6. SAMPLE history

_____ 7. Sphygmomanometer

_____ 8. Capillary refill

_____ 9. Bradycardia

_____ 10. Cyanosis

_____ 11. Diaphoretic

_____ 12. Hypertension

_____ 13. Hypotension

_____ 14. Sclera

_____ 15. Tachycardia

A. the pressure of the circulating blood against the walls of the arteries

B. characterized by profuse sweating

C. white portion of the eye

D. examination by touch

E. listening to sounds within the organs, usually with a stethoscope

F. the ability of the circulatory system to restore blood to the capillary blood vessels after it is squeezed out

G. blood pressure that is higher than normal range

H. a patient's history consisting of signs/symptoms, allergies, medications, pertinent past history, last oral intake, and events leading to the illness/injury

I. blood pressure that is lower than normal range

J. rapid heart rate

K. a blood pressure cuff

L. the process whereby blood enters an organ or tissue through its arteries and leaves through its veins, providing nutrients and oxygen and removing waste

M. slow heart rate

N. the pressure wave that is felt with the expansion and contraction of an artery

O. bluish-gray skin color caused by reduced blood-oxygen levels

Baseline Vital Signs and SAMPLE History

Multiple Choice

Read each item carefully, then select the best response.

_____ **1.** When assessing the patient, you will have to:

   A. visualize.

   B. auscultate.

   C. palpate.

   D. all of the above

_____ **2.** The reason that a patient or other individual calls 9-1-1 is called the:

   A. sign.

   B. symptom.

   C. chief complaint.

   D. primary problem.

_____ **3.** Signs include all of the following except:

   A. dizziness.

   B. marked deformities.

   C. external bleeding.

   D. wounds.

_____ **4.** A critical problem or deficit in any of the body's vital systems or functions will affect and be reflected by changes in the:

   A. respiratory system.

   B. circulatory system.

   C. central nervous system.

   D. all of the above

_____ **5.** The first set of vital signs that you obtain is called the:

   A. original vital signs.

   B. baseline vital signs.

   C. actual vital signs.

   D. real vital signs.

NOTES

_____ **6.** Besides pulse, respirations, and blood pressure, you should also include evaluation of:

A. level of consciousness.

B. pupillary reaction.

C. capillary refill in children.

D. all of the above

_____ **7.** What occurs during inspiration?

A. The chest rises up and out.

B. The phase is passive.

C. Carbon dioxide is released.

D. all of the above

_____ **8.** Assess breathing by:

A. watching for chest rise and fall.

B. feeling for air through the mouth and nose during exhalation.

C. listening for breath sounds with a stethoscope.

D. all of the above

_____ **9.** The normal range for adult respirations is _____ breaths/min.

A. 8 to 20

B. 15 to 30

C. 25 to 50

D. none of the above

_____ **10.** Normal breathing does not affect a patient's:

A. speech.

B. posture.

C. positioning.

D. all of the above

_____ **11.** In the _____ position, the patient sits leaning forward on outstretched arms with the head and chin thrust slightly forward.

A. Fowler's

B. tripod

C. sniffing

D. lithotomy

_____ **12.** In the _____ position, the patient sits upright with the head and chin thrust slightly forward.

A. Fowler's

B. tripod

C. sniffing

D. lithotomy

_____ **13.** Signs of labored breathing include all of the following except:

A. accessory muscle use.

B. dyspnea.

C. retractions.

D. gasping.

_____ **14.** The _____ is the pressure wave that occurs as each heartbeat causes a surge in the blood circulating through the arteries.

A. systolic pressure

B. diastolic pressure

C. pulse

D. ventricular pressure

_____ **15.** In responsive patients who are older than 1 year, you should palpate a pulse at the _____ artery.

    A. carotid

    B. femoral

    C. radial

    D. brachial

_____ **16.** In unresponsive patients who are older than 1 year, you should palpate a pulse at the _____ artery.

    A. carotid

    B. femoral

    C. radial

    D. brachial

_____ **17.** A pulse that is weak and _____ should be palpated and counted for a full minute.

    A. difficult to palpate

    B. irregular

    C. extremely slow

    D. all of the above

_____ **18.** When the interval between each ventricular contraction of the heart is short, the pulse is:

    A. slow.

    B. rapid.

    C. regular.

    D. irregular.

_____ **19.** The rhythm of cardiac contractions is considered _____ if the heart periodically has a premature or late beat or if a pulse beat is missed.

    A. slow

    B. rapid

    C. regular

    D. irregular

_____ **20.** When assessing the skin, you should evaluate:

    A. color.

    B. temperature.

    C. moisture.

    D. all of the above

_____ **21.** Perfusion may be assessed in the:

    A. fingernail beds.

    B. lips.

    C. conjunctiva.

    D. all of the above

_____ **22.** Poor peripheral circulation will cause the skin to appear:

    A. pale.

    B. ashen.

    C. gray.

    D. all of the above

_____23. Liver disease or dysfunction may cause _____, resulting in the patient's skin and sclera turning yellow.

    A. cyanosis

    B. jaundice

    C. diaphoresis

    D. lack of perfusion

_____24. The skin will feel cool when the patient:

    A. is in early shock.

    B. has mild hypothermia.

    C. has inadequate perfusion.

    D. all of the above

_____25. Capillary refill reflects the patient's perfusion and is often affected by the patient's:

    A. body temperature.

    B. position.

    C. medications.

    D. all of the above

_____26. With adequate perfusion, the color in the nail bed should be restored to its normal pink within _____ seconds when checking capillary refill.

    A. 1½

    B. 2

    C. 2½

    D. 3

_____27. Adequate _____ is necessary to maintain proper circulation and perfusion of the vital organ cells.

    A. blood pressure

    B. pulse

    C. capillary refill

    D. body temperature

_____28. A decrease in blood pressure may indicate:

    A. loss of blood.

    B. loss of vascular tone.

    C. a cardiac pumping problem.

    D. all of the above

_____29. When blood pressure drops, the body compensates to maintain perfusion to the vital organs by:

    A. decreasing the pulse rate.

    B. decreasing the blood flow to the skin and extremities.

    C. decreasing the respiratory rate.

    D. dilating the arteries.

_____30. Blood pressure is usually measured through:

    A. auscultation.

    B. palpation.

    C. visualization.

    D. rationalization.

_____ **31.** When obtaining a blood pressure by palpation, you should place your fingertips on the _____ artery.

   A. carotid

   B. brachial

   C. radial

   D. posterior tibial

_____ **32.** You must assume that a patient who has a critically _____ can no longer compensate sufficiently to maintain adequate perfusion.

   A. low blood pressure

   B. high blood pressure

   C. low pulse rate

   D. high pulse rate

_____ **33.** The patient's level of responsiveness reflects the status of the:

   A. peripheral nervous system.

   B. central nervous system.

   C. peripheral perfusion.

   D. distal perfusion.

_____ **34.** The Glasgow Coma Scale evaluates all of the following except:

   A. eye opening.

   B. verbal response.

   C. distal circulation.

   D. motor response.

_____ **35.** The diameter and reactivity to light of the patient's pupils reflect the status of the brain's:

   A. perfusion.

   B. oxygenation.

   C. condition.

   D. all of the above

_____ **36.** You should reassess vital signs:

   A. every 15 minutes in a stable patient.

   B. every 5 minutes in an unstable patient.

   C. after every medical intervention.

   D. all of the above

_____ **37.** In the mnemonic "SAMPLE," the "P" stands for:

   A. pupillary response.

   B. pulse rate.

   C. pertinent past history.

   D. pain level.

Vocabulary www.OECzone.com vocab explorer

Define the following terms using the space provided.

  1. Glasgow Coma Scale:

_____

_____

_____

2. AVPU scale:

_____

_____

_____

3. Chief complaint:

_____

_____

_____

4. Stridor:

_____

_____

_____

Fill-in

Read each item carefully, then complete the statement by filling in the missing word.

1. _____ is the amount of air that is exchanged with each breath.

2. The _____ is the delicate membrane lining the eyelids and covering the exposed surface of the eye.

3. By using your _____ powers, you will be able to interpret the meaning and implications of your findings and the information that you have gathered while assessing the patient.

4. The severity of a _____ is subjective because it is based on the patient's interpretation and tolerance.

5. A patient who is breathing without assistance is said to have _____.

6. _____ are the key signs that are used to evaluate the patient's initial general condition.

7. When assessing respirations, you must determine the rate, _____, and depth of the patient's breathing.

8. When you can actually see the effort of the patient's breathing, it is described as

_____.

9. If you can hear bubbling or gurgling, the patient probably has _____ in the airway.

10. The condition of the patient's skin can tell you a lot about the patient's peripheral circulation and _____, blood oxygen levels, and body temperature.

True/False

If you believe the statement to be more true than false, write the letter "T" in the space provided. If you believe the statement to be more false than true, write the letter "F."

1. _____ A pulse is an indicator of the condition of the heart.

2. _____ A blood pressure determined by palpation is less accurate than if determined by auscultation.

3. _____ Only the diastolic pressure can be measured by the palpation method.

4. _____ Labored breathing can be described as increased breathing effort, grunting, and use of accessory muscles.

5. _____ A conscious patient is likely to alter his or her breathing if he or she is aware that you are evaluating it.

6. _____ The pulse is most commonly palpated at the femoral artery.

7. _____ The normal pulse range for a newborn is 140 to 160 beats/min.

8. _____ To assess skin color in an infant, you should look at the palms of the hands and soles of the feet.

9. _____ Cyanosis indicates a need for oxygen.

10. _____ The skin will feel hot when the patient is in profound shock or has hypothermia.

11. _____ Normal reaction to a bright light shone in one eye is pupil constriction in only that eye.

12. _____ Normal respirations in an adult are 15 to 30 breaths/min.

Short Answer

Complete this section with short written answers using the space provided.

1. Name the seven basic vital signs.

_____

_____

_____

_____

_____

_____

_____

2. List four abnormal skin colors.

_____

_____

_____

_____

3. Name five factors to be considered when assessing adequate or inadequate breathing.

_____

_____

_____

_____

4. Define systolic blood pressure.

_____

_____

_____

5. Define diastolic blood pressure.

_____

_____

_____

6. Name the three factors to consider when assessing a patient's pulse.

_____

_____

_____

7. Name the three factors to consider when assessing a patient's skin.

_____

_____

_____

8. Describe the process for assessing capillary refill.

_____

_____

_____

9. Define the acronym PEARRL.

_____

_____

_____

10. Explain the difference between a sign and a symptom.

_____

_____

_____

Word Fun www.OECzone.com vocab explorer

The following crossword puzzle is an activity to reinforce correct spelling and understanding of medical terminology associated with emergency care. Use the clues in the column to complete the puzzle.

CLUES

Across

1. Heartbeat, respirations, BP, etc.

3. Circulation within the organs

5. Acronym used to assess LOR

9. BP lower than normal

11. Pressure against the wall of arteries

13. Harsh, high-pitched inspiratory sound

14. Coma scale

Down

2. Listening

4. Yellow

6. Objective finding

7. Bluish

8. BP higher than normal

10. Cardiac pressure wave

12. Subjective finding

Calls to the Scene

The following case scenarios provide an opportunity to explore the concerns associated with patient management. Read each scenario, then answer each question in detail.

1. You are dispatched to the ski lodge cafeteria to an elderly man who is not feeling well. He is very warm to the touch. He tells you he had some nausea and vomiting this morning and feels dizzy.

   How would you best manage this patient?

   _____

   _____

   _____

   _____

   _____

   _____

   _____

   _____

2. Being a teacher with OEC training, you are called to the school's administrative office to see a sick child. Upon arrival, you find a 9-year-old girl lying on the bed in the office. She is flushed and appears weak. Closer inspection reveals a yellow tint to her sclera. The nurse tells you she has a history of liver disease.

   How would you best manage this patient?

   _____

   _____

   _____

   _____

   _____

   _____

   _____

   _____

   _____

3. You are hiking and meet up with an individual who has had a possible cardiac arrest. Family members tell you that the patient, a 57-year-old man, stopped breathing and had no pulse. They also tell you he has a cardiac history. They stopped CPR when he resumed breathing and regained a pulse, approximately 2 minutes before your arrival.

How would you best manage this patient?

_____

_____

_____

_____

_____

_____

_____

_____

1

Skill Drills [www.OECzone.com video clips]

Skill Drill 5-1: Obtaining a Blood Pressure by Auscultation or Palpation
Test your knowledge of this skill drill by placing the photos below in the correct order. Number the first step with a "1," the second step with a "2," etc.

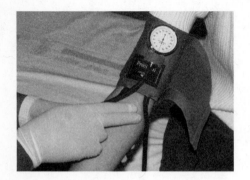

Palpate the brachial artery.

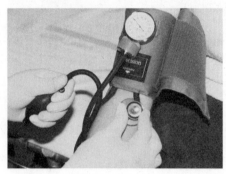

Close the valve and pump to 20 mm Hg above the point at which you stop hearing pulse sounds. Note the systolic and diastolic pressures as you let air escape slowly.

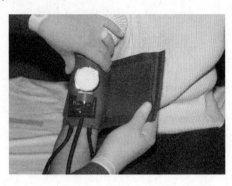

Apply the cuff snugly.

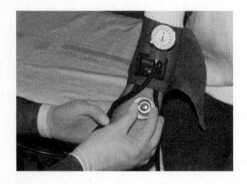

Place the stethoscope and grasp the ball-pump and turn-valve.

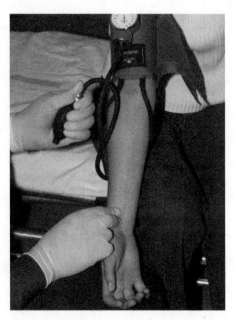

When using the palpation method, you should place your fingertips on the radial artery so that you feel the radial pulse.

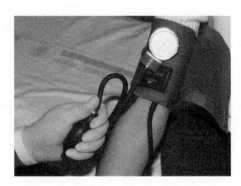

Open the valve and quickly release remaining air.

Notes

Workbook Activities

The following activities have been designed to help you. Your instructor may require you to complete some or all of these activities as a regular part of your OEC training program. You are encouraged to complete any activity that your instructor does not assign as a way to enhance your learning in the classroom.

Chapter Review

The following exercises provide an opportunity to refresh your knowledge of this chapter.

NOTES

Matching

Match each of the terms in the left column to the appropriate definition in the right column.

_____ **1.** Inhalation

_____ **2.** Exhalation

_____ **3.** Alveoli

_____ **4.** Automatic function

_____ **5.** Hypoxic drive

_____ **6.** Tidal volume

_____ **7.** Diaphragm

_____ **8.** Intercostal muscle

_____ **9.** Ventilation

_____ **10.** Larynx

_____ **11.** Hypoxia

_____ **12.** Cheyne-Stokes respirations

A. moves down slightly when it contracts

B. irregular breathing pattern with increased rate and depth, followed by apnea

C. active part of breathing

D. voice box

E. amount of air moved during one breath

F. raises ribs when it contracts

G. controls breathing during sleep

H. site of oxygen diffusion

I. thorax size decreases

J. insufficient oxygen for cells and tissues

K. backup system to control respiration

L. exchange of air between lungs and environment

Multiple Choice

Read each item carefully, then select the best response.

_____ **1.** What percentage of the air we breathe is made up of oxygen?

    A. 78%

    B. 12%

    C. 16 %

    D. 21%

C H A P T E R   6

Airway

_____ **2.** Regarding the maintenance of the airway in an unconscious adult, which of the following is false?

    A. Insertion of an oropharyngeal airway helps keep the airway open.

    B. The head tilt-chin lift maneuver should always be used to open the airway.

    C. Secretions should be suctioned from the mouth as necessary.

    D. Inserting a rigid suction catheter beyond the tongue may cause gagging.

_____ **3.** The normal respiratory rate for an adult is:

    A. about equal to the person's heart rate.

    B. 12 to 20 breaths per minute.

    C. faster when the person is sleeping.

    D. the same as in infants and children.

_____ **4.** All of the following conditions are associated with hypoxia except:

    A. heart attack.

    B. altered mental status.

    C. chest injury.

    D. hyperventilation syndrome.

_____ **5.** The brain stem normally triggers breathing by increasing respirations when:

    A. carbon dioxide levels increase.

    B. oxygen levels increase.

    C. carbon dioxide levels decrease.

    D. nitrogen levels decrease.

_____ **6.** Which of the following is not a sign of abnormal breathing?

    A. warm, dry skin

    B. speaking in two- or three-word sentences

    C. unequal breath sounds

    D. skin pulling in around the ribs during inspiration

_____ **7.** The proper technique for sizing an oropharyngeal airway before insertion is to measure the device from the:

    A. tip of the nose to the earlobe.

    B. bridge of the nose to the tip of the chin.

    C. corner of the mouth to the earlobe.

    D. center of the jaw to the earlobe.

_____ **8.** What is the most common problem you may encounter when using a BVM device?

    A. volume of the BVM device

    B. positioning of the patient's head

    C. environmental conditions

    D. maintaining an airtight seal

_____ **9.** When ventilating a patient with a BVM device, you should:

    A. look for inflation of the cheeks.

    B. look for signs of the patient breathing on his or her own.

    C. look for rise and fall of the chest.

    D. listen for gurgling.

_____ **10.** Suctioning the oral cavity of an adult should be accomplished within:

    A. 10 seconds.

    B. 5 seconds.

    C. 20 seconds.

    D. 15 seconds.

Labeling

www.OECzone.com
anatomy review

Label the following diagrams with the correct terms.

    1. Upper and Lower Airways

A. _____

B. _____

C. _____

D. _____

E. _____

F. _____

G. _____

H. _____

I. _____

J. _____

K. _____

L. _____

M. _____

N. _____

O. _____

P. _____

Q. _____

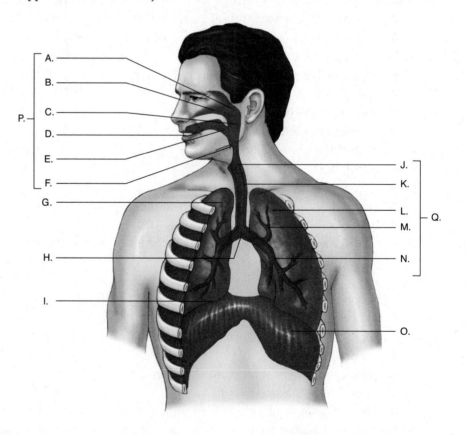

2. The Thoracic Cage

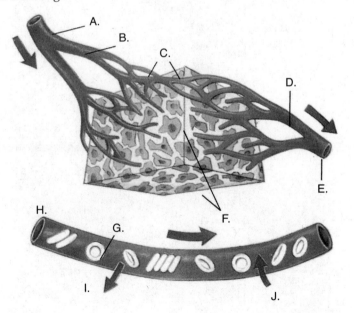

A. _____

B. _____

C. _____

D. _____

E. _____

F. _____

G. _____

H. _____

I. _____

J. _____

3. Cellular Exchange

A. _____

B. _____

C. _____

D. _____

E. _____

F. _____

G. _____

H. _____

I. _____

J. _____

4. Pulmonary Exchange
  Where arrows are shown, indicate which molecules are moving in that direction.

A. _____

B. _____

C. _____

D. _____

E. _____

F. _____

G. _____

H. _____

I. _____

J. _____

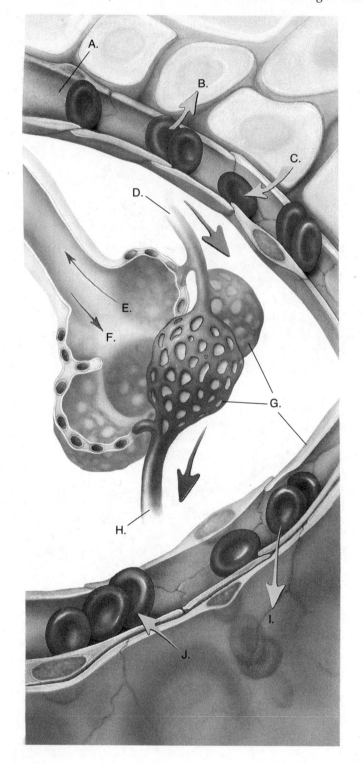

Vocabulary www.OECzone vocab explorer

Define the following terms using the space provided.

1. Gag reflex:

_____

_____

_____

2. Gastric distention:

_____

_____

_____

3. Bag-valve-mask device:

_____

_____

_____

Fill-in

Read each item carefully, then complete the statement by filling in the missing word(s).

1. Air enters the body through the _____.

2. In exhalation, air pressure in the lungs is _____ than the pressure outside.

3. The air we breathe contains _____% oxygen and _____% nitrogen.

4. The primary mechanism for triggering breathing is the level of

_____ in the blood.

5. During inhalation, the _____ and _____ contract, causing the thorax to enlarge.

6. The drive to breathe is triggered by _____ or _____ levels in arterial blood.

7. Insufficient oxygen in the cells and tissues is called _____.

True/False

If you believe the statement to be more true than false, write the letter "T" in the space provided. If you believe the statement to be more false than true, write the letter "F."

1. _____ Nasal airways keep the tongue from blocking the upper airway and facilitate suctioning of the oropharynx.

2. _____ Nasal cannulas can deliver a maximum of 44% oxygen at 6 L/min.

3. _____ Oral airways should be measured from the tip of the nose to the earlobe.

4. _____ Compressed gas cylinders pose no unusual risk.

5. _____ The pin-indexing system is used to ensure compatibility between pressure regulators and oxygen flowmeters.

Short Answer

Complete this section with short written answers using the space provided.

1. List the five early signs of hypoxia.

_____

_____

_____

_____

_____

2. What are the normal respiratory rates for adults, children, and infants?

_____

_____

_____

3. How can you avoid gastric distention while performing artificial ventilation?

_____

_____

_____

4. List the six steps for providing one-rescuer artificial ventilation with a BVM device.

_____

_____

_____

_____

_____

_____

5. List six signs of inadequate breathing.

_____

_____

_____

_____

_____

_____

6. What are accessory muscles? Name three.

_____

_____

_____

7. When should medical control be consulted before inserting a nasal airway?

_____

_____

_____

8. List the four steps in nasal airway insertion.

_____

_____

_____

9. What is the best suction tip for suctioning the pharynx, and why?

_____

_____

_____

10. What is the time limit for each episode of suctioning an adult?

_____

_____

_____

Word Fun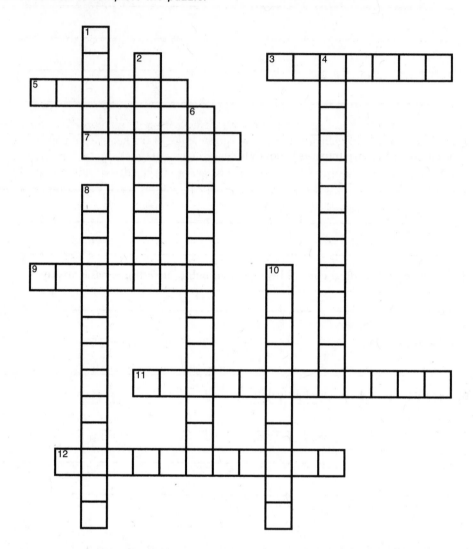

The following crossword puzzle is an activity provided to reinforce correct spelling and understanding of medical terminology associated with emergency care. Use the clues in the column to complete the puzzle.

CLUES

Across

3. Requires more than normal effort

5. Dying, gasping respirations

7. Larynx, nose, mouth, throat

9. Not enough O_2

11. Face piece attached to a reservoir

12. Exchange of air between lungs and outside

Down

1. Opening in neck connected to trachea

2. Mechanism that causes retching

4. Limits exposure to body fluids

6. Airway inserted in nostril

8. Airway inserted in mouth

10. Diaphragm relaxes

Calls to the Scene

The following case scenarios provide an opportunity to explore the concerns associated with patient management. Read each scenario, then answer each question in detail.

1. You are dispatched to an incident in a wooded area off a difficult trail. Your patient is a 38-year-old woman who struck her face against a tree. There is a large laceration on her nose and several teeth are missing. Though unconscious, she has vomited a large amount of food and blood, which is pooling in her mouth. You note gurgling noises as she attempts to breathe.

How would you best manage this patient?

_____

_____

_____

_____

_____

_____

_____

_____

_____

_____

2. You are dispatched to a private cabin adjacent to a mountain resort. You arrive to find an 83-year-old man sitting upright on the edge of his bed gasping for air. A family member states that the patient woke this morning feeling "ill" and having a difficult time breathing. The patient acknowledges a history of emphysema, but takes no prescriptions for the problem. He states that he "can't get enough air."

How would you best manage this patient?

_____

_____

_____

_____

_____

_____

_____

_____

3. You have been called to the Slopeside Lodge and directed to one of the rental units. When you arrive, the mother meets you at the door with her 1-year-old daughter in her arms. The mother states that she left the kids' room to answer the telephone and returned to find the child motionless on the floor next to a spilled jar of marbles. You note that the child remains motionless and there are no signs of respirations. The child is cyanotic.

How would you best manage this patient?

_____

_____

_____

_____

_____

_____

_____

_____

_____

_____

_____

Skill Drills

Skill Drill 6-1: Positioning an Unconscious Patient

Test your knowledge of this skill drill by placing the photos below in the correct order. Number the first step with a "1," the second step with a "2," etc.

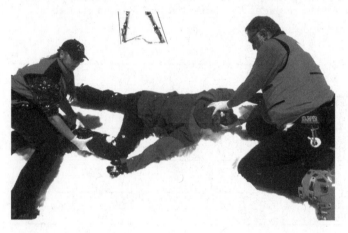

Have your partner place his or her hand on the patient's far shoulder and hip.

_____

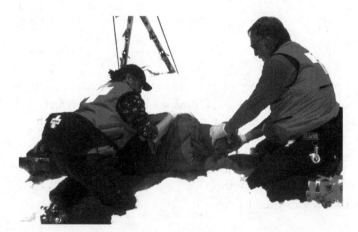

Open and assess the patient's airway and breathing status.

_____

(continued)

2

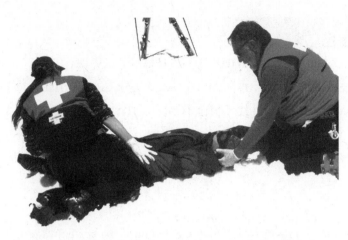

Support the head while your partner straightens the patient's legs.

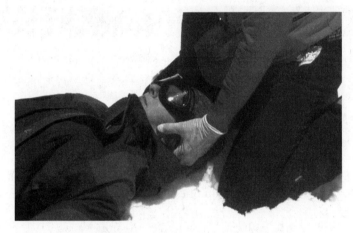

Roll the patient as a unit with the person at the head calling the count to begin the move.

Workbook Activities

The following activities have been designed to help you. Your instructor may require you to complete some or all of these activities as a regular part of your OEC training program. You are encouraged to complete any activity that your instructor does not assign as a way to enhance your learning in the classroom.

Chapter Review

The following exercises provide an opportunity to refresh your knowledge of this chapter.

■ NOTES ■

Matching

Match each of the terms in the left column to the appropriate definition in the right column.

_____ **1.** Triage	**A.** lining of the eyelid
_____ **2.** Distal	**B.** nearer to the tips of the extremities
_____ **3.** Subcutaneous emphysema	**C.** the six pain questions
_____ **4.** Hemorrhage	**D.** high-pitched sound in the upper airway
_____ **5.** Conjunctiva	**E.** a crackling sound
_____ **6.** Crepitus	**F.** examine by touch
_____ **7.** Hypothermia	**G.** urgent measure that interrupts assessment
_____ **8.** Chief complaint	**H.** the way in which a patient responds to external stimuli
_____ **9.** Radiating pain	**I.** pain not identified as being specific to a single location
_____ **10.** Localized pain	**J.** internal body temperature falls below 95°F
_____ **11.** Intervention	**K.** air under the skin
_____ **12.** Stridor	**L.** profuse bleeding
_____ **13.** OPQRST	**M.** the reason a patient called for help
_____ **14.** Palpate	**N.** pain easily identified as being specific to a single location
_____ **15.** Responsiveness	**O.** a process of identifying the severity of each patient's condition; sorting

Patient Assessment

Multiple Choice

Read each item carefully, then select the best response.

_____ **1.** The scene size-up consists of all of the following except:
   A. determining mechanism of injury.
   B. requesting additional assistance.
   C. determining level of responsiveness.
   D. PPE/BSI.

_____ **2.** Possible dangers you may observe during the scene size-up include:
   A. oncoming traffic.
   B. unstable surfaces.
   C. downed electrical lines.
   D. all of the above

_____ **3.** Proper assessment procedures begin with:
   A. splinting fractures.
   B. making accurate observations.
   C. cleaning wounds.
   D. completing incident reports.

_____ **4.** The characteristics of injury or illness that a patient tells you about are called:
   A. impressions.
   B. signs.
   C. symptoms.
   D. facts.

_____ **5.** You can use the mechanism of injury as a guide to predict the potential for a serious injury by evaluating:

  A. the amount of force applied to the body.

  B. the length of time the force was applied.

  C. the areas of the body that are involved.

  D. all of the above

_____ **6.** Every unresponsive, injured patient must be considered to have:

  A. a spine injury.

  B. a brain injury.

  C. internal injuries

  D. a blocked airway.

_____ **7.** The purpose of the initial assessment is to:

  A. determine what circumstances caused the accident.

  B. determine how many patients will need to be assisted.

  C. immediately identify and treat life-threatening emergencies.

  D. determine if an ambulance or helicopter will be needed.

_____ **8.** Clear or blood-tinged fluid draining from the nose or ears may be an indication of:

  A. spinal injury.

  B. cerebrovascular attack.

  C. heart attack.

  D. skull fracture.

_____ **9.** In order to quickly determine the nature of illness, talk with:

  A. the patient.

  B. family members.

  C. bystanders.

  D. all of the above

_____ **10.** When considering the need for additional resources, questions to ask include all of the following, except:

  A. How many patients are there?

  B. How extreme are weather conditions?

  C. Who contacted EMS?

  D. Does the scene pose a threat to you or your patient's safety?

_____ **11.** The initial assessment includes evaluation of all of the following except:
  A. mental status.
  B. pupils.
  C. airway.
  D. circulation.

_____ **12.** An altered mental status may be caused by:
  A. brain trauma.
  B. hypoxemia.
  C. hypoglycemia.
  D. all of the above

_____ **13.** All of the following are signs of inadequate breathing except:
  A. tightness in the chest.
  B. two- to three-word dyspnea.
  C. use of accessory muscles.
  D. nasal flaring.

_____ **14.** Airway obstruction in an unresponsive patient is most commonly due to:
  A. vomitus.
  B. the tongue.
  C. dentures.
  D. food.

_____ **15.** Signs of airway obstruction in an unconscious patient include:
  A. obvious trauma, blood, or other obstruction.
  B. noisy breathing.
  C. extremely shallow or absent breathing.
  D. all of the above

_____ **16.** The _____ of the patient's pulse will give you a general idea of the overall status of the patient's cardiac function.
  A. rate
  B. rhythm
  C. strength
  D. all of the above

_____ **17.** Which of the following statements about the focused history and physical exam is true?
  A. It is automatic and almost instantaneous.
  B. It identifies injuries that are not immediately life threatening.
  C. It is a quick check for major injuries.
  D. It starts with opening the airway.

_____ **18.** To test for paralysis in the extremities of the responsive patient, the rescuer should check for:
  A. movement and sensation.
  B. pain, by doing a sternal rub.
  C. pain, by using a pin or other sharp object.
  D. reaction to hot and cold.

3

_____ **19.** Assessing the _____ is one of the most important and readily accessible ways of evaluating circulation.

   A. pulse

   B. respirations

   C. skin

   D. capillary refill

_____ **20.** Skin color depends on:

   A. pigmentation.

   B. blood oxygen levels.

   C. the amount of blood circulating through the vessels of the skin.

   D. all of the above

_____ **21.** Cyanosis is defined as a bluish discoloration of the skin, fingernails, and mucous membranes that occurs:

   A. because of chemical dependence.

   B. because of preexisting asthma.

   C. only when a patient has carbon monoxide poisoning.

   D. because the blood is not properly oxygenated.

_____ **22.** If a patient has inadequate circulation, you must take immediate action to do all of the following except:

   A. restore or improve circulation.

   B. apply an AED.

   C. control severe bleeding.

   D. improve oxygen delivery to the tissues.

_____ **23.** While initial care is important, it is essential to remember that immediate _____ is one of the keys to the survival of any high-priority patient.

   A. airway control

   B. bleeding control

   C. transport

   D. application of oxygen

_____ **24.** Goals of the focused history and physical exam include:

   A. identifying the patient's chief complaint.

   B. understanding the specific circumstances surrounding the chief complaint.

   C. directing further physical examination.

   D. all of the above

_____25. Understanding the _____ helps you to understand the severity of the patient's problem and provide invaluable information to hospital staff as well.
  A. chief complaint
  B. mechanism of injury
  C. physical exam
  D. focused history

_____26. A weak, slow pulse may be a sign of:
  A. normal sleep.
  B. diabetic coma.
  C. hypothermia.
  D. early shock.

_____27. An integral part of the rapid trauma assessment is evaluation using the mnemonic:
  A. AVPU.
  B. DCAP-BTLS.
  C. OPQRST.
  D. SAMPLE.

_____28. It is particularly important to evaluate the neck before:
  A. log rolling the patient.
  B. examining the chest.
  C. covering it with a cervical collar.
  D. checking for the presence of a carotid pulse.

_____29. To check for motor function, you should ask the patient:
  A. to wiggle his or her fingers or toes.
  B. to identify which extremity you are touching.
  C. if he or she can feel your touch.
  D. all of the above

_____30. The "E" in SAMPLE stands for:
  A. eating habits.
  B. emergency medications.
  C. events leading up to the episode.
  D. episodes experienced previously.

_____31. Patients who require a complete rapid trauma assessment, coupled with short scene time and immediate transport to definitive care, include all of the following except a patient who:
  A. experienced a significant mechanism of injury.
  B. complained of neck pain after being hit from the rear.
  C. is unresponsive or disoriented.
  D. is extremely intoxicated from drugs or alcohol.

■ **NOTES** ■

_____**32.** The "S" in the mnemonic OPQRST stands for:
  A. signs.
  B. symptoms.
  C. severity.
  D. syncope.

_____**33.** A patient who points to a single place for his or her pain has what is known as:
  A. diffuse pain.
  B. localized pain.
  C. radiating pain.
  D. referred pain.

_____**34.** When assessing a chief complaint of chest pain, you should evaluate:
  A. skin color.
  B. pulse.
  C. breath sounds.
  D. all of the above

_____**35.** Baseline vital signs provide useful information about the:
  A. overall functions of the patient's heart.
  B. overall functions of the patient's lungs.
  C. patient's stability.
  D. all of the above

_____**36.** If you have successfully stabilized the ABCs on any patient who is unresponsive, confused, or unable to relate the chief complaint adequately, you should:
  A. try to obtain information from family members.
  B. perform a rapid assessment.
  C. look for clues from medication bottles.
  D. transport immediately.

_____**37.** When performing a detailed physical exam, depending on what is learned, you should be prepared to:
  A. return to the initial assessment if a potentially life-threatening condition is identified.
  B. provide treatment for problems that were identified during the exam.
  C. modify any treatment that is underway on the basis of any new information.
  D. all of the above

_____**38.** When performing a detailed physical exam, check the neck for:
  A. subcutaneous emphysema.
  B. jugular vein distention.
  C. crepitus.
  D. all of the above

_____**39.** The purpose of the ongoing assessment is to ask and answer the following questions except:
  A. Is treatment improving the patient's condition?
  B. What is the patient's diagnosis?
  C. Has an already identified problem gotten better? Worse?
  D. What is the nature of any newly identified problems?

_____**40.** When reevaluating any interventions you started, take a moment to ensure that:

    A. oxygen is still flowing.

    B. backboard straps are still tight.

    C. bleeding has been controlled.

    D. all of the above

Vocabulary www.OECzone.com vocab explorer

Define the following terms using the space provided.

1. Intervention:

_____

_____

_____

2. Recovery position:

_____

_____

_____

3. Mechanism of injury:

_____

_____

_____

4. Golden Hour:

_____

_____

_____

3

Fill-in

Read each item carefully, then complete the statement by filling in the missing word(s).

1. The best way to reduce your risk of exposure is to follow _____ (BSI) precautions.

2. _____, _____, and _____ are three features to be checked when taking a pulse.

3. The _____ _____ is based on your immediate assessment of the environment, the presenting signs and symptoms, mechanism of injury in a trauma patient, and the patient's chief complaint.

4. The first steps in caring for any patient focus on finding and treating the most

_____ illnesses and injuries.

5. With an unresponsive patient or one with a decreased level of consciousness,

the _____ should immediately be assessed.

6. If a patient seems to have difficulty breathing, you should immediately

_____ the airway.

7. Correct identification of high-priority patients is an essential aspect of the

_____ and helps to improve patient outcome.

True/False

If you believe the statement to be more true than false, write the letter "T" in the space provided. If you believe the statement to be more false than true, write the letter "F."

1. _____ Responsiveness is evaluated with the mnemonic DCAP-BTLS.

2. _____ The detailed physical exam is normally performed in a warm environment.

3. _____ An ongoing assessment is not necessary for stable patients.

4. _____ Distinguishing between medical and trauma patients is less important than identifying and treating their problems appropriately.

5. _____ The apparent absence of a palpable pulse in a responsive patient is not caused by cardiac arrest.

6. _____ Sometimes injuries are missed because the rescuer did not do a systematic examination.

7. _____ A rapid body survey is not necessary for a patient without a significant mechanism of injury.

Short Answer

Complete this section with short written answers using the space provided.

1. List four objectives of patient assessment.

_____

_____

_____

_____

2. What is the single goal of initial assessment?

_____

_____

_____

3. What is the general impression based on?

_____

_____

_____

4. What do the letters ABC stand for in the assessment process?

_____

_____

_____

3

5. What are the three goals of the focused history and physical exam?

_____

_____

_____

6. List the elements of DCAP-BTLS.

_____

_____

_____

Word Fun

The following crossword puzzle is an activity provided to reinforce correct spelling and understanding of medical terminology associated with emergency care. Use the clues in the column to complete the puzzle.

Across
1. Rattling, moist sounds
4. Body substance isolation
5. Pain assessment acronym
6. Grating or grinding
8. Mechanism of injury
10. Below 95° F

Down
1. Distal discomfort or pain
2. Acronym for history
3. Involuntary muscle contraction, to protect
7. Coarse breath sounds
9. Pain in a single area

Calls to the Scene

The following case scenarios provide an opportunity to explore the concerns associated with patient management. Read each scenario, then answer each question in detail.

1. You get called to the scene of an unresponsive patient who has a facial laceration. How would you best manage this patient?

_____

_____

_____

_____

_____

_____

_____

_____

_____

2. You arrive on the scene where there is a 20-year-old snowboarder in the terrain park just below a jump. He complains of an injured shoulder.

How would you best manage this patient?

_____

_____

_____

_____

_____

_____

_____

_____

_____

3. You are called to the cafeteria where a 30-year-old man reportedly fainted and is now responsive and sitting in a chair.

How would you best manage this patient?

_____

_____

_____

_____

_____

_____

_____

_____

_____

Skill Drills

Skill Drill 7-1: Performing a Rapid Body Survey

Test your knowledge of this skill drill by placing the photos below in the correct order.
Number the first step with a "1," the second step with a "2," etc.

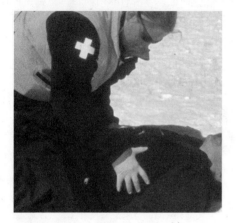

_____

Assess the chest.

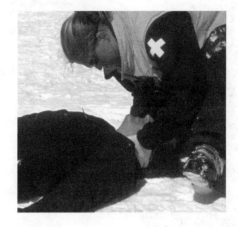

_____

Assess the neck.

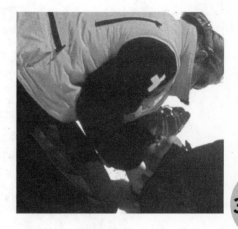

_____

Assess the head.

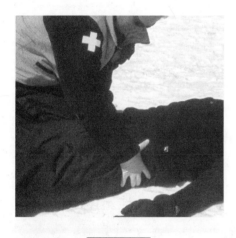

_____

Assess the pelvis.

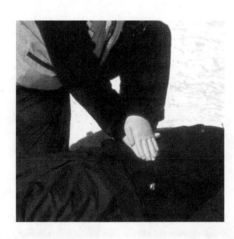

_____

Assess the abdomen.

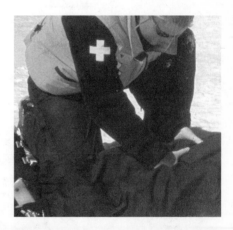

_____

Assess the lower extremities.

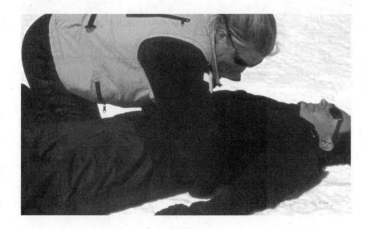

_____

Assess the back.

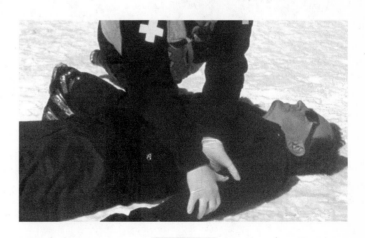

_____

Assess the upper extremities.

Skill Drill 7-2: Performing a Focused History and Physical Exam —
Responsive Trauma Patient
Test your knowledge of this skill drill by placing the photos below in the correct order.
Number the first step with a "1," the second step with a "2," etc.

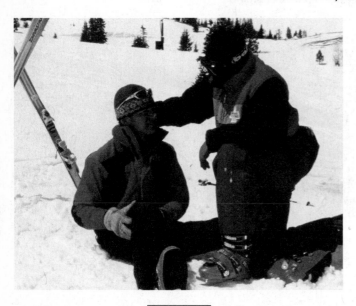

_____

Assess the patient's head, neck and back if a loss of
responsiveness or spine or head injury is suspected.

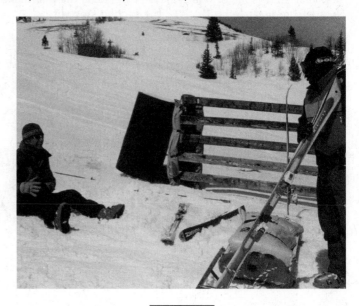

_____

Ensure scene safety and patient responsiveness. Recheck
ABCs.

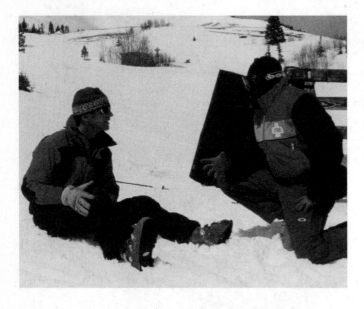

_____

Institute BSI precautions and obtain the patient's consent
for treatment.

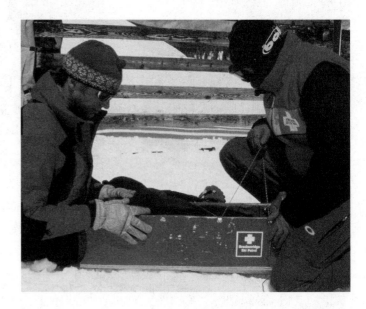

_____

Splint and/or provide appropriate care of injuries.

(continued)

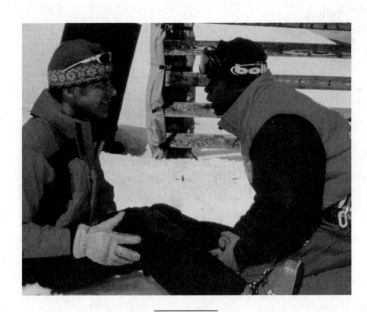

Determine the patient's chief complaint.

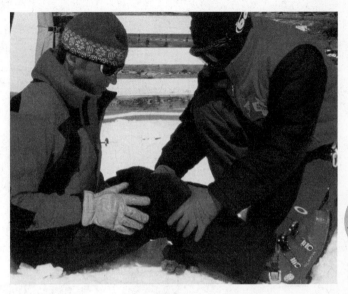

Perform a focused assessment of the injured site (chief complaint).

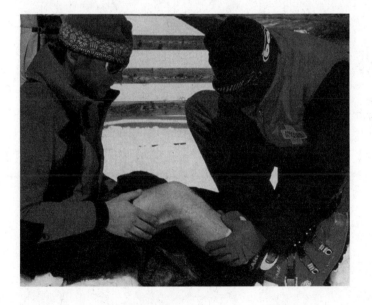

Expose only what is necessary to determine the essential emergency care.

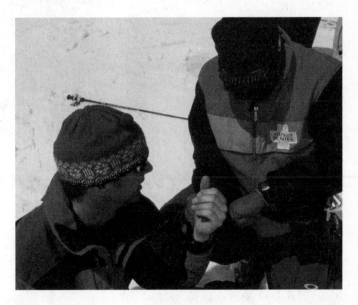

Assess the patient's pulse, skin temperature, and breathing rate. Obtain a SAMPLE history.

Skill Drill 7-4: Performing the Detailed Physical Exam
Test your knowledge of this skill drill by placing the photos below in the correct order. Number the first step with a "1," the second step with a "2," etc.

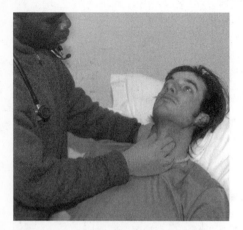

_____

Palpate the neck, front and back.

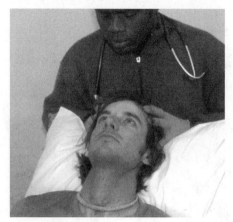

_____

Observe and palpate the head.

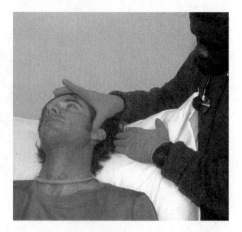

_____

Check the ears for drainage or blood.

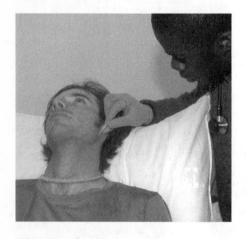

_____

Look behind the ear for Battle's sign.

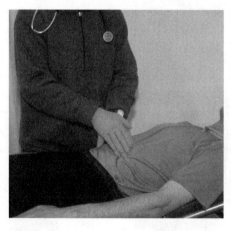

_____

Gently palpate the abdomen.

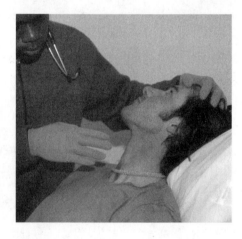

_____

Observe for jugular vein distention.

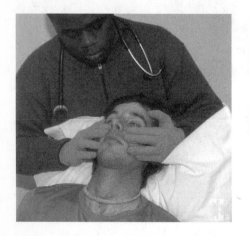

_____

Palpate the zygomas and maxillae.

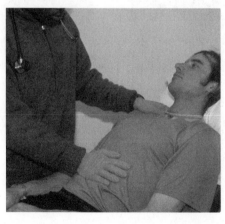

_____

Inspect the chest and observe breathing motion.

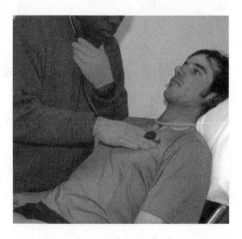

_____

Listen to anterior breath sounds (midaxillary, midclavicular).

(continued)

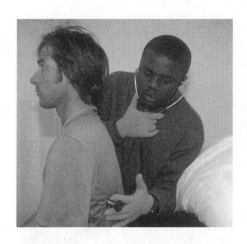

Listen to posterior breath sounds (bases, apices).

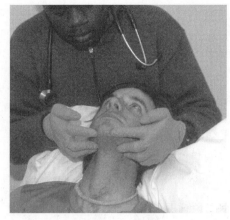

Palpate the mandible.

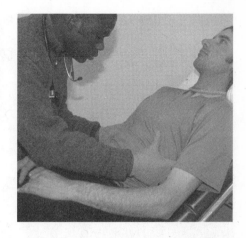

Gently palpate the ribs.

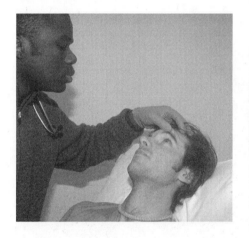

Inspect the eyelids and the area around the eyes.

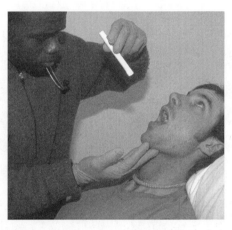

Assess the mouth.

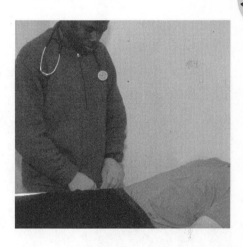

Observe the abdomen and pelvis.

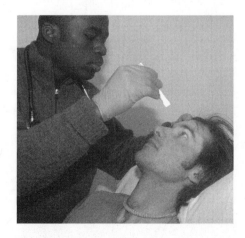

Examine the eyes for redness, contact lenses. Check pupil function.

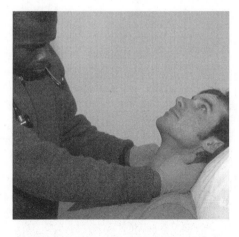

Inspect the neck.

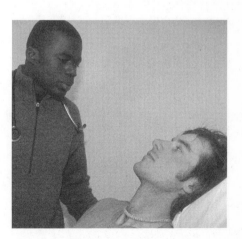

Observe the patient's face.

(continued)

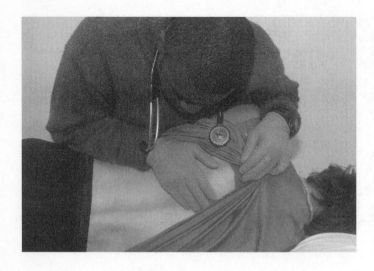

Log roll the patient. Inspect and palpate the back.

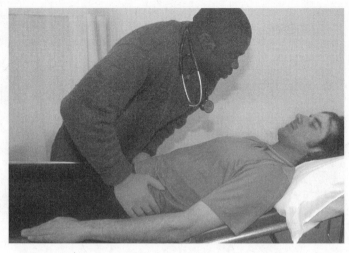

Gently press the iliac crests.

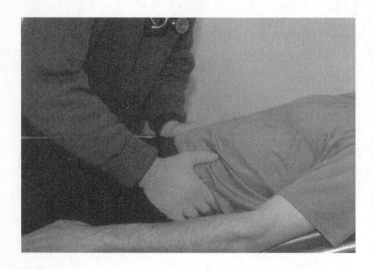

Gently compress the pelvis from the sides.

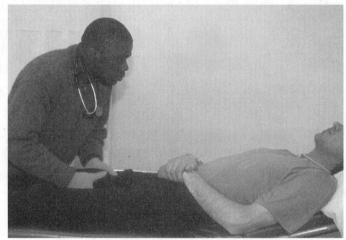

Assess the lower extremities.

(continued)

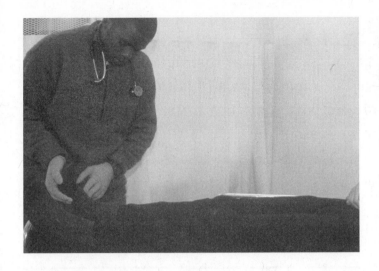

Assess distal circulation, motor, and sensory function in the lower extremities.

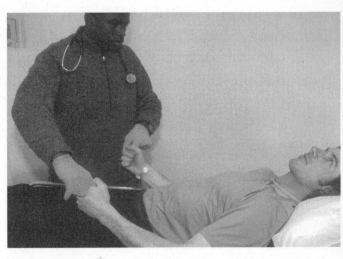

Assess distal circulation, motor, and sensory functions in the upper extremities.

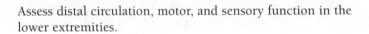
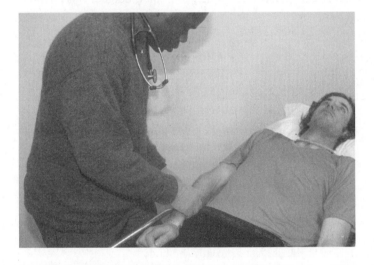

Assess the upper extremities.

Workbook Activities

The following activities have been designed to help you. Your instructor may require you to complete some or all of these activities as a regular part of your OEC training program. You are encouraged to complete any activity that your instructor does not assign as a way to enhance your learning in the classroom.

Chapter Review

The following exercises provide an opportunity to refresh your knowledge of this chapter.

NOTES

Matching

Match each of the terms in the left column to the appropriate definition in the right column.

_____ 1. Pulmonary artery   **A.** mass of blood in the soft tissues beneath the skin

_____ 2. Heart   **B.** formation of clot to plug opening in injured blood vessel and stop blood flow

_____ 3. Ventricle   **C.** upper chamber

_____ 4. Aorta   **D.** a congenital condition in which a patient lacks one or more of the blood's normal clotting factors

_____ 5. Atrium   **E.** hollow muscular organ

_____ 6. Pulmonary vein   **F.** largest artery in the body

_____ 7. Coagulation   **G.** a condition in which low blood volume results in inadequate perfusion

_____ 8. Ecchymosis   **H.** oxygenated blood travels through this

_____ 9. Epistaxis   **I.** bruising

_____ 10. Hematoma   **J.** deoxygenated blood travels through this

_____ 11. Hemophilia   **K.** lower chamber

_____ 12. Hemorrhage   **L.** bleeding

_____ 13. Hypovolemic shock   **M.** nosebleed

Multiple Choice

Read each item carefully, then select the best response.

_____ 1. The function of the blood is to _____ all of the body's cells and tissues.

   A. deliver oxygen to

   B. deliver nutrients to

   C. carry waste products away from

   D. all of the above

Bleeding

_____ **2.** The cardiovascular system consists of:
   A. a pump.
   B. a container.
   C. fluid.
   D. all of the above

_____ **3.** Blood leaves each chamber of a normal heart through a(n):
   A. vein.
   B. artery.
   C. one-way valve.
   D. capillary.

_____ **4.** Blood enters the right atrium from the:
   A. coronary arteries.
   B. lungs.
   C. vena cava.
   D. coronary veins.

_____ **5.** Blood enters the left atrium from the:
   A. coronary arteries.
   B. lungs.
   C. vena cava.
   D. coronary veins.

_____ **6.** The only arteries in the body to carry deoxygenated blood are the:
   A. pulmonary arteries.
   B. coronary arteries.
   C. femoral arteries.
   D. subclavian arteries.

_____ **7.** The _____ is the thickest chamber of the heart.
   A. right atrium
   B. right ventricle
   C. left atrium
   D. left ventricle

_____ **8.** The _____ link(s) the arterioles and the venules.

A. aorta

B. capillaries

C. vena cava

D. valves

_____ **9.** At the arterial end of the capillaries, the muscles dilate and constrict in response to conditions such as:

A. fright.

B. a specific need for oxygen.

C. a need to dispose of metabolic wastes.

D. all of the above

_____ **10.** Blood contains all of the following except:

A. white cells.

B. plasma.

C. cerebrospinal fluid.

D. platelets.

_____ **11.** _____ is the circulation of blood within an organ or tissue in adequate amounts to meet the cells' current needs for oxygen, nutrients, and waste removal.

A. Anatomy

B. Perfusion

C. Physiology

D. Conduction

_____ **12.** The _____ only require(s) a minimal blood supply when at rest.

A. lungs

B. kidneys

C. muscles

D. heart

_____ **13.** The term _____ means constantly adapting to changing conditions.

A. perfusion

B. conduction

C. dynamic

D. autonomic

_____ **14.** _____ is inadequate tissue perfusion.

A. Shock

B. Hyperperfusion

C. Hypertension

D. Contraction

_____ **15.** The brain and spinal cord cannot go for more than _____ minutes without perfusion, or the nerve cells will be permanently damaged.

A. 30 to 45

B. 12 to 20

C. 8 to 10

D. 4 to 6

_____ **16.** The body will not tolerate an acute blood loss of greater than _____ of blood volume.

    A. 10%

    B. 20%

    C. 30%

    D. 40%

_____ **17.** If the typical adult loses more than 1 L of blood, significant changes in vital signs such as _____ will occur.

    A. increased heart rate

    B. increased respiratory rate

    C. decreased blood pressure

    D. all of the above

_____ **18.** _____ is a condition in which low blood volume results in inadequate perfusion and even death.

    A. Hypovolemic shock

    B. Metabolic shock

    C. Septic shock

    D. Psychogenic shock

_____ **19.** You should consider bleeding to be serious if all of the following conditions are present, except:

    A. rapid blood loss

    B. no mechanism of injury.

    C. a poor general appearance.

    D. signs and symptoms of shock.

_____ **20.** Significant blood loss demands your immediate attention as soon as you have managed:

    A. fractures.

    B. extrication.

    C. the airway.

    D. none of the above

_____ **21.** The process of blood clotting and plugging the hole is called:

    A. conglomeration.

    B. configuration.

    C. coagulation.

    D. coalition.

_____ **22.** Even though the body is very efficient at controlling bleeding on its own, it may fail in situations such as:

    A. when medications interfere with normal clotting.

    B. when damage to the vessel may be so large that a clot cannot completely block the hole.

    C. when only part of the vessel wall is cut, preventing it from constricting.

    D. all of the above

_____23. A lack of one or more of the blood's clotting factors is called:
  A. a deficiency.
  B. hemophilia.
  C. platelet anomaly.
  D. anemia.

_____24. The first step in controlling bleeding is:
  A. direct pressure.
  B. maintaining the airway.
  C. BSI precautions.
  D. elevation.

_____25. When applying a bandage to hold a dressing in place, stretch the bandage tight enough to control bleeding, but not so tight as to decrease _____ to the extremity.
  A. blood flow
  B. pulses
  C. oxygen
  D. CRTs

_____26. If bleeding continues after applying a pressure dressing, you should do all of the following except:
  A. remove the dressing and apply another sterile dressing.
  B. apply manual pressure through the dressing.
  C. add more gauze pads over the first dressing.
  D. secure both dressings tighter with a roller bandage.

_____27. When using an air splint to control bleeding in a fractured extremity, you should reassess the _____ frequently.
  A. airway
  B. breathing
  C. circulation in the injured extremity
  D. fracture site

_____28. A tourniquet is rarely needed to control bleeding and often _____ problems.
  A. resolves
  B. decreases
  C. creates
  D. all of the above

_____29. When applying a tourniquet, make sure you:
  A. use the narrowest bandage possible to minimize the area restricted.
  B. cover the tourniquet with a bandage.
  C. do not pad underneath the tourniquet.
  D. do not loosen the tourniquet after you have applied it.

_____ **30.** Bleeding from the nose, ears, and/or mouth may be the result of:

    A. a skull fracture.

    B. sinusitis.

    C. coagulation disorders.

    D. all of the above

_____ **31.** You should not attempt to stop the blood flow from the nose or ears following a head injury because:

    A. it should be collected to be reinfused at the hospital.

    B. it could collect within the head and increase the pressure in the brain.

    C. it is contaminated.

    D. you could fracture the skull with the pressure needed to staunch the flow of blood.

_____ **32.** When treating a patient with signs and symptoms of hypovolemic shock and no outward signs of bleeding, always consider the possibility of bleeding into the:

    A. thoracic cavity.

    B. abdomen.

    C. skull.

    D. chest.

_____ **33.** Nontraumatic internal bleeding may be caused by:

    A. an ulcer.

    B. a ruptured ectopic pregnancy.

    C. an aneurysm.

    D. all of the above

_____ **34.** The most common symptom of internal abdominal bleeding is:

    A. bruising around the abdomen.

    B. distention of the abdomen.

    C. rigidity of the abdomen.

    D. acute pain in the abdomen.

_____ **35.** Signs and symptoms of internal bleeding in both trauma and medical patients include:

    A. hematochezia.

    B. melena.

    C. hemoptysis.

    D. all of the above

_____ **36.** The first sign of hypovolemic shock is a change in:

    A. respirations.

    B. heart rate.

    C. mental status.

    D. blood pressure.

3

Labeling www.OECzone.com anatomy review

Label the following diagrams with the correct terms. Where arrows appear, indicate the substance and its origin and destination.

1. The Left and Right Sides of the Heart

A. _____

B. _____

C. _____

D. _____

E. _____

F. _____

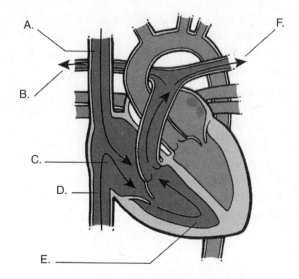

A. _____

B. _____

C. _____

D. _____

E. _____

F. _____

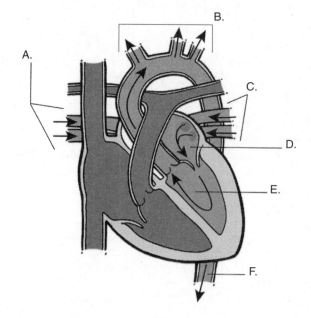

2. Perfusion

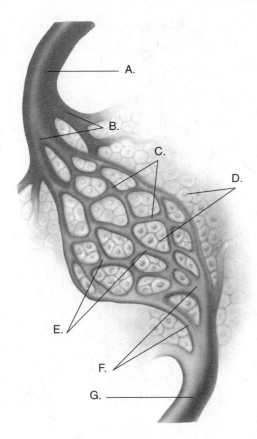

A. _____

B. _____

C. _____

D. _____

E. _____

F. _____

G. _____

3

3. Arterial Pressure Points

A. _____

B. _____

C. _____

D. _____

E. _____

F. _____

G. _____

H. _____

I. _____

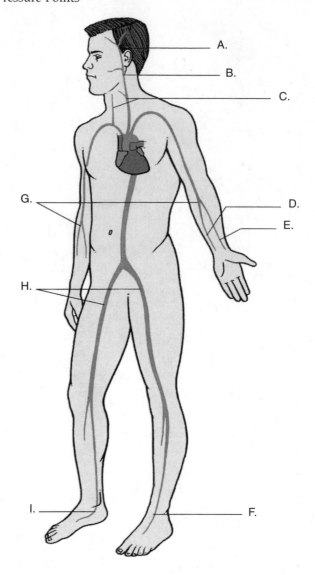

Vocabulary

Define the following terms using the space provided.

1. Perfusion:

_____

_____

_____

2. Shock:

_____

_____

_____

3. Melena:

_____

_____

_____

4. Hematemesis:

_____

_____

_____

5. Hemoptysis:

_____

_____

_____

Fill-in

Read each item carefully, then complete the statement by filling in the missing word.

1. The circulation of blood in adequate amounts to meet cellular needs is called

   _____.

2. The heart is a(n) _____ muscle, which is controlled by the autonomic nervous system.

3. Exchange of oxygen and carbon dioxide occurs in the _____.

4. Shock is a condition related to _____.

5. Blood returning to the heart from the lower body is first collected in the

   _____ vena cava.

6. The four major components of blood are _____, _____,

   _____, and _____.

7. The left ventricle receives _____ blood while the right ventricle

   receives _____ blood.

8. During a state of shock, the autonomic nervous system directs blood away from

   some organs and distributes it to the _____.

9. The brain and spinal cord generally cannot go longer than _____ minutes without adequate perfusion, or permanent nerve cell damage may occur.

True/False

If you believe the statement to be more true than false, write the letter "T" in the space provided. If you believe the statement to be more false than true, write the letter "F."

1. _____ Venous blood tends to spurt and is difficult to control.

2. _____ The human body is tolerant of blood losses greater than 20% of blood volume.

3. _____ The first step in preparing to treat a bleeding patient is BSI.

4. _____ A properly applied tourniquet should be loosened by the rescuer every ten minutes.

5. _____ A patient who has swallowed a lot of blood may become nauseated and vomit.

6. _____ If a wound continues to bleed after it is bandaged, you should remove the bandage and start over again.

Short Answer

Complete this section with short written answers in the space provided.

1. Describe how the autonomic nervous system responds to severe bleeding.

_____

_____

_____

2. Describe the characteristics of bleeding from each type of vessel (artery, vein, capillary).

_____

_____

_____

3. List, in the proper sequence, the methods in which a rescuer should attempt to control external bleeding.

_____

_____

_____

4. List ten signs and symptoms of hypovolemic shock.

_____

_____

_____

_____

_____

_____

_____

_____

_____

5. List, in the proper sequence, the general outdoor emergency care for patients with internal bleeding.

_____

_____

_____

Word Fun www.OECzone.com vocab explorer

The following crossword puzzle is an activity provided to reinforce correct spelling and understanding of medical terminology associated with emergency care. Use the clues in the column to complete the puzzle.

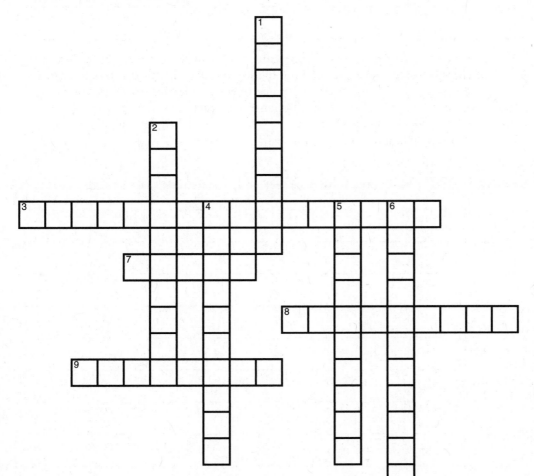

Across

3. Low blood volume, inadequate perfusion

7. Circulatory system failure

8. Circulation of blood within the body

9. Mass of blood in soft tissues

Down

1. Nosebleed

2. Lacks normal clotting factors

4. Discoloration of skin from closed wound

5. Bleeding

6. Formation of clots to stop bleeding

3

Calls to the Scene

The following case scenarios provide an opportunity to explore the concerns associated with patient management. Read each scenario, then answer each question in detail.

1. You are dispatched to the children's ski school for an 8-year-old boy who has a laceration to his left wrist with uncontrollable hemorrhaging. The blood is steady, but not spurting, and dark in color.

   How would you best manage this patient?

   _____

   _____

   _____

   _____

   _____

   _____

   _____

   _____

   _____

2. A motor vehicle crash has been reported on the winding road up to the resort. There is major damage to the front of the vehicle where the driver is restrained. She is a 23-year-old woman with no pertinent medical history according to a passenger in the vehicle. She is responsive to pain and showing signs of hypo-volemic shock. Her only visible injury is a bruise to her right upper quadrant.

   How would you best manage this patient?

   _____

   _____

   _____

   _____

   _____

   _____

   _____

   _____

   _____

3. A ski shop employee was trying to lift skis onto a display rack using a stool instead of a ladder. He leaned too far, and fell to the floor, cutting the inside of his arm on a ski. There is continuous bleeding from an arterial laceration, with blood on the patient, skis, and floor.

How would you best manage this patient?

_____

_____

_____

_____

_____

_____

_____

_____

_____

Skill Drills

Skill Drill 8-1: Controlling External Bleeding
Test your knowledge of this skill drill by filling in the correct words in the photo captions.

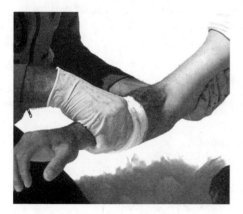

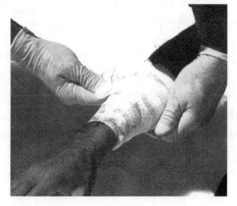

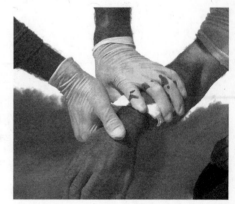

1. Apply _____
_____ over the wound.
Elevate the injury above the
_____ of the _____ if
no _____ is suspected.

2. Apply a _____
_____.

3. Apply pressure at the appropriate
_____ _____
while continuing to hold
_____ _____
and _____.

Workbook Activities

The following activities have been designed to help you. Your instructor may require you to complete some or all of these activities as a regular part of your OEC training program. You are encouraged to complete any activity that your instructor does not assign as a way to enhance your learning in the classroom.

Chapter Review

The following exercises provide an opportunity to refresh your knowledge of this chapter.

◼ NOTES ◼

Matching

Match each of the terms in the left column to the appropriate definition in the right column.

_____ 1. Shock
_____ 2. Perfusion
_____ 3. Sphincters
_____ 4. Autonomic nervous system
_____ 5. Blood pressure
_____ 6. Anaphylaxis
_____ 7. Septic shock
_____ 8. Syncope
_____ 9. Compensated shock

A. severe allergy
B. hypoperfusion
C. regulates involuntary body functions
D. early stage of shock
E. provides a rough measure of perfusion
F. severe bacterial infection
G. sufficient circulation to meet cell needs
H. regulate blood flow in capillaries
I. fainting

Multiple Choice

Read each item carefully, then select the best response.

_____ 1. Which of the following statements about shock is true?
   A. It refers to a state of collapse and failure of the cardiovascular system.
   B. It results in the inadequate flow of blood to the body's cells.
   C. It results in failure to rid cells of metabolic wastes.
   D. all of the above

_____ 2. Blood flow through the capillary beds is regulated by:
   A. systolic pressure.
   B. the capillary sphincters.
   C. perfusion.
   D. diastolic pressure.

Shock

_____ **3.** The autonomic nervous system regulates involuntary functions such as:

A. sweating.

B. digestion.

C. constriction and dilation of capillary sphincters.

D. all of the above

_____ **4.** Regulation of blood flow is determined by:

A. oxygen intake.

B. systolic pressure.

C. cellular need.

D. diastolic pressure.

_____ **5.** Perfusion requires having a working cardiovascular system as well as adequate:

A. oxygen exchange in the lungs.

B. glucose levels in the blood.

C. waste removal.

D. all of the above

_____ **6.** The action of the hormones stimulates _____ to maintain pressure in the system and, as a result, perfusion of all vital organs.

A. an increase in heart rate

B. an increase in the strength of cardiac contractions

C. vasoconstriction in nonessential areas

D. all of the above

_____ **7.** Basic causes of shock include:

A. poor pump function.

B. blood or fluid loss.

C. blood vessel dilation.

D. all of the above

_____ **8.** Noncardiovascular causes of shock include respiratory insufficiency and:

A. sepsis.

B. hypothermia.

C. anaphylaxis.

D. hypovolemia.

_____ **9.** When the heart no longer functions well, a major effect is the backup of blood into the lungs called pulmonary:

A. edema.

B. overload.

C. cessation.

D. failure.

_____ **10.** _____ develops when the heart muscle can no longer generate enough pressure to circulate the blood to all organs.

A. Pump failure

B. Cardiogenic shock

C. Myocardial infarction

D. Congestive heart failure

_____ **11.** Damage to the _____ may cause significant injury to the part of the nervous system that controls the size and muscular tone of the blood vessels.

A. cervical vertebrae

B. skull

C. spinal cord

D. peripheral nerves

_____ **12.** Neurogenic shock usually results from damage to the spinal cord at which level?

A. cervical

B. thoracic

C. lumbar

D. sacral

_____ **13.** Septic shock results from _____, in combination with the loss of plasma through the injured vessel walls.

A. pump failure

B. massive vasoconstriction

C. widespread dilation

D. increased volume

_____ **14.** Which of the following statements about septic shock is true?

A. There is an insufficient volume of fluid in the container.

B. The fluid that has leaked out often collects in the respiratory system.

C. There is a larger-than-normal vascular bed to contain the smaller-than-normal volume of intravascular fluid.

D. all of the above

_____ **15.** Neurogenic shock is caused by:

A. a radical change in the size of the vascular system.

B. massive vasoconstriction.

C. low volume.

D. fluid collecting around the spinal cord causing compression of the cord.

_____ **16.** Hypovolemic shock is a result of:

A. widespread vasodilation.

B. low volume.

C. massive vasoconstriction.

D. pump failure.

_____ **17.** An insufficient concentration of _____ in the blood can produce shock as rapidly as vascular causes.

   A. oxygen

   B. hormones

   C. epinephrine

   D. histamine

_____ **18.** In anaphylactic shock, the combination of poor oxygenation and poor perfusion is a result of:

   A. widespread vascular dilation.

   B. low volume.

   C. massive vasoconstriction.

   D. pump failure.

_____ **19.** Causes of syncope include:

   A. fear.

   B. the sight of blood.

   C. cardiac arrhythmias.

   D. all of the above

_____ **20.** In shock, the last measurable factor to change is normally:

   A. mental status.

   B. blood pressure.

   C. pulse rate.

   D. respirations.

_____ **21.** Anaphylactic shock is caused by:

   A. grating bone ends.

   B. toxemia during pregnancy.

   C. sexually transmitted diseases.

   D. an allergic reaction to a substance.

_____ **22.** When treating a suspected shock patient, vital signs should be recorded approximately every _____ minutes.

   A. 2

   B. 5

   C. 10

   D. 15

_____ **23.** The Golden Hour refers to the first 60 minutes after:

   A. medical help arrives on scene.

   B. transport begins.

   C. the injury occurs.

   D. 9-1-1 is called.

_____ **24.** Signs of cardiogenic shock include all of the following except:

   A. cyanosis.

   B. strong, bounding pulse.

   C. nausea.

   D. anxiety.

_____ **25.** Primary treatment of shock includes:

   A. securing and maintaining an airway.

   B. providing respiratory support.

   C. assisting ventilations.

   D. all of the above

_____ **26.** When assessing the patient who has psychogenic shock, be sure to consider possible _____ if the patient fell.

A. extremity fractures

B. cervical spine injury

C. paralysis

D. pelvic fractures

Vocabulary www.OECzone.com vocab explorer

Define the following terms using the space provided.

1. Edema:

_____

_____

_____

2. Hypothermia:

_____

_____

_____

3. Shock:

_____

_____

_____

4. Autonomic nervous system:

_____

_____

_____

5. Cyanosis:

_____

_____

_____

6. Dehydration:

_____

_____

_____

7. Sensitization:

_____

_____

_____

Fill-in

Read each item carefully, then complete the statement by filling in the missing word(s).

1. _____ refers to the failure of the cardiovascular system.

2. Pressure in the arteries during cardiac _____ is known as systolic pressure.

3. In shock conditions, the body redirects blood from _____ organs to _____ organs.

4. Blood pressure is a rough measurement of _____.

5. The cardiovascular system consists of the _____, _____, and _____.

6. Inadequate circulation that does not meet the body's needs is known as _____.

7. _____ are circular muscle walls in capillaries, causing the walls to _____ and _____.

8. _____ pressure occurs during cardiac relaxation, while _____ pressure occurs during cardiac contractions.

9. _____ pressure is the pressure in the blood vessels at any one time.

10. The autonomic nervous system controls the _____ actions of the body.

True/False

If you believe the statement to be more true than false, write the letter "T" in the space provided. If you believe the statement to be more false than true, write the letter "F."

1. _____ Life-threatening allergic reactions can occur in response to almost any substance in which a patient has been sensitized.

2. _____ Bleeding is the most common cause of shock following an injury.

3. _____ Shock occurs when oxygen and nutrients cannot get to the body's cells.

4. _____ A person in shock, left untreated, will most likely survive.

5. _____ Compensated shock is related to the last stages of shock.

6. _____ An injection of epinephrine is the only really effective treatment for anaphylactic shock.

7. _____ Septic shock is a combination of vessel and content failure.

Short Answer

Complete this section with short written answers using the space provided.

1. List the causes, signs and symptoms, and treatment of anaphylactic shock.

_____

_____

_____

2. List the causes, signs and symptoms, and treatment of cardiogenic shock.

_____

_____

_____

3. List the causes, signs and symptoms, and treatment of hypovolemic shock.

_____

_____

_____

4. List the causes, signs and symptoms, and treatment of respiratory insufficiency.

_____

_____

_____

5. List the causes, signs and symptoms, and treatment of neurogenic shock.

_____

_____

_____

6. List the causes, signs and symptoms, and treatment of psychogenic shock.

_____

_____

_____

7. List the causes, signs and symptoms, and treatment of septic shock.

_____

8. List the three basic physiologic causes of shock.

Word Fun www.OECzone vocab explorer

The following crossword puzzle is an activity provided to reinforce correct spelling and understanding of medical terminology associated with emergency care. Use the clues in the column to complete the puzzle.

CLUES

Across

7. Fainting
8. Circular muscles
9. Caused by severe infection
10. Fluid in the extracellular spaces
11. Caused by inadequate heart function

Down

1. Severe allergic reaction
2. Caused by paralysis of nerves
3. Caused by loss of blood and fluids
4. Body temperature below 95°F
5. Circulation of blood in adequate amounts
6. Difficulty breathing
12. Lack of oxygen

3

Calls to the Scene

The following case scenarios provide an opportunity to explore the concerns associated with patient management. Read each scenario, then answer each question in detail.

1. You witness a rollover motor vehicle crash on Interstate 10. You stop to lend assistance. You come upon a 17-year-old boy who was ejected and is found supine beside the vehicle. He is responsive to pain, respirations are 14 and nonlabored, and he has no radial pulses. His carotid pulse is 72 and weak. His skin is warm and dry. He has no motor function or sensation in his extremities. How would you best manage this patient?

_____

_____

_____

_____

_____

_____

_____

_____

_____

2. An alumni reunion is being held at a retreat center in the California mountains. A structure fire erupted in one of the resident buildings. A 72-year-old woman was severely burned in the fire. Her respirations are 28 and shallow, she is unresponsive, and has no radial pulses. She is pale and diaphoretic where she is not burned.

How would you best manage this patient?

_____

_____

_____

_____

_____

_____

_____

_____

3. Hiking on the Arizona Trail, you come upon a 16-year-old girl who has been stung by a bee. Her mother tells you she is severely allergic to bees. She is responsive to voice, covered in hives, and is wheezing audibly. She has a very weak radial pulse and is blue around the lips.

How would you best manage this patient?

_____

_____

_____

_____

_____

_____

_____

_____

3

Skill Drills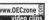

Test your knowledge of this skill drill by placing the photos below in the correct order. Number the first step with a "1," the second step with a "2," etc.

Skill Drill 9-1: Treating Shock

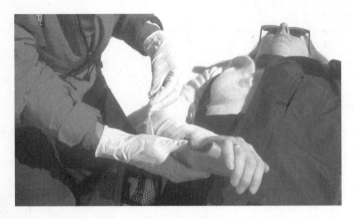

_____

Splint any broken bones or joint injuries.

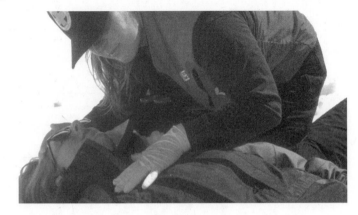

_____

Keep the patient supine, open the airway, and check breathing and pulse.

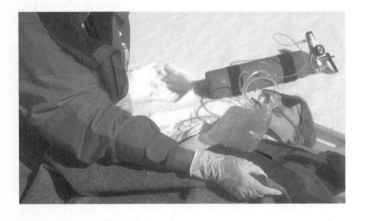

_____

Give high-flow oxygen if you have not already done so, and place blankets under and over the patient.

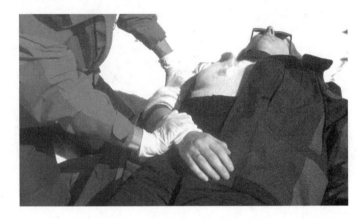

_____

Control obvious external bleeding.

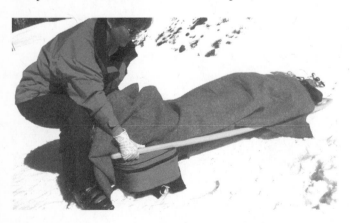

_____

If no fractures are suspected, elevate the legs 6" to 12".

Notes

Workbook Activities

The following activities have been designed to help you. Your instructor may require you to complete some or all of these activities as a regular part of your OEC training program. You are encouraged to complete any activity that your instructor does not assign as a way to enhance your learning in the classroom.

Chapter Review

The following exercises provide an opportunity to refresh your knowledge of this chapter.

■ NOTES ■

Matching

Match each of the terms in the left column to the appropriate definition in the right column.

_____ 1. Asthma

_____ 2. Pulmonary edema

_____ 3. Epiglottitis

_____ 4. Emphysema

_____ 5. Pleural effusion

_____ 6. Pneumothorax

_____ 7. Dyspnea

_____ 8. Pneumonia

_____ 9. Hypoxia

_____ 10. Bronchitis

_____ 11. Hyperventilation

_____ 12. Allergen

_____ 13. Embolus

A. irritation of the major lung passageways

B. acute spasm of the bronchioles, associated with excessive mucus production and sometimes spasm of the bronchiolar muscles

C. accumulation of air in the pleural space

D. fluid build-up within the alveoli and lung tissue

E. an infectious disease of the lung that damages lung tissue

F. a substance that causes an allergic reaction

G. difficulty breathing

H. bacterial infection that can produce severe swelling

I. a blood clot or other substance in the circulatory system that travels to a blood vessel where it causes blockage

J. disease of the lungs in which the alveoli stretch, lose elasticity, and are destroyed

K. rapid or deep breathing that lowers blood carbon dioxide levels below normal

L. fluid outside of the lung

M. condition in which the body's cells and tissues do not have enough oxygen

Respiratory Emergencies

Multiple Choice

Read each item carefully, then select the best response.

_____ 1. When treating a patient with dyspnea, you must be prepared to treat the:
  A. symptoms.
  B. underlying problem.
  C. patient's anxiety.
  D. all of the above

_____ 2. The oxygen-carbon dioxide exchange takes place in the:
  A. trachea.
  B. bronchial tree.
  C. alveoli.
  D. blood.

_____ 3. Oxygen-carbon dioxide exchange may be hampered if the:
  A. pleural space is filled with air or excess fluid.
  B. alveoli are damaged.
  C. air passages are obstructed.
  D. all of the above

_____ 4. If carbon dioxide levels in the arterial blood drop too low, a person automatically breathes:
  A. normally.
  B. rapidly and deeply.
  C. slower and shallowly.
  D. rapidly and shallowly.

_____ 5. If carbon dioxide levels in the arterial blood rise above normal, a person automatically breathes:
  A. normally.
  B. rapidly and deeply.
  C. slower and shallowly.
  D. rapidly and shallowly.

NOTES

_____ **6.** Which of the following signs indicates adequate breathing?

    A. a normal rate and depth

    B. pale or cyanotic skin

    C. pursed lips and nasal flaring

    D. cool, damp skin

_____ **7.** The level of carbon dioxide in the arterial blood can rise as a result of:

    A. emphysema.

    B. chronic bronchitis.

    C. cardiovascular disease.

    D. all of the above

_____ **8.** The second stimulus that develops in patients with normally high levels of carbon dioxide responds to:

    A. increased oxygen levels.

    B. decreased oxygen levels.

    C. increased carbon dioxide levels.

    D. decreased carbon dioxide levels.

_____ **9.** _____ is a sign of hypoxia to the brain.

    A. Altered mental status

    B. Decreased heart rate

    C. Decreased respiratory rate

    D. Delayed capillary refill time

_____ **10.** An obstruction to the exchange of gases between the alveoli and the capillaries may result from:

    A. epiglottitis.

    B. pneumonia.

    C. a cold.

    D. all of the above

_____ **11.** Pulmonary edema can develop quickly after a major:

    A. heart attack.

    B. episode of syncope.

    C. brain injury.

    D. all of the above

_____ **12.** The _____ is the narrowest point in a child's airway.

    A. carina

    B. trachea

    C. epiglottis

    D. larynx

_____ **13.** In addition to a major heart attack, pulmonary edema may also be produced by:

    A. inhaling large amounts of smoke.

    B. traumatic injuries to the chest.

    C. inhaling toxic chemical fumes.

    D. all of the above

_____ **14.** Chronic oxygenation problems from bronchitis can lead to:

    A. cerebral edema.

    B. upper airway obstruction.

    C. right-sided heart failure.

    D. fluid retention.

_____ **15.** _____ is a loss of the elastic material around the air spaces as a result of chronic stretching of the alveoli when bronchitic airways obstruct easy expulsion of gases.

   A. Emphysema

   B. Bronchitis

   C. Pneumonia

   D. Diphtheria

_____ **16.** Most patients with chronic obstructive pulmonary disease will:

   A. chronically produce sputum.

   B. have a chronic cough.

   C. have difficulty expelling air from their lungs.

   D. all of the above

_____ **17.** The patient with chronic obstructive pulmonary disease usually presents with:

   A. an increased blood pressure.

   B. a green or yellow productive cough.

   C. a decreased heart rate.

   D. all of the above

_____ **18.** A pneumothorax caused by a medical condition without any injury is known as a:

   A. tension pneumothorax.

   B. subcutaneous pneumothorax.

   C. spontaneous pneumothorax.

   D. none of the above

_____ **19.** Asthma produces a characteristic _____ as patients attempt to exhale through partially obstructed air passages.

   A. rhonchi

   B. stridor

   C. wheezing

   D. rattle

_____ **20.** An allergic response to certain foods or some other allergen may produce an acute:

   A. bronchodilation.

   B. asthma attack.

   C. vasoconstriction.

   D. insulin release.

_____ **21.** Treatment for anaphylaxis and acute asthma attacks includes:

   A. epinephrine.

   B. high-flow oxygen.

   C. antihistamines.

   D. all of the above

_____ **22.** A collection of fluid outside the lungs on one or both sides of the chest is called a:

   A. spontaneous pneumothorax.

   B. subcutaneous emphysema.

   C. pleural effusion.

   D. tension pneumothorax.

4

_____23. Always consider _____ in patients who were eating just before becoming short of breath:

    A. upper airway obstruction

    B. anaphylaxis

    C. lower airway obstruction

    D. bronchoconstriction

_____24. Pulmonary emboli may occur as a result of:

    A. damage to the lining of the vessels.

    B. a tendency for blood to clot unusually fast.

    C. slow blood flow in the lower extremity.

    D. all of the above

_____25. _____ is defined as overbreathing to the point that the level of arterial carbon dioxide falls below normal.

    A. Reactive airway syndrome

    B. Hyperventilation

    C. Tachypnea

    D. Pleural effusion

_____26. Slowing of respirations after administration of oxygen to a patient with chronic obstructive pulmonary disease does not necessarily mean that the patient no longer needs the oxygen; he or she may need:

    A. insulin.

    B. even more oxygen.

    C. mouth-to-mouth resuscitation.

    D. none of the above

_____27. Aspiration of vomit into the lungs may cause:

    A. croup.

    B. alkalosis.

    C. pneumonia.

    D. bronchitis.

_____28. Questions to ask during the focused history and physical examination include which of the following?

    A. What has the patient already done for the breathing problem?

    B. Does the patient use a prescribed inhaler?

    C. Does the patient have any allergies?

    D. all of the above

_____29. The problem in asthma is getting the air:

    A. to diffuse through mucus.

    B. past the carina.

    C. into the narrowed trachea.

    D. out of the lungs.

_____30. Contraindications to helping a patient self-administer any metered-dose inhaler medication include:

    A. not obtaining permission from medical control.

    B. noticing that the inhaler is not prescribed for this patient.

    C. noticing that the patient has already had the maximum prescribed dose.

    D. all of the above

_____ **31.** Possible side effects of over-the-counter cold medications may include:

    A. agitation.

    B. increased heart rate.

    C. increased blood pressure.

    D. all of the above

_____ **32.** A prolonged asthma attack that is unrelieved by epinephrine may progress into a condition known as:

    A. pleural effusion.

    B. status epilepticus.

    C. status asthmaticus.

    D. reactive airway disease.

Labeling www.OECzone.com anatomy review

Label the following diagrams with the correct terms.

The Upper Airway

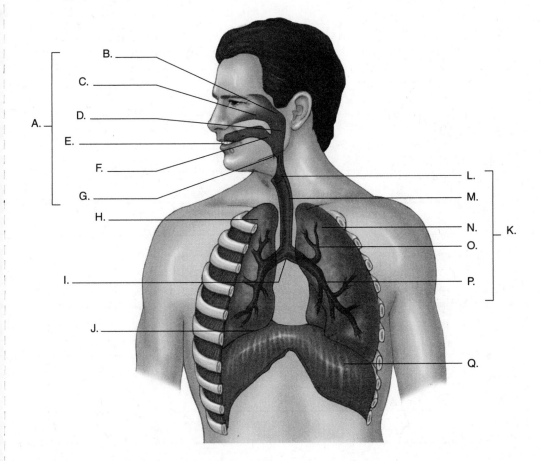

A. _____

B. _____

C. _____

D. _____

E. _____

F. _____

G. _____

H. _____

I. _____

J. _____

K. _____

L. _____

M. _____

N. _____

O. _____

P. _____

Q. _____

Vocabulary www.OECzone.com vocab explorer

Define the following terms using the space provided.

1. Stridor:

_____

_____

_____

2. Croup:

_____

_____

_____

3. Rales:

_____

_____

_____

4. Rhonchi:

_____

_____

_____

5. Diphtheria:

_____

_____

_____

6. Chronic obstructive pulmonary disease (COPD):

_____

_____

_____

Fill-in

Read each item carefully, then complete the statement by filling in the missing word(s).

1. The level of _____ bathing the brain stem stimulates respiration.

2. The level of _____ in the blood is a secondary stimulus for respiration.

3. _____ entering the alveoli passes into the capillaries, which carry

_____ back to the heart.

4. Carbon dioxide and oxygen are exchanged in the _____.

5. Air enters the body through the _____.

6. Abnormal breathing is indicated by a rate slower than _____ breaths/min or

faster than _____ breaths/min.

7. During respiration, oxygen is provided to the blood, and _____ is removed from it.

True/False

If you believe the statement to be more true than false, write the letter "T" in the space provided. If you believe the statement to be more false than true, write the letter "F."

1. _____ Chronic bronchitis is characterized by spasm and narrowing of the bronchioles due to exposure to allergens.

2. _____ With pneumothorax, the lung collapses because the negative vacuum pressure in the pleural space is lost.

3. _____ Anaphylactic reactions occur only in patients with a previous history of asthma or allergies.

4. _____ Decreased breath sounds in asthma occur because fluid in the pleural space has moved the lung away from the chest wall.

5. _____ Pulmonary emboli are difficult to diagnose.

6. _____ COPD most often results from cigarette smoking.

7. _____ Asthma and COPD are characterized by long inspiratory times.

Short Answer

Complete this section with short written answers using the space provided.

1. List five characteristics of normal breathing.

_____

_____

_____

_____

_____

2. List the five most common mechanisms occurring in lung disorders.

_____

_____

_____

_____

_____

3. Under what conditions should you not assist a patient with a metered-dose inhaler?

_____

_____

_____

4. Describe chronic bronchitis.

_____

_____

_____

5. List five signs of inadequate breathing.

_____

_____

_____

_____

_____

6. Explain carbon dioxide retention.

_____

_____

_____

Word Fun www.OECzone.com vocab explorer

The following crossword puzzle is an activity provided to reinforce correct spelling and understanding of medical terminology associated with emergency care. Use the clues provided to complete the puzzle.

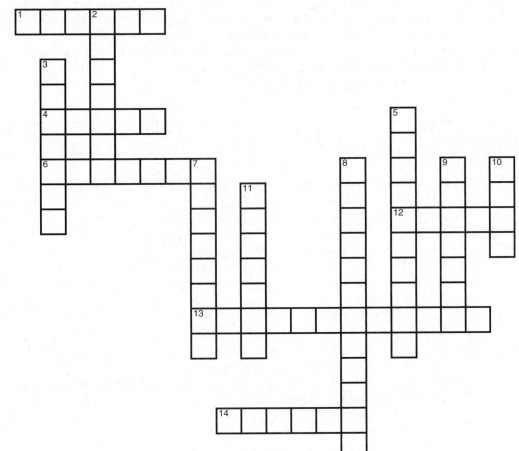

■ C L U E S ■

Across

1. High-pitched, whistling sound

4. Crackling, rattling sounds

6. Difficulty breathing

12. Barking cough

13. Inflammation of leaf-shaped airway cover

14. Muscle spasm in small airways

Down

2. Traveling clot

3. Harsh, high-pitched sound

5. Irritation of major airways

7. Substance causing a reaction

8. Air in pleural space

9. Coarse sounds from mucus in airways

10. Slow process of chronic disruption of airways

11. Low oxygen

Calls to the Scene

The following case scenarios will give you an opportunity to explore the concerns associated with patient management. Read each scenario, then answer each question in detail.

1. Three school-aged friends were skiing very close together coming down the hill and collided with each other. They think this is all kind of a joke. However, one person has stress-induced asthma and is having an attack as the rescuer arrives. Vital signs present with a pulse of 112 beats/min and labored respirations.

How would you best manage this patient?

_____

_____

_____

_____

_____

_____

_____

2. You find a 24-year-old woman in the lodge hotel who is visibly upset and breathing rapidly. She is complaining of numbness and tingling in her hands and feet, as well as dyspnea. Family members tell you that they found her this way and that she has a history of panic attacks. The patient assures you that this is not a panic attack and that it is hard for her to breathe.

How would you best manage this patient?

_____

_____

_____

_____

_____

_____

_____

3. You come upon a skier who reports that he has twisted his knee. Your examination convinces you that he has probably sprained it. He also complains of shortness of breath, tingling in the fingers and toes, and dizziness. His respirations are more than 20 breaths/min. He has voiced anxiety about getting off the hill and appears frightened.

How would you best manage this patient?

_____

_____

_____

_____

_____

_____

Skill Drills

www.OECzone.com video clips

Test your knowledge of this skill drill by filling in the correct words in the photo captions.

Skill Drill 10-1: Assisting a Patient with a Metered-Dose Inhaler

1. Check to see if you have the right _____, the right _____, and the right _____.

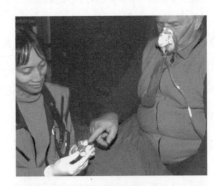

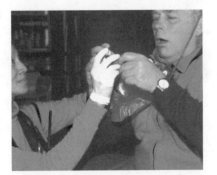

2. Remove oxygen mask.
Hand inhaler to the patient. Instruct the patient about breathing and _____

_____.

Use a _____ if the patient has one.

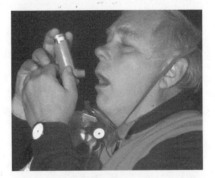

3. Instruct the patient to press the inhaler and inhale.
Instruct the patient about _____

_____.

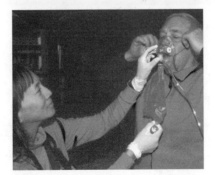

4. Reapply _____.
After a few _____, have the patient repeat the _____ if order/protocol allows.

Workbook Activities

The following activities have been designed to help you. Your instructor may require you to complete some or all of these activities as a regular part of your OEC training program. You are encouraged to complete any activity that your instructor does not assign as a way to enhance your learning in the classroom.

Chapter Review

The following exercises provide an opportunity to refresh your knowledge of this chapter.

■ NOTES ■

Matching

Match each of the terms in the left column to the appropriate definition in the right column.

_____ **1.** Atria

_____ **2.** Coronary arteries

_____ **3.** Atrioventricular (AV) node

_____ **4.** Myocardium

_____ **5.** Sinus node

_____ **6.** Venae cavae

_____ **7.** Ventricles

_____ **8.** Aorta

_____ **9.** Atherosclerosis

_____ **10.** Ischemia

_____ **11.** Pedal edema

_____ **12.** Infarction

_____ **13.** Tachycardia

_____ **14.** Asystole

A. absence of all heart electrical activity

B. swelling of feet and ankles

C. calcium and cholesterol buildup inside blood vessels

D. blood vessels that supply blood to the myocardium

E. lack of oxygen

F. heart muscle

G. lower chambers of the heart

H. tissue death

I. rapid heart rhythm, more than 100 beats/min

J. carry oxygen-poor blood back to the heart

K. upper chambers of the heart

L. body's main artery

M. electrical impulses begin here

N. electrical impulses slow here to allow blood to move from the atria to the ventricles

Cardiovascular Emergencies

Multiple Choice

Read each item carefully, then select the best response.

_____ 1. The number of deaths attributed to cardiovascular disease can be reduced with:
   A. better public awareness.
   B. early access.
   C. public access defibrillation.
   D. all of the above

_____ 2. The aorta receives its blood supply from the:
   A. right atria.
   B. left atria.
   C. right ventricle.
   D. left ventricle.

_____ 3. Blood enters into the right atrium from the body through the:
   A. vena cava.
   B. aorta.
   C. pulmonary artery.
   D. pulmonary vein.

_____ 4. The only veins in the body to carry oxygenated blood are the:
   A. external jugular veins.
   B. pulmonary veins.
   C. subclavian veins.
   D. inferior vena cava.

_____ 5. Normal electrical impulses originate in the sinus node, just above the:
   A. atria.
   B. ventricles.
   C. AV junction.
   D. Bundle of His.

_____ **6.** Dilation of the coronary arteries will _____ blood flow.

　　A. shut off

　　B. increase

　　C. decrease

　　D. regulate

_____ **7.** At the level of the navel, the aorta divides into two main branches called the right and left _____ arteries.

　　A. femoral

　　B. renal

　　C. iliac

　　D. sacral

_____ **8.** The _____ are tiny blood vessels about one cell thick.

　　A. arterioles

　　B. venules

　　C. capillaries

　　D. ventricles

_____ **9.** _____ carry oxygen to the body's tissues and then remove carbon dioxide.

　　A. Red blood cells

　　B. White blood cells

　　C. Platelets

　　D. Veins

_____ **10.** _____ is (are) a mixture of water, salts, nutrients, and proteins.

　　A. Platelets

　　B. Cerebrospinal fluid

　　C. Plasma

　　D. all of the above

_____ **11.** _____ is the maximum pressure exerted by the left ventricle as it contracts.

　　A. Cardiac output

　　B. Diastolic blood pressure

　　C. Systolic blood pressure

　　D. Stroke volume

_____ **12.** Atherosclerosis can lead to a complete _____ of a coronary artery.

　　A. occlusion

　　B. disintegration

　　C. dilation

　　D. contraction

_____ **13.** The lumen of an artery may be partially or completely blocked by the blood-clotting system due to a _____ that exposes the inside of the atherosclerotic wall.

　　A. tear

　　B. crack

　　C. clot

　　D. rupture

_____ **14.** Tissues downstream from a blood clot will suffer from lack of oxygen. If blood flow is resumed in a short time, the _____ tissues will recover.

A. dead

B. ischemic

C. necrosed

D. dry

_____ **15.** Risk factors for myocardial infarction include all of the following except:

A. male gender.

B. high blood pressure.

C. stress.

D. increased activity level.

_____ **16.** When, for a brief period of time, heart tissues do not get enough oxygen, the pain is called:

A. AMI.

B. angina.

C. ischemia.

D. CAD.

_____ **17.** Angina pain may be felt in the:

A. arms.

B. midback.

C. epigastrium.

D. all of the above

_____ **18.** Angina may be associated with:

A. shortness of breath.

B. nausea.

C. sweating.

D. all of the above

_____ **19.** Because oxygen supply to the heart is diminished with angina, the _____ can be compromised and the person is at risk for significant cardiac rhythm problems.

A. circulation

B. cardiac output

C. electrical system

D. vasculature

_____ **20.** An acute myocardial infarction is more likely to occur in the larger, thick-walled left ventricle, which needs more _____ than the right ventricle.

A. oxygen and glucose

B. force to pump

C. blood and oxygen

D. electrical activity

4

_____ **21.** The pain of AMI differs from the pain of angina because it:
   A. may be caused by exertion.
   B. is usually relieved by rest.
   C. does not resolve in a few minutes.
   D. all of the above

_____ **22.** Consequences of AMI may include:
   A. cardiogenic shock.
   B. congestive heart failure.
   C. sudden death.
   D. all of the above

_____ **23.** Sudden death is usually the result of _____, in which the heart fails to generate an effective blood flow.
   A. AMI
   B. atherosclerosis
   C. PVCs
   D. cardiac arrest

_____ **24.** Disorganized, ineffective quivering of the ventricles is known as:
   A. ventricular fibrillation.
   B. asystole.
   C. ventricular stand still.
   D. ventricular tachycardia.

_____ **25.** In _____, often caused by a heart attack, the problem is that the heart lacks enough power to force the proper volume of blood through the circulatory system.
   A. asystole
   B. cardiogenic shock
   C. ventricular fibrillation
   D. angina

_____ **26.** Causes of congestive heart failure include all of the following except:
   A. chronic hypotension.
   B. heart valve damage.
   C. a myocardial infarction.
   D. longstanding high blood pressure.

_____ **27.** Signs and symptoms of shock include all of the following except:
   A. elevated heart rate.
   B. pale, clammy skin.
   C. air hunger.
   D. elevated blood pressure.

_____ **28.** In patients with congestive heart failure, changes in heart function occur, including:
   A. a decrease in heart rate.
   B. enlargement of the left ventricle.
   C. enlargement of the right ventricle.
   D. a decrease in blood pressure.

_____**29.** Fluid that collects in the feet and legs is called:

    A. pedal edema.

    B. pulmonary edema.

    C. cerebral edema.

    D. tibial edema.

_____**30.** Physical findings of AMI include skin that is _____ because of poor cardiac output and the loss of perfusion.

    A. pink

    B. white

    C. gray

    D. red

_____**31.** To assess chest pain, use the mnemonic:

    A. AVPU.

    B. OPQRST.

    C. SAMPLE.

    D. CHART.

_____**32.** Nitroglycerin may be in the form of a:

    A. skin patch.

    B. spray.

    C. pill.

    D. all of the above

_____**33.** _____ are inserted when the electrical control system of the heart is so damaged that it cannot function properly.

    A. Stents

    B. Pacemakers

    C. Balloon angioplasties

    D. AEDs

_____**34.** When the battery wears out in a pacemaker, the patient may experience:

    A. syncope.

    B. dizziness.

    C. weakness.

    D. all of the above

_____35. The computer inside the AED is specifically programmed to recognize rhythms that require defibrillation to most commonly correct:

A. asystole.

B. ventricular tachycardia.

C. ventricular fibrillation.

D. supraventricular tachycardia.

_____36. You should apply the AED only to unresponsive patients with no:

A. significant medical problems.

B. cardiac history.

C. pulse.

D. brain activity.

_____37. _____ usually refers to a state of cardiac arrest despite an organized electrical complex.

A. Asystole

B. Pulseless electrical activity

C. Ventricular fibrillation

D. Ventricular tachycardia

_____38. The links in the chain of survival include all of the following except early:

A. access and CPR.

B. ACLS.

C. administration of nitroglycerin.

D. defibrillation.

_____39. An AED may fail to function properly as a result of:

A. the batteries not working.

B. improper maintenance.

C. operator error.

D. all of the above

Labeling

Label the following diagrams with the correct terms.

1. The Right and Left Sides of the Heart
Where arrows appear, indicate the substance and its origin and destination.

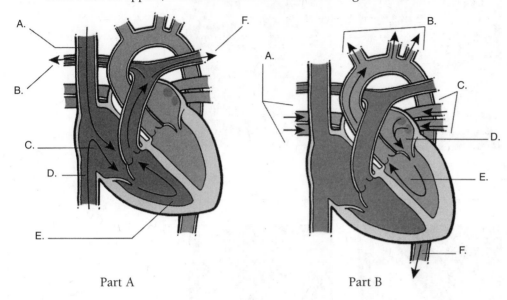

Part A   Part B

2. Electrical Conduction

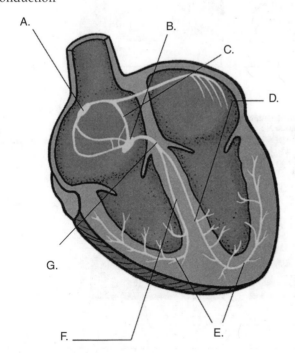

Part A

A. _____

B. _____

C. _____

D. _____

E. _____

F. _____

Part B

A. _____

B. _____

C. _____

D. _____

E. _____

F. _____

A. _____

B. _____

C. _____

D. _____

E. _____

F. _____

G. _____

3. Pulse Points

State the name of the artery that is being assessed at each pulse point below.

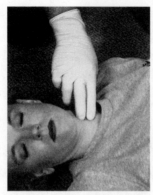

A._____

_____

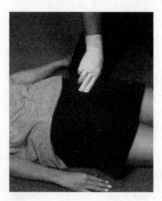

B._____

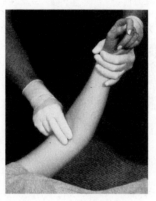

C._____

_____

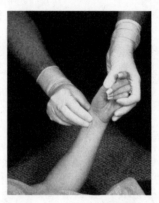

D._____

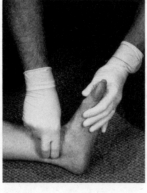

E._____

_____

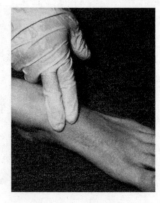

F._____

_____

Vocabulary

Define the following terms using the space provided.

1. Angina pectoris:

_____

_____

_____

2. Ventricular fibrillation:

_____

_____

_____

3. Cardiogenic shock:

_____

_____

_____

4. Acute myocardial infarction (AMI):

_____

_____

_____

5. Cardiac arrest:

_____

_____

_____

6. Congestive heart failure (CHF):

_____

_____

_____

Fill-in

Read each item carefully, then complete the statement by filling in the missing word.

1. The heart is divided down the middle by a wall called the _____.

2. The _____ is the largest artery.

3. The _____ ventricle pumps blood in through the pulmonary circulation.

4. Electrical impulses spread from the _____ node to the ventricles.

5. Blood supply to the heart is increased by _____ of the coronary arteries.

6. _____ cells remove carbon dioxide from the body's tissues.

7. _____ blood pressure reflects the pressure on the walls of the arteries when the ventricle is at rest.

8. The heart has _____ chambers.

9. The _____ side of the heart is more muscular because it must pump blood into the aorta and all the other arteries of the body.

True/False

If you believe the statement to be more true than false, write the letter "T" in the space provided. If you believe the statement to be more false than true, write the letter "F."

1. _____ The right side of the heart pumps oxygen-rich blood to the body.

2. _____ In the normal heart, the need for increased blood flow to the myocardium is easily met by an increase in heart rate.

3. _____ Atherosclerosis results in narrowing of the lumen of coronary arteries.

4. _____ Infarction is a temporary interruption of the blood supply to the tissues.

5. _____ Angina can result from a spasm of the artery.

6. _____ The pain of angina and the pain of AMI are easily distinguishable.

7. _____ CPR can be performed on a patient being transported in a toboggan.

8. _____ If an AED malfunctions during use, you must report that problem to the manufacturer and the Department of Human Resources.

9. _____ Angina occurs when the heart's need for oxygen exceeds its supply.

10. _____ White blood cells are the most numerous and help the blood to clot.

Short Answer

Complete this section with short written answers in the space provided.

1. Define angina pectoris.

_____

_____

_____

2. List three complications of myocardial infarction.

_____

_____

_____

3. List the signs and symptoms for a patient with a heart attack.

_____

_____

_____

4. List six safety considerations for operating an AED.

_____

_____

_____

_____

_____

_____

5. List three ways in which AMI pain differs from angina pain.

_____

_____

_____

6. List three serious consequences of AMI.

_____

_____

_____

7. Name at least five signs and symptoms associated with AMI.

_____

_____

_____

_____

_____

■ **CLUES** ■

Across

1. Less than 60 beats/min
5. Greater than 100 beats/min
6. Lower chamber
7. Lack of oxygen to tissues
8. Widening
9. Absence of electrical activity

Down

2. Irregular heart rhythm
3. To shock the heart
4. Blockage
9. Main artery of body

Word Fun

www.OECzone vocab explorer

The following crossword puzzle is an activity provided to reinforce correct spelling and understanding of medical terminology associated with emergency care. Use the clues in the column to complete the puzzle.

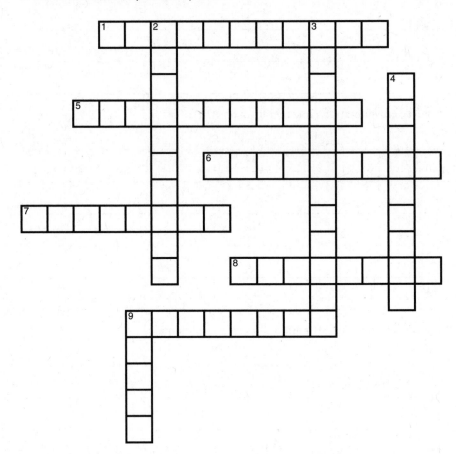

Calls to the Scene

The following case scenarios provide an opportunity to explore the concerns associated with patient management. Read each scenario, then answer each question in detail.

1. You are dispatched to the residence of a 58-year-old man complaining of chest pain. He states that it feels like "somebody is standing on my chest." He sat down when it started and took a nitroglycerin tablet. He is still a little nauseated and sweaty, but feels better. He is very anxious.

   How would you best manage this patient?

   _____

   _____

   _____

_____

_____

_____

_____

_____

_____

2. You are called to the restaurant at the top of the mountain for a 38-year-old man complaining of indigestion. His friends tell you that the pain started suddenly and he clutched his chest and vomited. He insists that he will be all right and that it is probably something he ate. He is pale and diaphoretic.

How would you best manage this patient?

_____

_____

_____

_____

_____

_____

_____

_____

3. A 24-year-old woman complains of a sudden severe headache and collapses to the ground. She is unresponsive and her left pupil is fixed and dilated. What is most likely to cause this condition?

How would you best manage this patient?

_____

_____

_____

_____

_____

_____

Skill Drills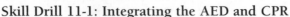

Skill Drill 11-1: Integrating the AED and CPR

Test your knowledge of this skill drill by placing the photos below in the correct order. Number the first step with a "1," the second step with a "2," etc.

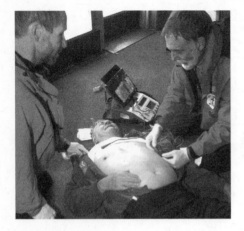

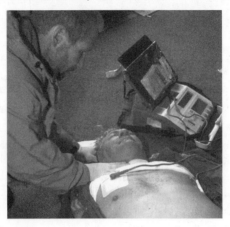

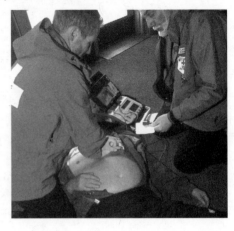

Check pulse.
If pulse is present, check breathing.

If pulseless, begin CPR.
Prepare the AED pads.
Turn on the AED; begin narrative if needed.

Apply AED pads.
Stop CPR.

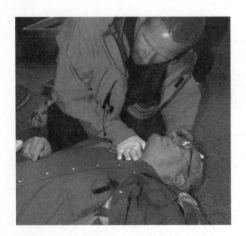

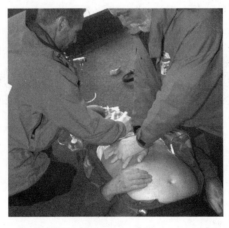

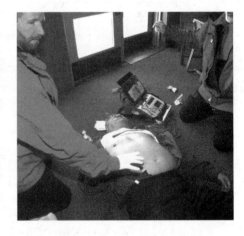

If breathing adequately, give oxygen and transport. If not, open airway, ventilate, and transport.
If no pulse, perform CPR for 1 minute.
Clear the patient and analyze again.
If necessary, repeat one cycle of up to three shocks.
Transport and call medical control.
Continue to support breathing or perform CPR, as needed.

Verbally and visually clear the patient.
Push the Analyze button if there is one.
Wait for the AED to analyze rhythm.
If no shock advised, perform CPR for 1 min.
If shock advised, recheck that all are clear and push the Shock button.
Push the Analyze button, if needed, to analyze rhythm again.
Press Shock if advised (second shock).
Push the Analyze button, if needed, to analyze rhythm again.
Press Shock if advised (third shock).

Stop CPR if in progress.
Assess responsiveness.
Check breathing and pulse.
If unresponsive and not breathing adequately, give two slow ventilations.

Notes

Workbook Activities

The following activities have been designed to help you. Your instructor may require you to complete some or all of these activities as a regular part of your OEC training program. You are encouraged to complete any activity that your instructor does not assign as a way to enhance your learning in the classroom.

Chapter Review

The following exercises provide an opportunity to refresh your knowledge of this chapter.

NOTES

Matching

Match each of the terms in the left column to the appropriate definition in the right column.

_____ **1.** Brain stem

_____ **2.** Foramen magnum

_____ **3.** Spinal nerves

_____ **4.** Cerebrum

_____ **5.** Cranial nerves

_____ **6.** Cerebellum

_____ **7.** Embolism

_____ **8.** Aneurysm

_____ **9.** Status epilepticus

_____ **10.** Hypoglycemia

_____ **11.** Aphasia

_____ **12.** Berry aneurysm

_____ **13.** Dysarthria

A. slurred, hard to understand speech

B. the back part of this area of the brain processes sight

C. weakness in an artery wall

D. controls most basic functions of the body

E. exit at each vertebra and carry messages to and from the body

F. the area of the brain that controls muscle and body coordination

G. hole in the base of the skull

H. low blood glucose

I. innervate eyes, ears, face

J. clot that forms elsewhere and travels to the site of damage

K. weakness in a blood vessel that resembles a tiny balloon

L. inability to produce or understand speech

M. seizures that recur every few minutes

Multiple Choice

Read each item carefully, then select the best response.

_____ **1.** Seizures may occur as a result of:

   A. metabolic problems.

   B. brain tumor.

   C. a recent or old head injury.

   D. all of the above

Neurologic Emergencies

_____ **2.** The _____ controls the most basic functions of the body, such as breathing, blood pressure, swallowing, and pupil constriction.

A. brain stem

B. cerebellum

C. cerebrum

D. spinal cord

_____ **3.** At each vertebra in the neck and back, _____ nerves, called spinal nerves, branch out from the spinal cord and carry signals to and from the body.

A. two

B. three

C. four

D. five

_____ **4.** Brain disorders include all of the following except:

A. coma.

B. infection.

C. hypoglycemia.

D. tumor.

_____ **5.** When blood flow to a particular part of the brain is cut off by a blockage inside a blood vessel, the result is:

A. a hemorrhagic stroke.

B. atherosclerosis.

C. an ischemic stroke.

D. a cerebral embolism.

_____ **6.** Patients who are at the highest risk of hemorrhagic stroke are those who have:

A. untreated hypertension.

B. an aneurysm.

C. a berry aneurysm.

D. atherosclerosis.

_____ **7.** Patients with a subarachnoid hemorrhage typically complain of a sudden severe:

   A. bout of dizziness.

   B. headache.

   C. altered mental status.

   D. thirst.

_____ **8.** The plaque that builds up in atherosclerosis obstructs blood flow and interferes with the vessel's ability to:

   A. constrict.

   B. dilate.

   C. diffuse.

   D. exchange gases.

_____ **9.** A transient ischemic attack (TIA), or mini-stroke, is the name given to a stroke when symptoms go away on their own in less than:

   A. 30 minutes.

   B. 1 hour.

   C. 12 hours.

   D. 24 hours.

_____ **10.** Seizures characterized by unconsciousness and a generalized severe twitching of all the body's muscles that lasts several minutes or longer is called a:

   A. grand mal seizure.

   B. petit mal seizure.

   C. focal motor seizure.

   D. febrile seizure.

_____ **11.** Metabolic seizures may be due to:

   A. epilepsy.

   B. a brain tumor.

   C. high fevers.

   D. hypoglycemia.

_____ **12.** When assessing a patient with a history of seizure activity, it is important to:

   A. determine whether this episode differs from any previous ones.

   B. recognize the postictal state.

   C. look for other problems associated with the seizure.

   D. all of the above

_____ **13.** Signs and symptoms of possible seizure activity include:

   A. altered mental status.

   B. incontinence.

   C. rapid and deep respirations.

   D. all of the above

_____ **14.** Common causes of altered mental status include all of the following except:

   A. body temperature abnormalities.

   B. hypoxemia.

   C. unequal pupils.

   D. hypoglycemia.

_____ 15. The principle difference between a patient who has had a stroke and a patient with hypoglycemia almost always has to do with the:

    A. pupillary response.

    B. mental status.

    C. blood pressure.

    D. capillary refill time.

_____ 16. Consider the possibility of _____ in a patient who has had a seizure.

    A. brain injury

    B. hyperglycemia

    C. hypoglycemia

    D. hypertension

_____ 17. Low oxygen levels in the bloodstream will affect the entire brain, causing:

    A. anxiety.

    B. restlessness.

    C. confusion.

    D. all of the above

_____ 18. Patients with _____ may have trouble understanding speech but can speak clearly.

    A. aphasia

    B. receptive aphasia

    C. expressive aphasia

    D. dysarthria

_____ 19. The following conditions may simulate a stroke except:

    A. hyperglycemia.

    B. a postictal state.

    C. hypoglycemia.

    D. subdural bleeding.

_____ 20. When assessing a patient with a possible cerebrovascular accident, you should check the _____ first.

    A. pulse

    B. airway

    C. pupils

    D. blood pressure

_____ 21. Indications that the patient can understand you include:

    A. pressure of the hand.

    B. efforts to speak.

    C. nodding the head.

    D. all of the above

_____ 22. Key physical tests for patients suspected of having a stroke include tests of:

    A. speech.

    B. neck movement.

    C. leg movement.

    D. all of the above

4

_____23. A patient with a Glasgow Coma Scale score of 12 has:

A. no dysfunction.

B. mild dysfunction.

C. moderate to severe dysfunction.

D. severe dysfunction.

_____24. To transport the patient with a suspected stroke, the patient should be placed in _____ position.

A. Trendelenburg's

B. Fowler's

C. a comfortable

D. a lithotomy

_____25. Following a major seizure, you should anticipate:

A. a decreased heart rate.

B. rapid, deep respirations.

C. respiratory arrest.

D. a return to normal mental status within 5–10 minutes.

_____26. Assess the mental status using the mnemonic:

A. OPQRST.

B. SAMPLE.

C. AVPU.

D. PEARRL.

_____27. Even a patient who has a history of chronic epilepsy that is controlled with medications may have an occasional seizure, commonly referred to as a(n) _____ seizure.

A. chronic

B. generalized

C. absence

D. breakthrough

Labeling

Label the following diagrams with the correct terms.

1. Brain

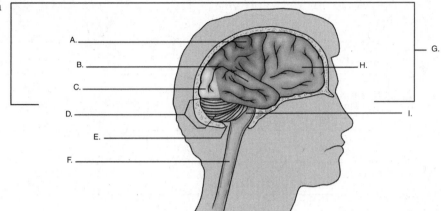

A. _____

B. _____

C. _____

D. _____

E. _____

F. _____

G. _____

H. _____

I. _____

2. Spinal Cord

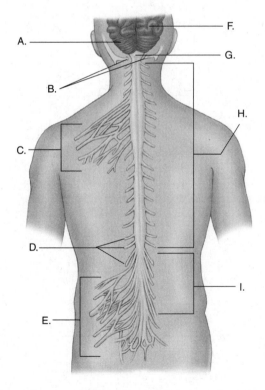

A. _____

B. _____

C. _____

D. _____

E. _____

F. _____

G. _____

H. _____

I. _____

4

Vocabulary www.OECzone.com vocab explorer

Define the following terms listed using the space provided.

1. Cerebrovascular accident (CVA):

_____

_____

2. Ischemic stroke:

_____

_____

_____

3. Transient ischemic attack (TIA):

_____

_____

_____

4. Hemorrhagic stroke:

_____

_____

_____

5. Generalized seizure:

_____

_____

_____

6. Absence seizure:

_____

_____

_____

7. Atherosclerosis:

_____

_____

_____

8. Cerebral embolism:

_____

_____

_____

9. Febrile seizure:

_____

_____

_____

10. Thrombosis:

_____

_____

_____

Fill-in

Read each item carefully, then complete the statement by filling in the missing word(s).

1. There are _____ cranial nerves.

2. Playing the piano is coordinated by the _____.

3. The front part of the cerebrum controls _____.

4. The cranial nerves run to the _____.

5. The brain is divided into _____ major parts.

6. All messages traveling to and from the brain travel along _____.

7. Each hemisphere of the cerebrum controls activities on the _____ side of the body.

8. The _____ is the largest part of the brain.

9. _____ is a loss of bowel and bladder control and can be due to a generalized seizure.

10. The _____ is the body's computer.

11. Onset of _____ bleeding is usually very rapid after injury.

12. Weakness on one side of the body is known as _____.

13. No matter what the cause, you should consider _____ to be an emergency that requires immediate attention, even when it appears that the cause may simply be alcohol intoxication or a minor crash or fall.

True/False

If you believe the statement to be more true than false, write the letter "T" in the space provided. If you believe the statement to be more false than true, write the letter "F."

1. _____ The postictal state following a seizure commonly lasts only about 3 to 5 minutes.

2. _____ Metabolic seizures result from an area of abnormality in the brain.

3. _____ Febrile seizures result from sudden high fevers and are generally well tolerated by children.

4. _____ Hemiparesis is the inability to speak or understand speech.

5. _____ The dura covers the brain.

6. _____ Unconscious stroke patients are usually unable to speak or hear.

7. _____ Right-sided facial droop is most likely an indication of a problem in the right cerebral hemisphere.

Short Answer

Complete this section with short written answers using the space provided.

1. List and describe the three key tests for assessing stroke.

_____

_____

_____

2. Why is prompt transport of stroke patients critical?

_____

_____

_____

3. What are some techniques for cooling a child with a febrile seizure?

_____

_____

_____

4. Describe the characteristics of a postictal state.

_____

_____

_____

5. What is the difference between infarcted and ischemic cells?

_____

_____

_____

6. List three conditions that may simulate stroke.

_____

_____

_____

Word Fun

www.OECzone.com
vocab explorer

The following crossword puzzle is an activity provided to reinforce correct spelling and understanding of medical terminology associated with emergency care. Use the clues in the column to complete the puzzle.

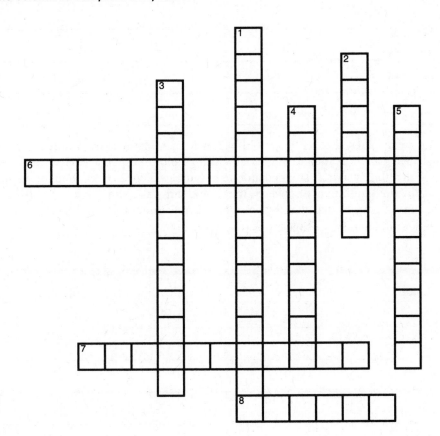

CLUES

Across

  6. Cholesterol and calcium build-up

  7. One-sided weakness

  8. Loss of brain function

Down

  1. Related to high temperatures, particularly with children

  2. Inability to pronounce words clearly

  3. Low blood glucose level

  4. Clotting of a vessel

  5. Inability to speak

4

Calls to the Scene

The following case scenarios will give you an opportunity to explore the concerns associated with patient management. Read each scenario, then answer each question in detail.

1. A 24-year-old woman complains of a sudden severe headache and collapses to the ground. She is unresponsive. Her left pupil is fixed and dilated.

   How would you best manage this patient?

   _____

   _____

   _____

   _____

   _____

   _____

   _____

   _____

2. You are dispatched to a 36-year-old man who had seizure activity at least an hour ago. The patient is incontinent, cold, clammy, and unresponsive. His friends tell you that the "shaking" stopped and he has not awakened. They thought he might just be tired until they discovered they could not wake him. He has no history of seizure activity. He has diabetes for which he takes medication.

   How would you best manage this patient?

   _____

   _____

   _____

   _____

   _____

   _____

   _____

   _____

3. A middle-aged woman is walking from the parking lot to the ticket office. She slips on an icy patch on the walkway. As she falls, her skis hit her face and she bangs her head on the ground. The patient doesn't remember the fall, but is conscious and eager to get on with her day of skiing. She has some point tenderness on the back of her head and a small laceration on her face.

How would you best manage this patient?

_____

_____

_____

_____

_____

_____

_____

_____

_____

4

Workbook Activities

The following activities have been designed to help you. Your instructor may require you to complete some or all of these activities as a regular part of your OEC training program. You are encouraged to complete any activity that your instructor does not assign as a way to enhance your learning in the classroom.

Chapter Review

The following exercises provide an opportunity to refresh your knowledge of this chapter.

■ NOTES ■

Matching

Match each of the terms in the left column to the appropriate definition in the right column.

_____ **1.** Aneurysm   **A.** acute, intermittent cramping abdominal pain

_____ **2.** Colic   **B.** vomiting

_____ **3.** Emesis   **C.** swelling or enlargement of a weakened arterial wall

_____ **4.** Peritonitis   **D.** inflammation of the peritoneum

_____ **5.** Polydipsia   **E.** altered level of consciousness caused by insufficient glucose in the blood

_____ **6.** Insulin   **F.** excessive thirst persisting for a long period of time

_____ **7.** Diabetic coma   **G.** extremely high blood glucose level

_____ **8.** Insulin shock   **H.** hormone that enables glucose to enter the cells

_____ **9.** Glucose   **I.** primary fuel, along with oxygen, for cellular metabolism

_____ **10.** Hyperglycemia   **J.** state of unconsciousness resulting from several problems, including ketoacidosis, dehydration, and hyperglycemia

_____ **11.** Allergic reaction   **K.** substance that counteracts the effect of venom from a bite or sting

_____ **12.** Wheezing   **L.** raised, swollen area on skin resulting from an insect bite or allergic reaction

_____ **13.** Wheal   **M.** an exaggerated immune response to any substance

_____ **14.** Antivenin   **N.** a high-pitched, whistling breath sound usually resulting from blockage of the airway and typically heard on expiration

_____ **15.** Antidote   **O.** drug or agent with actions similar to morphine

_____ **16.** Ingestion   **P.** may result from eating improperly canned food

_____ **17.** Opioid   **Q.** a substance that will counteract the effects of a particular poison

_____ **18.** Botulism   **R.** taking a substance by mouth

Common Medical Emergencies

Multiple Choice

Read each item carefully, then select the best response.

_____ **1.** Distention of the abdomen is gauged by:

    A. visualization.

    B. auscultation.

    C. palpation.

    D. the patient's complaint of pain around the umbilicus.

_____ **2.** The _____ are found in the retroperitoneal space.

    A. stomach and gallbladder

    B. kidneys, genitourinary structures, and large vessels

    C. liver and pancreas

    D. adrenal glands and uterus

_____ **3.** A patient with peritonitis may present with rapid, shallow breaths resulting from:

    A. hypovolemia.

    B. ileus.

    C. pain.

    D. inflammation.

_____ **4.** Common signs and symptoms of irritation or inflammation of the peritoneum may include:

    A. a quiet patient who is resting comfortably.

    B. hypertension and tachycardia.

    C. rebound tenderness and fever.

    D. Kussmaul respirations.

_____ **5.** When assessing a patient with severe abdominal pain, you should anticipate the development of _____ and treat the patient when it is evident.

    A. fever

    B. appendicitis

    C. hypovolemic shock

    D. pancreatitis

_____ **6.** Diabetes is a metabolic disorder in which the hormone _____ is missing or ineffective.

    A. estrogen

    B. adrenalin

    C. insulin

    D. epinephrine

_____ **7.** Insulin is produced by the:

    A. adrenal glands.

    B. hypothalamus.

    C. spleen.

    D. pancreas.

_____ **8.** Factors that may contribute to diabetic coma include:

    A. infection.

    B. alcohol consumption.

    C. insufficient insulin.

    D. all of the above

_____ **9.** The sweet or fruity odor on the breath of a patient with diabetes is caused by _____ in the blood.

    A. acetone

    B. ketones

    C. alcohol

    D. insulin

_____ **10.** The onset of hypoglycemia can occur within:

    A. seconds.

    B. minutes.

    C. hours.

    D. days.

_____ **11.** Without _____, or with very low levels, brain cells rapidly suffer permanent damage.

    A. epinephrine

    B. ketones

    C. bicarbonate

    D. glucose

_____ **12.** Diabetic coma may develop as a result of:

    A. too little insulin.

    B. too much insulin.

    C. overhydration.

    D. metabolic alkalosis.

_____ **13.** Always suspect hypoglycemia in any patient with:

    A. Kussmaul respirations.

    B. an altered mental status.

    C. nausea and vomiting.

    D. all of the above

_____ **14.** The most important step in caring for the unresponsive patient with diabetes is to:

    A. give oral glucose immediately.

    B. perform a focused assessment.

    C. open the airway.

    D. obtain a SAMPLE history.

_____ **15.** Determination of diabetic coma or insulin shock should be:

    A. made before transport of the patient.

    B. made before administration of oral glucose.

    C. determined by a urine glucose test.

    D. based on your knowledge of the signs and symptoms of each condition.

_____ **16.** Contraindications for the use of oral glucose include:

    A. unconsciousness.

    B. known alcoholism.

    C. insulin shock.

    D. all of the above

_____ **17.** When reassessing the patient with diabetes after administration of oral glucose, watch for:

    A. airway problems.

    B. seizures.

    C. sudden loss of consciousness.

    D. all of the above

_____ **18.** Signs and symptoms associated with hypoglycemia include:

    A. warm, dry skin.

    B. rapid, weak pulse.

    C. Kussmaul respirations.

    D. anxious or combative behavior.

_____ **19.** Signs of dehydration include:

    A. good skin turgor.

    B. elevated blood pressure.

    C. sunken eyes.

    D. all of the above

_____ **20.** Patients with diabetes who complain of "not feeling so well" should:

    A. have their glucose level checked.

    B. have a rapid trauma assessment completed.

    C. be rapidly transported to the closest medical facility.

    D. immediately be given oral glucose.

_____ **21.** A patient in insulin shock or a diabetic coma may appear to be:

    A. having a heart attack.

    B. perfectly normal.

    C. intoxicated.

    D. having a stroke.

_____ **22.** Important questions to ask when questioning the ill patient with diabetes include which of the following?

    A. Have you eaten normally today?

    B. Do you take medication for diabetes?

    C. Have you taken your normal dose of insulin (or pills) today?

    D. all of the above

_____ **23.** _____ may be substituted for oral glucose for a patient in insulin shock.

    A. Honey

    B. Synthetic sweetening compounds

    C. A diet drink

    D. Sugar-free candy

————24. Steps for assisting a patient with administration of an EpiPen include:

    A. taking body substance isolation precautions.

    B. placing the tip of the auto-injector against the medial part of the patient's thigh.

    C. recapping the injector before placing it in the trash.

    D. all of the above

————25. Rocky Mountain spotted fever and Lyme disease are both spread through the tick's:

    A. saliva.

    B. blood.

    C. hormones.

    D. all of the above

————26. Signs of envenomation by a pit viper include:

    A. swelling.

    B. severe burning pain at the site of the injury.

    C. ecchymosis.

    D. all of the above

————27. Removal of a tick should be accomplished by:

    A. suffocating it with gasoline.

    B. burning it with a lighted match to cause it to release its grip.

    C. using fine tweezers to pull it straight out of the skin.

    D. suffocating it with Vaseline.

————28. The wasp's stinger is unbarbed, meaning that it can:

    A. be removed easily.

    B. inflict multiple stings.

    C. inject more venom with each sting.

    D. penetrate deeper.

————29. Anaphylaxis is not always life threatening, but it typically involves:

    A. multiple organ systems.

    B. wheezing.

    C. urticaria.

    D. all of the above

————30. Signs and symptoms of insect stings or bites include:

    A. swelling.

    B. wheals.

    C. localized heat.

    D. all of the above

————31. Questions to ask when obtaining a history from a patient who appears to have an allergic reaction include:

    A. whether the patient has a history of allergies.

    B. what the patient was exposed to.

    C. how the patient was exposed.

    D. all of the above

————32. Treatment of a snake bite from a pit viper includes:

    A. calming the patient.

    B. providing BLS as needed if the patient shows no sign of envenomation.

    C. marking the skin with a pen over the swollen area to note whether swelling is spreading.

    D. all of the above

_____33. Epinephrine, whether made by the body or by a drug manufacturer, works rapidly to:

A. raise the pulse rate and blood pressure.

B. inhibit an allergic reaction.

C. dilate the bronchioles.

D. all of the above

_____34. If a patient suspected of having an allergic reaction has no signs of respiratory distress or shock, you should:

A. place the patient in a supine position.

B. continue with the focused assessment.

C. administer epinephrine via an EpiPen auto-injector before signs and symptoms develop.

D. all of the above

_____35. Treatment for ingestion of poisonous plants includes:

A. assessing the ABCs.

B. taking the plant to the emergency department.

C. prompt transport.

D. all of the above

_____36. Alcohol is a powerful central nervous system depressant that:

A. sharpens the sense of awareness.

B. slows reflexes.

C. increases reaction time.

D. all of the above

_____37. Signs and symptoms of staphylococcal food poisoning include:

A. difficulty in speaking.

B. nausea, vomiting, and diarrhea.

C. blurred vision.

D. all of the above

_____38. Inhalant effects range from mild drowsiness to coma, but unlike most other sedative-hypnotics, these agents may often cause:

A. seizures.

B. vomiting.

C. swelling of the tongue.

D. all of the above

_____39. A person who has been using marijuana rarely needs transport to the hospital. Exceptions may include someone who is:

A. hallucinating.

B. very anxious.

C. paranoid.

D. all of the above

_____40. Which of the following statements about carbon monoxide is true?

A. It is odorless.

B. It produces severe hypoxia.

C. It does not damage or irritate the lungs.

D. all of the above

_____41. Localized signs and symptoms of absorbed poisoning include:

A. a history of exposure.

B. burns and irritation of the skin.

C. dyspnea.

D. all of the above

NOTES

4

_____42. Poisoning by injection is almost always the result of:

   A. repetitive bee stings.

   B. pit viper envenomation.

   C. deliberate drug overdose.

   D. homicide.

_____43. Treatment for inhaled poisons includes:

   A. moving the patient into fresh air.

   B. applying a self-contained breathing apparatus to the patient.

   C. covering the patient to prevent spread of the poison.

   D. all of the above

_____44. Ingestion of an opiate, sedative, or barbituate can cause depression of the CNS and:

   A. paralysis of the extremities.

   B. dilation of the pupils.

   C. carpopedal spasms.

   D. slow breathing.

_____45. The most important treatment for poisoning is administering _____ and/or physically removing the poisonous agent.

   A. administering a specific antidote

   B. high-flow oxygen

   C. a diluting agent

   D. syrup of ipecac

Labeling www.OECzone.com anatomy review

Label the following diagrams with the correct terms.

   1. Solid Organs

A. _____

B. _____

C. _____

D. _____

E. _____

F. _____

G. _____

H. _____

2. Hollow Organs

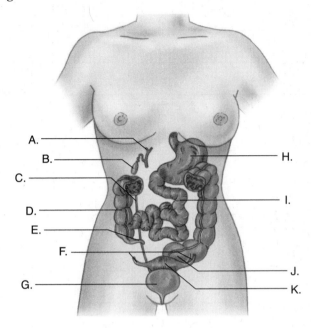

A. _____

B. _____

C. _____

D. _____

E. _____

F. _____

G. _____

H. _____

I. _____

J. _____

K. _____

3. Retroperitoneal Organs

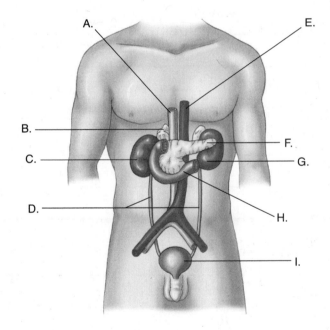

A. _____

B. _____

C. _____

D. _____

E. _____

F. _____

G. _____

H. _____

I. _____

Vocabulary   www.OECzone.com vocab explorer

Define the following terms using the space provided.

1. Acute abdomen:

_____

_____

_____

2. *Giardia lamblia:*

_____

_____

_____

3. Anaphylaxis:

_____

_____

_____

4. Histamine:

_____

_____

_____

5. Epinephrine:

_____

_____

_____

6. Envenomation:

_____

_____

_____

7. Hallucinogen:

_____

_____

_____

8. Substance abuse:

_____

_____

_____

Fill-in

Read each item carefully, then complete the statement by filling in the missing word(s).

1. A patient in insulin shock needs _____ immediately, and a patient in

a diabetic coma needs _____ and IV fluid therapy.

2. Wheezing occurs because excessive fluid and mucus are secreted into the

_____ _____.

3. The stinger of the honeybee is _____, so the bee cannot withdraw it.

4. Your ability to recognize and manage the many signs and symptoms of allergic

reactions may be the only thing standing between a patient and _____

_____.

5. When dealing with exposure to chemicals, treatment focuses on support:

assessing and maintaining the patient's _____.

6. If the patient has a chemical agent in the eyes, you should irrigate them quickly

and thoroughly, at least _____ for acid substances and

_____ for alkalis.

7. Opioid analgesics are central nervous system depressants and can cause severe

_____.

8. Approximately 80% of all poisoning is by _____, including plants,
contaminated food, and most drugs.

9. Phosphorus and elemental sodium _____ when they come in contact
with water.

True/False

If you believe the statement to be more true than false, write the letter "T" in the space provided. If you believe the statement to be more false than true, write the letter "F."

1. _____ Referred pain is a result of connections between ligaments in the abdominal and chest cavities.

2. _____ It is important to accurately diagnose the cause of acute abdominal pain in order to properly treat the patient.

3. _____ When palpating the abdomen, always start with the quadrant where the patient complains of the most severe pain.

4. _____ If blood glucose levels remain low, a patient may lose consciousness or have permanent brain damage.

5. _____ Diabetic emergencies can occur when a patient's blood glucose level gets too high or when it drops too low.

6. _____ Patients with diabetes may require insulin to control their blood glucose.

4

7. _____ Ice should be promptly applied to any insect sting or snake bite with swelling.

8. _____ The pain of coelenterate stings may respond to flushing with cold water.

9. _____ Allergic reactions can occur in response to almost any substance.

10. _____ For a patient who appears to have an allergic reaction, give 100% oxygen via nasal cannula.

11. _____ Systemic symptoms of envenomation by coelenterates include headache, dizziness, and hypotension.

12. _____ Abdominal pain in women is usually related to the menstrual cycle and is rarely serious.

13. _____ Activated charcoal is a standard of care in all ingestion poisonings.

14. _____ Inhaled chlorine produces profound hypoxia without lung irritation.

15. _____ Patients with opioid overdose typically have pinpoint pupils.

Short Answer

Complete this section with short written answers using the space provided.

1. Should a rescuer attempt to diagnose the cause of abdominal pain? Why or why not?

_____

_____

_____

2. List the general emergency care for patients with acute abdomen.

_____

_____

_____

3. If a patient with diabetes was "fine" 2 hours ago and now is unconscious and unresponsive, which diabetes-related condition would you suspect and why?

_____

_____

_____

4. What are five stimuli that most often cause allergic reactions?

_____

_____

_____

_____

_____

5. What are the common respiratory and circulatory signs or symptoms of an allergic reaction?

_____

_____

_____

6. What is the general treatment for a snake bite?

_____

_____

_____

7. What are the steps in treating a coelenterate envenomation?

_____

_____

_____

8. What are four routes of contact for poisoning?

_____

_____

_____

9. What five questions should you ask a patient with possible poisoning?

_____

_____

_____

_____

_____

4

━━■ CLUES ■━━

Across

3. Excessive thirst
4. Acute cramping abdominal pain
7. Harsh, high-pitched airway sounds
8. Disease that starts early in life, generally requires daily injections
9. Chemical substance produced by a gland
12. Involuntary muscle contractions for protection
13. Lack of appetite
14. Paralysis of the bowels

Down

1. Used to neutralize or counteract a poison
2. Abrasion of stomach or small intestine
3. Excessive urination
5. Responsible for allergy symptoms
6. Substance whose chemical action causes damage
9. Protrusion of a loop of an organ
10. Vomiting
11. Poison or harmful substance

Word Fun www.OECzone.com vocab explorer

The following crossword puzzle is an activity provided to reinforce correct spelling and understanding of medical terminology associated with emergency care. Use the clues in the column to complete the puzzle.

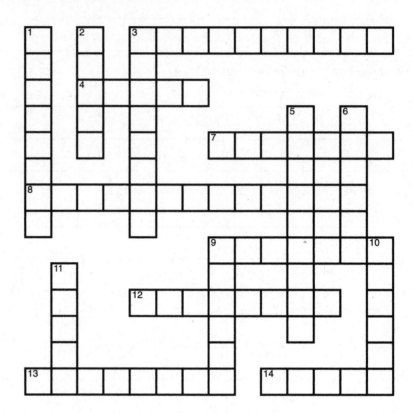

Calls to the Scene

The following case scenarios provide an opportunity to explore the concerns associated with patient management. Read each scenario, then answer each question in detail.

1. You are dispatched to a restaurant where a 28-year-old woman is complaining of a sudden onset of nausea and vomiting with severe right lower quadrant pain. The patient is doubled over in pain and is pale with clammy skin.

   What problem would you suspect and how would you treat this patient?

   _____

   _____

   _____

   _____

   _____

   _____

_____

_____

_____

2. You stop at a minor motor vehicle crash. The police officer on scene tells you it is a one-car wreck involving a tree, and the driver is "not acting right." The driver, a 33-year-old man, appears intoxicated but there is no smell of alcohol. He has no visible injuries.

How would you best manage this patient?

_____

_____

_____

_____

_____

_____

_____

_____

_____

_____

3. You are called to a slopeside restaurant for a person who is having difficulty breathing. Upon arrival, you find a 22-year-old woman with facial edema, cyanosis around the lips, audible wheezing, and urticaria on her face and upper body. Her boyfriend tells you she ate shrimp and she is allergic to them. He also tells you she has some medicine in her purse and hands you an EpiPen prescribed to her.

How would you best manage this patient?

_____

_____

_____

_____

_____

_____

_____

_____

_____

_____

4. You are called to a slopeside child care center where a toddler has been found chewing on the leaves of an unknown plant. The supervisor tells you she thinks the plant may be poisonous and they were not sure what they should do. His mother has been called and will meet you at the hospital.

How would you best manage this patient?

_____

_____

_____

_____

_____

_____

_____

_____

_____

Skill Drills www.OECzone.com video clips

Skill Drill 13-1: Administering Glucose
Test your knowledge of this skill drill by filling in the correct words in the photo captions.

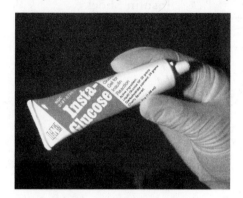

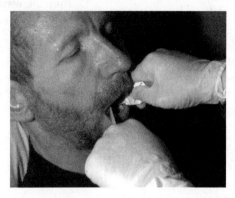

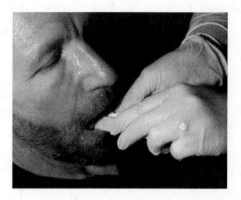

1. Make sure that the tube of glucose is intact and has not _____.

2. Squeeze the entire tube of oral glucose onto the _____ _____ of a _____ _____ or tongue depressor.

3. Open the patient's _____. Place the tongue depressor on the _____ _____ between the cheek and the gum with the _____ _____ next to the cheek.

Skill Drill 13-2: Using an Auto-Injector
Test your knowledge of this skill drill by filling in the correct words in the photo captions.

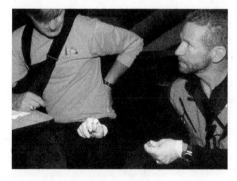

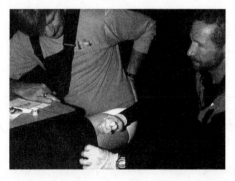

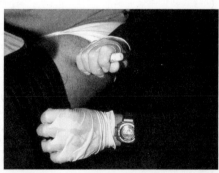

1. Remove the auto-injector's _____ _____.

2. Place the tip of the auto-injector against the _____ thigh.

3. Help the patient push the _____ firmly against the _____ and hold it in place until all the medication is injected.

Comparison Table

Complete the following table on the characteristics of diabetic emergencies.

	Diabetic Coma	Insulin Shock
History Food intake Insulin dosage Onset Skin Infection		
Gastrointestinal Tract Thirst Hunger Vomiting		
Respiratory System Breathing Odor of breath		
Cardiovascular System Blood pressure Pulse		
Nervous System Consciousness		
Urine Sugar Acetone		
Treatment Response		

Notes

Workbook Activities

The following activities have been designed to help you. Your instructor may require you to complete some or all of these activities as a regular part of your OEC training program. You are encouraged to complete any activity that your instructor does not assign as a way to enhance your learning in the classroom.

Chapter Review

The following exercises provide an opportunity to refresh your knowledge of this chapter.

■ NOTES ■

Matching

Match each of the terms in the left column to the appropriate definition in the right column.

_____ 1. Camber

_____ 2. Compression

_____ 3. Dorsiflex

_____ 4. Rotational fall

_____ 5. Inversion

_____ 6. FOOSH

A. To flex the foot upward

B. The arch formed by a ski or snowboard placed on a flat surface

C. Forcing the leg outward at the knee

D. Trauma caused by an impact between a body part and a blunt object

E. Fall onto outstretched hand

F. Reversal of normal relationship

Multiple Choice

Read each item carefully, then select the best response.

_____ 1. Which accident type averages 89 deaths per year in the United States?

A. skiing/snowboarding

B. lightning strikes

C. bathtub falls

D. automobile collisions

_____ 2. With new ski boot designs, which injuries are relatively uncommon?

A. knee sprains

B. hip contusions

C. ankle sprains and fractures

D. shoulder separations

_____ 3. Basic steps to injury prevention include:

A. good equipment.

B. good physical conditioning.

C. staying within your ability.

D. all of the above

Snowsports and Mountain Biking Emergencies

_____ **4.** The most common injury in bike riding is:

   A. abrasions.

   B. fractures.

   C. concussions.

   D. lacerations.

_____ **5.** Techniques and equipment used to transport injured cyclists over trails include:

   A. toboggans.

   B. snowmobiles.

   C. all-terrain vehicles.

   D. single-wheeled litters.

Vocabulary www.OECzone.com vocab explorer

Define the following terms using the space provided.

   1. Acromioclavicular separations:

   _____

   _____

   _____

   2. Anterior cruciate ligament (ACL):

   _____

   _____

   _____

   3. Medial collateral ligament (MCL):

   _____

   _____

   _____

4. Phantom foot syndrome:

_____

_____

_____

Fill-in

Read each item carefully, then complete the statement by filling in the missing word(s).

1. The most frequent upper body injury is _____.

2. The two basic types of ski accidents are _____ and _____.

3. Incident management includes keeping _____ of circumstances surrounding an incident.

4. _____ and _____ are two important factors in determining an individual's likelihood of injury.

5. Dislocations of the _____ are rare but signify a potential limb-threatening situation because of possible arterial damage.

6. Skier/snowboard deaths are largely due to _____ and _____ injuries resulting from collisions with trees or other stationary objects.

True/False

If you believe the statement to be more true than false, write the letter "T" in the space provided. If you believe the statement to be more false than true, write the letter "F."

1. _____ The number of accidents per 1,000 participants in bicycle riding is two.

2. _____ There is a greater number of deaths in snowsports accidents than lightning strikes.

3. _____ The snowsports industry continues to introduce new types of "sliding" equipment to enhance the sport.

4. _____ Skiers and snowboarders can lessen their chances of injury by following the responsibility code.

5. _____ Snowmobiles cannot be used to tow rescue devices.

6. _____ Off-road bicyclists are injured more often than road bicyclists.

Short Answer

Complete this section with short written answers using the space provided.

1. List common alpine skiing injuries.

_____

_____

_____

_____

_____

2. List common off-road bicycling injuries.

_____

_____

_____

_____

3. List common snowmobiling injuries.

_____

_____

_____

_____

4. Describe Raynaud's syndrome.

_____

_____

_____

_____

5. Describe skier's thumb.

_____

_____

_____

_____

_____

4

6. Describe skier's toe.

_____

_____

_____

_____

_____

7. Discuss snowboarder's ankle.

_____

_____

_____

_____

8. List ten methods for preventing snowsports emergencies.

_____

_____

_____

_____

_____

_____

_____

_____

_____

_____

Word Fun

www.OECzone.com
vocab explorer

The following crossword puzzle is an activity provided to reinforce correct spelling and understanding of medical terminology associated with emergency care. Use the clues in the column to complete the puzzle.

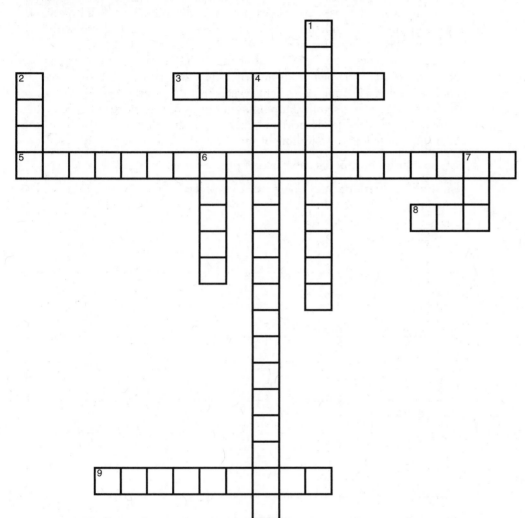

CLUES

Across

3. Twisting
5. Ski acts as lever pointing foot in opposite direction
8. Anterior cruciate ligament
9. Very short ski

Down

1. Common hand injury
2. National Mountain Bike Patrol
4. Joint between the clavicle and scapula
6. Fall on outstretched hand
7. Medial collateral ligament

4

Calls to the Scene

The following case scenarios will give you an opportunity to explore the concerns associated with patient management. Read each scenario, then answer each question.

1. While attempting an aerial maneuver on a terrain park's 9'-high spine feature, a teenage snowboarder loses his balance and attempts to break his fall by reaching down with his extended left hand. He lands very hard on his left side, with his left elbow flexed against his ribcage. He does not lose consciousness. Upon arriving at the scene, you find the rider lying on his left side in the fetal position. He complains of severe pain in his left rib cage and left wrist, and somewhat less pain in his midback. Your assessment reveals that the rider is alert and responsive, but he has significant point tenderness of the midback between the shoulder blades, deep tenderness and guarding of the left upper quadrant of the abdomen, and tenderness/swelling of the left wrist without deformity.

List the injuries of concern described in this scenario.

List, in order of priority, the emergency care procedures you would initiate in this scenario.

_____

_____

_____

_____

_____

_____

_____

_____

_____

2. On a very cold night near the end of the tubing session, a 9-year-old girl is riding on the outside lane of a large tubing park. Her tube ricochets repeatedly off the dividing lane berms at an increasing speed and then catapults over the outer berm, down an adjacent embankment, and into a stand of trees. When you arrive, the young girl is lying on her left side, supporting her partially flexed right arm across her chest and abdomen. She is sobbing and shivering violently, and you note that she is wearing jeans and a light windbreaker and has no hat. Your assessment reveals slow speech with slurred responses; palpable tenderness, swelling, and deformity of the right elbow; a right radial pulse that is diminished when compared to that on the left; and a weakened hand grasp on the right side. Her initial vital signs are a pulse of 108 beats/min and strong, and respirations of 20 breaths/min and shallow.

List the injuries of concern described in this scenario.

List, in order of priority, the emergency care procedures you would initiate in this scenario.

_____

_____

_____

_____

_____

_____

_____

_____

_____

_____

4

Workbook Activities

The following activities have been designed to help you. Your instructor may require you to complete some or all of these activities as a regular part of your OEC training program. You are encouraged to complete any activity that your instructor does not assign as a way to enhance your learning in the classroom.

Chapter Review

The following exercises provide an opportunity to refresh your knowledge of this chapter.

■ NOTES ■

Matching

Match each of the terms in the left column to the appropriate definition in the right column.

_____	**1.** Acute mountain sickness	**A.** slowing of heart rate caused by sudden immersion in cold water
_____	**2.** Evaporation	**B.** salts and other chemicals dissolved in body fluids
_____	**3.** Hyperthermia	**C.** cold-induced area of superficial blood vessel constriction
_____	**4.** Diving reflex	**D.** death from suffocation after submersion in water
_____	**5.** Core temperature	**E.** core temperature greater than 101°F
_____	**6.** Frostnip	**F.** condition when the entire body temperature falls
_____	**7.** Electrolytes	**G.** condition caused by lack of oxygen
_____	**8.** Hypothermia	**H.** heat loss resulting from sweating
_____	**9.** Ambient temperature	**I.** painful muscle spasms that occur after vigorous exercise
_____	**10.** Heat cramps	**J.** temperature of the surrounding environment
_____	**11.** Drowning	**K.** temperature of the central part of the body

C H A P T E R

Environmental Emergencies

Multiple Choice

Read each item carefully, then select the best response.

_____ **1.** Signs and symptoms of severe systemic hypothermia include all of the following except:

A. weak pulse.

B. coma.

C. confusion.

D. very slow respirations.

_____ **2.** Hypothermia is more common among:

A. elderly individuals.

B. infants and children.

C. individuals who are already ill.

D. all of the above

_____ **3.** To assess a patient's general temperature, pull back your glove and place the back of your hand on the patient's:

A. back, underneath the clothing.

B. forehead.

C. forearm, on the inside of the wrist.

D. neck, at the area where you check the carotid pulse.

_____ **4.** Never assume that a(n) _____, pulseless patient is dead.

A. apneic

B. cyanotic

C. cold

D. hyperthermic

_____ **5.** Management of hypothermia in the field consists of all of the following except:

A. stabilizing vital functions.

B. removing wet clothing.

C. preventing further heat loss.

D. massaging the cold extremities.

_____ **6.** It is necessary to assess the pulse of a hypothermic patient for at least _____, especially before considering CPR.

    A. 10 to 20 seconds

    B. several minutes

    C. 2 full minutes

    D. 60 to 75 minutes

_____ **7.** When exposed parts of the body become very cold but not frozen, the condition is called:

    A. frostnip.

    B. chilblains.

    C. immersion foot.

    D. all of the above

_____ **8.** Important factors in determining the severity of a local cold injury include all of the following except:

    A. the temperature to which the body part was exposed.

    B. a previous history of frostbite.

    C. the wind velocity during exposure.

    D. the duration of the exposure.

_____ **9.** Signs and symptoms of systemic hypothermia include:

    A. blisters and swelling.

    B. hard and waxy skin.

    C. altered mental status.

    D. local tissue damage.

_____ **10.** When the body is exposed to more heat energy than it loses, _____ result(s).

    A. hyperthermia

    B. heat cramps

    C. heat exhaustion

    D. heatstroke

_____ **11.** Contributing factors to the development of heat illnesses include:

    A. high air temperature.

    B. vigorous exercise.

    C. high humidity.

    D. all of the above

_____ **12.** Snowblindness is:

    A. the result of frostbitten eyelids.

    B. caused by moisture buildup, freezing the eyelids shut.

    C. a momentary condition manifested by exposure to sun reflections off snow.

    D. sunburn of the conjunctiva.

_____ **13.** Which of the following statements concerning heat cramps is not true?

    A. They only occur when it is hot outdoors.

    B. They may be seen in well-conditioned athletes.

    C. The exact cause of heat cramps is not well understood.

    D. Dehydration may play a role in the development of heat cramps.

_____ **14.** Signs and symptoms of heat exhaustion and associated hypovolemia include:

  A. cold, clammy skin with ashen pallor.

  B. dizziness, weakness, or faintness.

  C. normal vital signs.

  D. all of the above

_____ **15.** Be prepared to transport the patient to the hospital for aggressive treatment of hyperthermia if the patient's:

  A. symptoms do not clear up promptly.

  B. level of consciousness improves.

  C. temperature drops.

  D. all of the above

_____ **16.** Often, the first sign of heatstroke is:

  A. a change in behavior.

  B. an increase in pulse rate.

  C. an increase in respirations.

  D. hot, dry, flushed skin.

_____ **17.** The least common but most serious illness caused by heat exposure, occurring when the body is subjected to more heat than it can handle and normal mechanisms for getting rid of the excess heat are overwhelmed, is:

  A. hyperthermia.

  B. heat cramps.

  C. heat exhaustion.

  D. heatstroke.

_____ **18.** _____ is the body's attempt at self-preservation by preventing water from entering the lungs.

  A. Bronchoconstriction

  B. Laryngospasm

  C. Esophageal spasms

  D. Swelling in the oropharynx

_____ **19.** Treatment of drowning/near drowning begins with:

  A. opening the airway.

  B. ventilation with 100% oxygen via BVM device.

  C. suctioning the lungs to remove the water.

  D. rescue and removal from the water.

_____ **20.** If you are unsure whether or not a spinal injury has occurred, you should:

  A. stabilize and protect the patient's spine.

  B. provide mouth-to-mouth ventilation as you would in any other situation.

  C. ascertain whether or not there is a spinal injury.

  D. all of the above

_____ **21.** After removing a near-drowning patient from the water, it may be difficult to find a pulse because of:

  A. dilation of peripheral blood vessels.

  B. body temperature at the core.

  C. low cardiac output.

  D. all of the above

4

_____22. If a near-drowning patient has evidence of upper airway obstruction by foreign matter, attempt to clear it by:

    A. removing the obstruction manually.

    B. suction.

    C. using abdominal thrusts.

    D. all of the above

_____23. You must assume that spinal injury exists if the patient is conscious but complains of:

    A. weakness.

    B. numbness in the arms or legs.

    C. paralysis.

    D. all of the above

_____24. You should never give up on resuscitating a cold-water drowning victim because:

    A. when the patient is submerged in water colder than body temperature, heat is maintained in the body.

    B. the resulting hypothermia can protect vital organs from the lack of oxygen.

    C. the resulting hypothermia raises the metabolic rate.

    D. all of the above

_____25. If a patient with acute mountain sickness is unable to walk, the most common position in which to carry the patient is:

    A. prone.

    B. sitting.

    C. semiprone.

    D. supine.

_____26. Areas usually affected by descent problems include:

    A. the lungs.

    B. the skin.

    C. the joints.

    D. vision.

_____27. Potential problems associated with rupture of the lungs include:

    A. air emboli.

    B. pneumomediastinum.

    C. pneumothorax.

    D. all of the above

_____28. The organs most severely affected by air embolism are the:

    A. brain and spinal cord.

    B. brain and heart.

    C. heart and lungs.

    D. brain and lungs.

_____29. Treatment of hypothermia caused by cold-water immersion is the same as that of hypothermia caused by cold exposure, with the exception of:

    A. the use of humidified oxygen.

    B. There are no exceptions.

    C. clearing the patient's airway of foreign material.

    D. massaging the extremities.

Vocabulary www.OECzone.com vocab explorer

Define the following terms using the space provided.

1. HACE:

_____

_____

_____

2. Decompression sickness:

_____

_____

_____

3. Heat exhaustion:

_____

_____

_____

4. Frostbite:

_____

_____

_____

5. Near drowning:

_____

_____

_____

6. HAPE:

_____

_____

_____

4

Fill-in

Read each item carefully, then complete the statement by filling in the missing word.

1. Do not attempt to rewarm patients who have _____ hypothermia, because arrhythmias may develop unless patients are handled very carefully.

2. Most significant diving injuries occur during _____.

3. When treating a patient with frostbite, never attempt _____ if there is any chance that the part may freeze again before the patient reaches the hospital.

4. As with so many hazards, you cannot help others if you do not

   practice _____.

5. _____, a common effect of hypothermia, is the body's attempt to

   maintain heat.

6. The first priority upon locating an avalanche victim is _____.

7. If the patient is alert and responds appropriately, the hypothermia is _____.

True/False

If you believe the statement to be more true than false, write the letter "T" in the space provided. If you believe the statement to be more false than true, write the letter "F."

1. _____ To assess the skin temperature in a patient experiencing a generalized cold emergency, you should feel the patient's skin.

2. _____ Mild hypothermia occurs when the core temperature drops to 85°F.

3. _____ The body's most efficient heat regulating mechanisms are sweating and dilation of skin blood vessels.

4. _____ People who are at greatest risk for heat illnesses are the elderly and children.

5. _____ The signs and symptoms of exposure to heat can include moist, pale skin.

6. _____ The strongest stimulus for breathing is an elevation of oxygen in the blood.

7. _____ The altitude at which a person sleeps seems to be a more important factor in acclimatizing than the highest altitude reached during the day.

8. _____ The signs and symptoms of exposure to heat can include hot, dry skin.

Short Answer

Complete this section with short written answers using the space provided.

1. What are the steps in treating heatstroke?

_____

_____

_____

2. What is an air embolism and how does it occur?

_____

_____

_____

3. If caught outside in an electrical storm, what should you avoid?

_____

_____

_____

4. How should a frostbitten foot be treated?

_____

_____

_____

5. What are four "Do Nots" in relation to local cold injuries?

_____

_____

_____

6. What are the potential signs and symptoms of an air embolism?

_____

_____

_____

CLUES

Across

7. A burn caused by ultraviolet light
9. Salts and chemicals in body fluids
10. Excessive heat problem, may be fatal
11. Temperature greater than 101°F
12. Loss of heat to colder environment
13. The temperature of the surrounding environment

Down

1. Irritation of the skin exposed to wind
2. An electronic device that can emit and receive a signal. Used to assist rescues.
3. Death from suffocation by submersion in water
4. Tissue death caused by loss of blood supply
5. The temperature of the central part of the body
6. Damage to tissues exposed to cold
8. A fall in body core temperature to below 95°F

Word Fun www.OECzone vocab explorer

The following crossword puzzle is an activity provided to reinforce correct spelling and understanding of medical terminology associated with emergency care. Use the clues in the column to complete the puzzle.

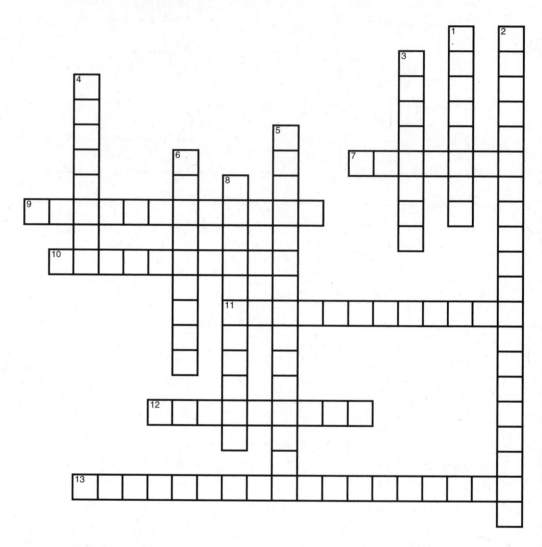

Calls to the Scene

The following case scenarios provide an opportunity to explore the concerns associated with patient management. Read each scenario, then answer each question in detail.

1. A middle-aged skier who lives in the southeastern United States was skiing for the first time in Colorado at an elevation of 10,000'. He stops at an aid station complaining of shortness of breath, severe fatigue after only four runs, headache, and nausea. The skier says he had "worked out at home" before the ski trip and thought he was in good shape.

How would you best manage this patient?

_____

_____

_____

_____

_____

_____

_____

_____

2. A person who was skiing on an intermediate nordic trail is reported missing. Two hours into the search, you find the missing skier, semiresponsive. You radio a snowmobile, which will take 30 minutes to arrive. The patient is lying semiprone, left side down. Her left arm is straight out from the body and will not bend. She is responsive only to painful stimulus secondary to hypothermia. Her hands and feet are frostbitten and she has a fractured left humerus. Her initial pulse is 58 beats/min and respirations are 10 breaths/min. Five minutes later, you take a second set of vital signs, which indicates a pulse of 54 beats/min and respirations of 12 breaths/min. A third set of vitals signs 10 minutes later indicates a pulse of 52 beats/min and respirations of 12 breaths/min.

How would you best manage this patient?

_____

_____

_____

_____

_____

_____

_____

3. You are working in an aid station for the annual marathon race. A racer comes in complaining of a sudden onset of abdominal cramps. It is very hot.

How would you best manage this patient?

_____

_____

_____

4

Skill Drills

Skill Drill 15-1: Treating for Heat Exhaustion

Test your knowledge of this skill drill by filling in the correct words in the photo captions.

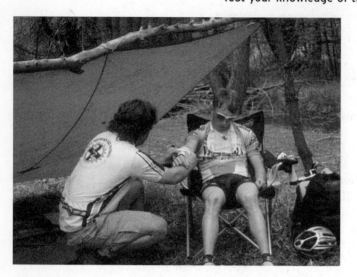

1. Remove _____ _____ .

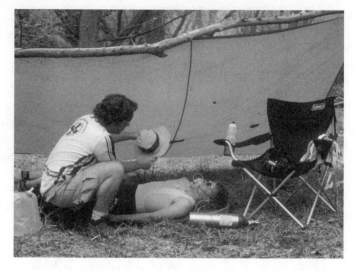

2. Move the patient to a _____ _____ .

Give _____ .

Place the patient in a _____ position, elevate the legs, and _____ the patient.

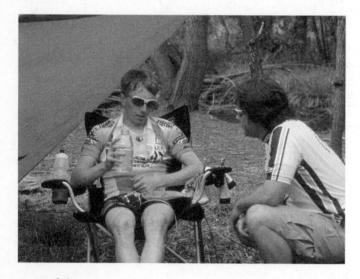

3. If the patient is _____ _____ , give an electrolyte solution by mouth.

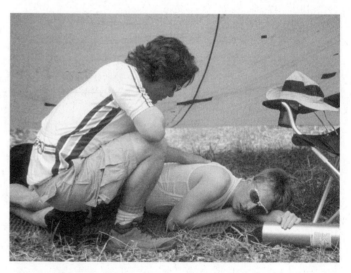

4. If nausea develops, _____ the patient on the side.

Skill Drill 15-2: Stabilizing a Patient with a Suspected Spinal Injury in the
Water
Test your knowledge of this skill drill by placing the photos below in the correct order.
Number the first step with a "1," the second step with a "2," etc.

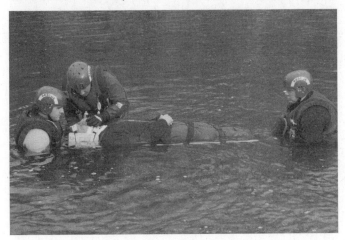

Secure the patient to the backboard.

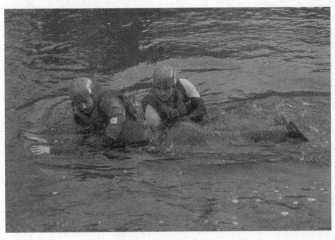

Turn the patient to a supine position by rotating the entire upper half of the body as a single unit.

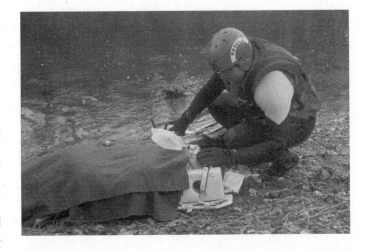

Cover the patient with a blanket and apply oxygen if breathing. Begin CPR if breathing and pulse are absent.

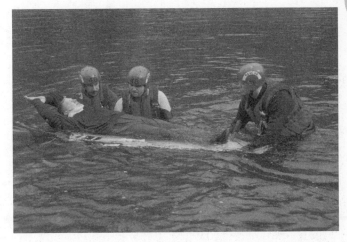

Float a buoyant backboard under the patient.

4

(continued)

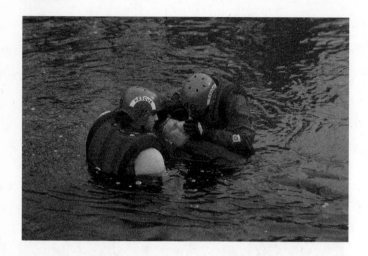

As soon as the patient is turned, begin artificial ventilation using the mouth-to-mouth method or a pocket mask.

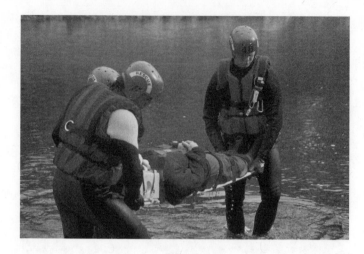

Remove the patient from the water.

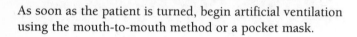

Notes

Workbook Activities

The following activities have been designed to help you. Your instructor may require you to complete some or all of these activities as a regular part of your OEC training program. You are encouraged to complete any activity that your instructor does not assign as a way to enhance your learning in the classroom.

Chapter Review

The following exercises provide an opportunity to refresh your knowledge of this chapter.

■ NOTES ■

Matching

Match each of the terms in the left column to the appropriate definition in the right column.

_____ **1.** Behavioral crisis

A. what you can see of a person's response to the environment; his or her actions

_____ **2.** Psychogenic

B. temporary or permanent dysfunction of the brain caused by a disturbance in brain tissue function

_____ **3.** Organic brain syndrome

C. any reaction to events that interferes with activities of daily living or is unacceptable to the patient or others

_____ **4.** Depression

D. a persistent mood of sadness, despair, or discouragement

_____ **5.** Functional disorder

E. abnormal operation of an organ that cannot be traced to an obvious change in structure or physiology of the organ

_____ **6.** Behavior

F. a symptom or illness caused by mental factors as opposed to physical ones

Multiple Choice

Read each item carefully, then select the best response.

_____ **1.** A psychological or behavioral crisis may be due to:
   A. mind-altering substances.
   B. the emergency situation.
   C. stress.
   D. all of the above

C H A P T E R 16

Behavioral Emergencies

_____ **2.** A normal reaction to a crisis situation would be:

   A. Monday morning blues that last until Friday.

   B. feeling "blue" after the break up of a long-term relationship.

   C. feeling depressed week after week with no discernible cause.

   D. all of the above

_____ **3.** The cause of a behavioral crisis experienced by an unmanageable patient may be:

   A. drug use.

   B. a history of mental illness.

   C. alcohol abuse.

   D. all of the above

_____ **4.** Learning to adapt to a variety of situations in daily life, including stresses and strains, is called:

   A. disruption.

   B. adjustment.

   C. behavior.

   D. functional.

_____ **5.** If the interruption of daily routine tends to recur on a regular basis, the behavior is also considered a _____ problem.

   A. mental health

   B. functional disorder

   C. behavioral

   D. psychogenic

_____ **6.** If an abnormal or disturbing pattern of behavior lasts for at least _____, it is regarded as a matter of concern from a mental health standpoint.

   A. 6 weeks

   B. 1 month

   C. 6 months

   D. 1 year

——————— **7.** A person who is no longer able to respond appropriately to the environment may be having what is called a psychological or ——————— emergency.
  A. psychiatric
  B. behavioral
  C. functional
  D. adjustment

——————— **8.** Mental disorders may be caused by a:
  A. social disturbance.
  B. chemical disturbance.
  C. biological disturbance.
  D. all of the above

——————— **9.** An altered mental status may arise from:
  A. an oxygen saturation of 98%.
  B. moderate temperatures.
  C. an inadequate blood flow to the brain.
  D. adequate glucose levels in the blood.

——————— **10.** Organic brain syndrome may be caused by:
  A. hypoglycemia.
  B. excessive heat or cold.
  C. lack of oxygen.
  D. all of the above

——————— **11.** An example of a functional disorder would be:
  A. schizophrenia.
  B. organic brain syndrome.
  C. Alzheimer's.
  D. all of the above

——————— **12.** When documenting abnormal behavior, it is important to:
  A. record detailed, subjective findings.
  B. avoid judgmental statements.
  C. avoid quoting the patient's own words.
  D. all of the above

——————— **13.** Safety guidelines for behavioral emergencies include:
  A. assessing the scene.
  B. being prepared to spend extra time.
  C. encouraging purposeful movement.
  D. all of the above

——————— **14.** In evaluating a situation that is considered a behavioral emergency, the first things to consider are:
  A. airway and breathing.
  B. scene safety and patient response.
  C. history of medications.
  D. respiratory and circulatory status.

——————— **15.** Psychogenic circumstances may include:
  A. severe depression.
  B. death of a loved one.
  C. a history of mental illness.
  D. all of the above

Vocabulary www.OECzone vocab explorer

Complete this section by defining the terms listed using the space provided.

1. Mental disorder:

_____

_____

_____

2. Activities of daily living (ADL):

_____

_____

_____

3. Altered mental status:

_____

_____

_____

4. Implied consent:

_____

_____

_____

Fill-in

Read each item carefully, then complete the statement by filling in the missing word.

1. _____ is what you can see of a person's response to the environment; his or her actions.

2. A _____ or emergency is any reaction to events that interferes with the activities of daily living or has become unacceptable to the patient, family, or community.

3. Chronic _____, or a persistent feeling of sadness or despair, may be a symptom of a mental or physical disorder.

4. _____ is a temporary or permanent dysfunction of the brain caused by a disturbance in the physical or physiologic functioning of the brain.

5. A behavioral crisis puts tremendous stress on a person's _____, including natural abilities and training.

True/False

If you believe the statement to be more true than false, write the letter "T" in the space provided. If you believe the statement to be more false than true, write the letter "F."

1. _____ Depression lasting 2 to 3 weeks after being fired from a job is a normal mental health response.

2. _____ Low blood glucose or lack of oxygen to the brain may cause behavioral changes, but not to the degree that a psychiatric emergency could exist.

3. _____ From a mental health standpoint, a pattern of abnormal behavior must last at least 3 months to be a matter of concern.

4. _____ A disturbed patient should always be transported with restraints.

5. _____ It is sometimes helpful to allow a patient with a behavioral emergency some time alone to calm down and collect his or her thoughts.

6. _____ It is important to avoid looking directly at the patient when dealing with a behavioral crisis.

7. _____ All individuals with mental health disorders are dangerous, violent, or otherwise unmanageable.

8. _____ When completing the documentation, it is important to record detailed, subjective findings that support the conclusion of abnormal behavior.

Short Answer

Complete this section with short written answers using the space provided.

1. What is the distinction between a behavioral crisis and a mental health problem?

_____

_____

2. What three major areas should be considered in evaluating the possible source of a behavioral crisis?

_____

_____

_____

3. List ten safety guidelines for dealing with behavioral emergencies.

_____

_____

_____

_____

_____

_____

_____

_____

_____

_____

Word Fun www.OECzone.com vocab explorer

The following crossword puzzle is a good way to review correct spelling and meaning of medical terminology associated with emergency care. Use the clues in the column to complete the puzzle.

Across

3. Reactions interfere with normal activities
5. Illness with psychological symptoms
6. Caused by mental factors; not physical
7. Persistent sadness; despair

Down

1. A change in behavior
2. No known physiologic reason for abnormality
4. Basic doings of a normal person

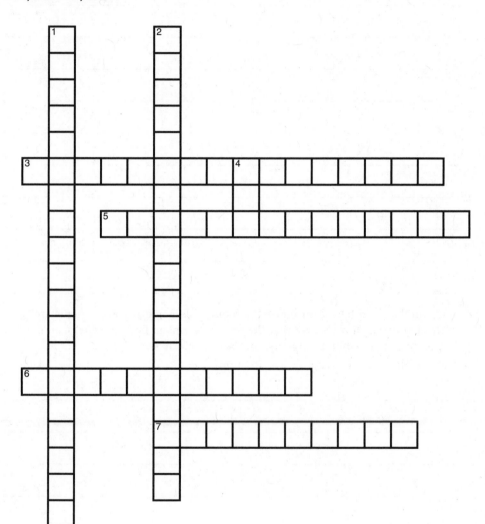

Calls to the Scene

The following case scenarios provide an opportunity to explore the concerns associated with patient management. Read each scenario, then answer each question in detail.

1. A ruckus has broken out in a local pub involving several men in their 20s. They appear to have had a large quantity of alcohol and you suspect that other drugs may also be involved. One of the men is exhibiting overly aggressive behavior and is yelling obscenities at anyone who comes near.

   How would you best manage this situation?

   _____

   _____

   _____

   _____

   _____

   _____

   _____

   _____

   _____

   _____

2. A death of a child has occurred on the mountain. Obviously, the parents are extremely upset. You observe that the mother seems to be incapable of responding reasonably during any interface with others.

   How would you best manage this situation?

   _____

   _____

   _____

   _____

   _____

   _____

   _____

   _____

   _____

   _____

Notes

Workbook Activities

The following activities have been designed to help you. Your instructor may require you to complete some or all of these activities as a regular part of your OEC training program. You are encouraged to complete any activity that your instructor does not assign as a way to enhance your learning in the classroom.

Chapter Review

The following exercises provide an opportunity to refresh your knowledge of this chapter.

NOTES

Matching

Match each of the terms in the left column to the appropriate definition in the right column.

_____ **1.** Cervix	**A.** an umbilical cord that is wrapped around the infant's neck
_____ **2.** Perineum	**B.** a fluid-filled, bag-like membrane inside the uterus that grows around the developing fetus
_____ **3.** Placenta	**C.** the area of skin between the vagina and the anus
_____ **4.** Amniotic sac	**D.** the neck of the uterus
_____ **5.** Fetus	**E.** Connects mother and infant
_____ **6.** Birth canal	**F.** the outermost part of a woman's reproductive system
_____ **7.** Uterus	**G.** the part of the infant that appears first
_____ **8.** Umbilical cord	**H.** the vagina and lower part of the uterus
_____ **9.** Vagina	**I.** a woman who has had more than one live birth
_____ **10.** Breech presentation	**J.** spontaneous abortion
_____ **11.** Limb presentation	**K.** delivery in which the presenting part is a single arm, leg, or foot
_____ **12.** Multipara	**L.** tissue that develops on the wall of the uterus and is connected to the fetus
_____ **13.** Nuchal cord	**M.** the hollow organ inside the female pelvis where the fetus grows
_____ **14.** Presentation	**N.** the developing baby in the uterus
_____ **15.** Miscarriage	**O.** delivery in which the buttocks come out first

CHAPTER 17

Obstetrics and Gynecological Emergencies

Multiple Choice

Read each item carefully, then select the best response.

_____ **1.** In the event of a nuchal cord, proper procedure is to:
   A. gently slip the cord over the infant's head or shoulder.
   B. clamp the cord and cut it before delivering the infant.
   C. clamp the cord and cut it, then gently unwind it from around the neck if wrapped around more than once.
   D. all of the above

_____ **2.** If the amniotic fluid is greenish instead of clear or has a foul odor, this is called:
   A. nuchal rigidity.
   B. meconium staining.
   C. placenta previa.
   D. bloody show.

_____ **3.** Meconium can cause all of the following except:
   A. a depressed newborn.
   B. rapid pulse rate.
   C. airway obstruction.
   D. aspiration.

_____ **4.** Once the head is delivered, the baby must be suctioned. This is accomplished by:
   A. suctioning the nose only.
   B. suctioning the nose, then the mouth.
   C. suctioning the mouth, then the nose.
   D. suctioning the mouth only.

_____ **5.** Once the entire infant is delivered, you should immediately:
   A. wrap it in a towel and place it on one side with the head lowered.
   B. be sure the head is covered and keep the neck in a neutral position.
   C. use a sterile gauze pad to wipe the infant's mouth, then suction again.
   D. all of the above

_____ **6.** You may help control bleeding by massaging the _____ after delivery of the placenta.

A. perineum

B. fundus

C. lower back

D. inner thighs

_____ **7.** The APGAR score should be calculated at _____ minutes after birth.

A. 1 and 5

B. 3 and 7

C. 2 and 10

D. 4 and 8

_____ **8.** Once the infant is delivered, feel for a brachial pulse or the pulsations in the umbilical cord. The pulse rate should be at least _____ beats/min; if not, you should begin artificial ventilations.

A. 60

B. 80

C. 100

D. 120

_____ **9.** When assisting ventilations in a newborn with a BVM device, the rate is _____ breaths/min.

A. 20 to 30

B. 30 to 50

C. 35 to 45

D. 40 to 60

_____ **10.** When performing CPR on a newborn, you should perform a combined total of _____ ventilations and compressions per minute.

A. 90

B. 100

C. 110

D. 120

_____ **11.** You cannot successfully deliver a _____ presentation in the field.

A. limb

B. breech

C. vertex

D. all of the above

_____ **12.** Care for a mother with a prolapsed cord includes:

A. positioning the mother to keep the weight of the infant off the cord.

B. high-flow oxygen and rapid transport.

C. using your hand to physically hold the infant's head off the cord.

D. all of the above

_____ **13.** The stages of labor include:

A. dilation of the cervix.

B. expulsion of the baby.

C. delivery of the placenta.

D. all of the above

_____ **14.** The first stage of labor begins with the onset of contractions and ends when:

    A. the infant is born.

    B. the cervix is fully dilated.

    C. the water breaks.

    D. the placenta is delivered.

_____ **15.** Signs of the beginning of labor include:

    A. the bloody show.

    B. contractions of the uterus.

    C. rupture of the amniotic sac.

    D. all of the above

_____ **16.** The second stage of labor begins when the cervix is fully dilated and ends when:

    A. the infant is born.

    B. the water breaks.

    C. the placenta delivers.

    D. the uterus stops contracting.

_____ **17.** You may safely use _____ to treat any heart or lung disease in the mother without harm to the fetus.

    A. epinephrine

    B. antihistamines

    C. oxygen

    D. all of the above

_____ **18.** The third stage of labor begins with the birth of the infant and ends with the:

    A. release of milk from the mother's breasts.

    B. cessation of uterine contractions.

    C. delivery of the placenta.

    D. cutting of the umbilical cord.

_____ **19.** The difference between preeclampsia and eclampsia is the onset of:

    A. seeing spots.

    B. seizures.

    C. swelling in the hands and feet.

    D. headaches.

_____ **20.** You should consider the possibility of a(n) _____ in women who have missed a menstrual cycle and complain of a sudden stabbing and usually unilateral pain in the lower abdomen.

    A. PID

    B. ectopic pregnancy

    C. miscarriage

    D. placenta abruptio

_____ **21.** Once labor has begun and delivery is imminent, it is important to:

    A. hold the mother's legs together.

    B. not let the mother go to the bathroom.

    C. restrict all movement of the mother.

    D. all of the above

4

_____**22.** Consider delivery of the fetus at the scene when:

    A. delivery can be expected within a few minutes.

    B. when a natural disaster, or other problem, makes it impossible to reach the hospital.

    C. no transportation is available.

    D. all of the above

_____**23.** When in doubt about the possibility of an imminent delivery, you should:

    A. go for help if you are alone.

    B. insert two fingers into the vagina to feel for the head.

    C. contact medical control for further guidance.

    D. all of the above

_____**24.** _____ is a condition of late pregnancy that also involves headache, visual changes, and swelling of the hands and feet.

    A. Pregnancy-induced hypertension (preeclampsia)

    B. Placenta previa

    C. Placenta abruptio

    D. Supine hypotension syndrome

_____**25.** Low blood pressure resulting from compression of the inferior vena cava by the weight of the fetus when the mother is supine is called:

    A. pregnancy-induced hypertension.

    B. placenta previa.

    C. placenta abruptio.

    D. supine hypotensive syndrome.

_____**26.** _____ is a situation in which the umbilical cord comes out of the vagina before the infant.

    A. Eclampsia

    B. Placenta previa

    C. Placenta abruptio

    D. Prolapsed cord

_____**27.** Premature separation of the placenta from the wall of the uterus is known as:

    A. eclampsia.

    B. placenta previa.

    C. placenta abruptio.

    D. prolapsed cord.

_____**28.** _____ is a condition in which the placenta develops over and covers the cervix.

    A. Eclampsia

    B. Placenta previa

    C. Placenta abruptio

    D. Prolapsed cord

_____**29.** _____ is heralded by the onset of convulsions, or seizures, resulting from severe hypertension in the pregnant woman.

    A. Eclampsia

    B. Placenta previa

    C. Placenta abruptio

    D. Supine hypotensive syndrome

Tables

Complete the following table for the APGAR scoring system by listing the characteristics for each score.

Area of Activity	Score		
	2	1	0
Appearance			
Pulse			
Grimace or Irritability			
Activity or Muscle Tone			
Respiration			

4

Labeling www.OECzone.com anatomy review

Label the following diagram with the correct terms.

1. Anatomic Structures of the Pregnant Woman

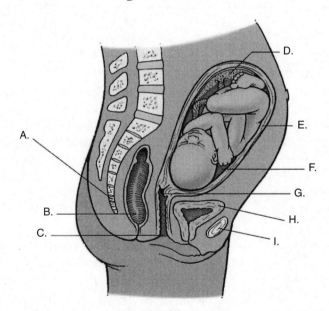

A. _____

B. _____

C. _____

D. _____

E. _____

F. _____

G. _____

H. _____

I. _____

Vocabulary www.OECzone vocab explorer

Define the following terms using the space provided.

1. Primigravida:

_____

_____

_____

2. Multigravida:

_____

_____

_____

3. Ectopic pregnancy:

_____

_____

_____

4. Crowning:

_____

_____

_____

5. APGAR score:

_____

_____

_____

6. Bloody show:

_____

_____

_____

Fill-in

Read each item carefully, then complete the statement by filling in the missing word(s).

1. After delivery, the _____, or afterbirth, separates from the uterus and is delivered.

2. The umbilical cord contains two _____ and one _____.

3. The amniotic sac contains about _____ of amniotic fluid, which helps to insulate and protect the floating fetus as it develops.

4. A full-term pregnancy is from _____ to _____ weeks, counting from the first day of the last menstrual cycle.

5. The pregnancy is divided into three _____ of about 3 months each.

6. There is a high potential of exposure to the rescuer due to _____ released during childbirth.

7. The leading cause of maternal death in the first trimester is internal hemorrhage into the abdomen following rupture of an _____.

8. In serious trauma, the only chance to save the infant is to adequately _____ the mother.

9. During the delivery, be careful that you do not poke your fingers into the infant's eyes or into the two soft spots, called _____, on the head.

True/False

If you believe the statement to be more true than false, write the letter "T" in the space provided. If you believe the statement to be more false than true, write the letter "F."

1. _____ The small mucous plug from the cervix that is discharged from the vagina, often at the beginning of labor, is called a bloody show.

2. _____ Crowning occurs when the baby's head obstructs the birth canal, preventing normal delivery.

3. _____ Labor begins with the rupture of the amniotic sac and ends with the delivery of the baby's head.

4. _____ A woman who is having her first baby is called a multigravida.

5. _____ Once labor has begun, it can be slowed by holding the patient's legs together.

6. _____ Delivery of the buttocks before the baby's head is called a breech delivery.

7. _____ After delivery, the baby should be kept at the same level as the mother's vagina until after the cord is cut.

8. _____ The placenta and cord should be properly disposed of in a biohazard container after delivery.

9. _____ The umbilical cord may be gently pulled to aid in delivery of the placenta.

10. _____ A limb presentation occurs when the baby's arm, leg, or foot is emerging from the vagina first.

11. _____ Multiple births may have more than one placenta.

Short Answer

Complete this section with short written answers using the space provided.

1. What are some possible causes of vaginal hemorrhage in early and late pregnancy?

_____

_____

_____

2. In what position should pregnant patients who are not delivering be transported and why?

_____

_____

_____

3. List three signs that indicate the beginning of labor.

_____

_____

_____

4. Under what three circumstances should you consider delivering the patient at the scene?

_____

_____

_____

5. Once the baby's head emerges, what actions should be taken to prevent too rapid a delivery?

_____

_____

_____

6. Why is it important to avoid pushing on the fontanels?

_____

_____

_____

7. How can you help decrease perineal tearing?

_____

_____

_____

8. What are the two situations in which a rescuer may insert his or her fingers into a patient's vagina?

_____

_____

_____

Word Fun

The following crossword puzzle is an activity provided to reinforce correct spelling and understanding of medical terminology associated with emergency care. Use the clues in the column to complete the puzzle.

Across

3. Fluid-filled bag for developing fetus

6. Umbilicus wrapped around baby's neck

8. Develops over and covers the cervix

9. Rating of newborn on 5 factors

Down

1. Buttocks first

2. Previously given birth

4. Head showing during labor

5. Convulsions from hypertension in pregnant woman

7. Area of skin between anus and vagina, subject to tearing during birth process

Calls to the Scene

The following case scenarios provide an opportunity to explore the concerns associated with patient management. Read each scenario, then answer each question in detail.

1. You are called to a 27-year-old woman, primigravida, in her 28th week of gestation. Her husband tells you she has a history of preeclampsia and suddenly started having convulsions. She is voice responsive and very lethargic. Her blood pressure is 230/180 mm Hg.

   How would you best manage this patient?

   _____

   _____

   _____

   _____

   _____

   _____

   _____

   _____

   _____

2. A 24-year-old woman who is 12 weeks' pregnant is complaining of "spotting." The patient tells you that her last pregnancy ended in a miscarriage at 8 weeks. This is her second pregnancy. She denies any pain and vital signs are within normal limits.

   How would you best manage this patient?

   _____

   _____

   _____

   _____

   _____

   _____

   _____

   _____

3. You are in an emergency situation with a 32-year-old woman who is 38 weeks' pregnant and delivery is imminent. Transportation to a medical facility via EMS access will be delayed at least 30 minutes. As the infant starts to crown, you notice that the amniotic sac is still intact.

How would you best manage this patient?

_____

_____

_____

_____

_____

_____

_____

4

Skill Drills www.OECzone.com video clips

Skill Drill 17-1: Delivering the Baby

Test your knowledge of this skill drill by placing the photos below in the correct order. Number the first step with a "1," the second step with a "2," etc. Also, fill in the correct words in the photo captions.

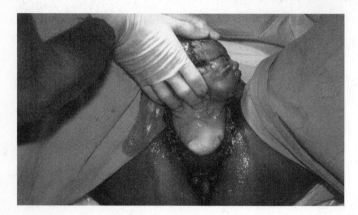

_____

Support the head and upper body as the _____ _____ delivers, guiding the head _____ if needed.

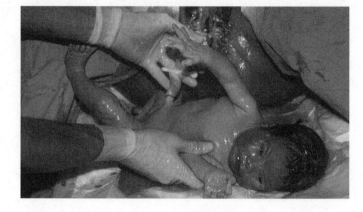

_____

Place clamps _____" to _____" apart and _____ between them.

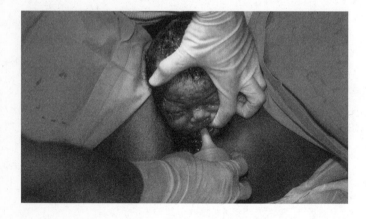

_____

Support the _____ parts of the head with your hands as it emerges.
Suction fluid from the _____, then _____.

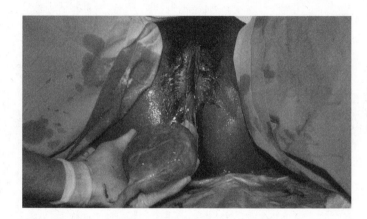

_____

Allow the _____ to deliver itself. Do not pull on the _____ to speed delivery.

(continued)

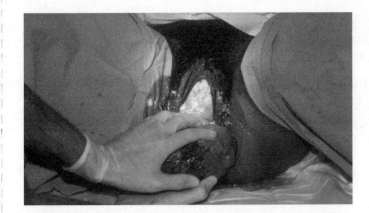

_____

As the _____ _____ appears, guide the head _____ slightly, if needed to deliver the _____.

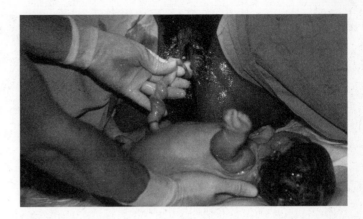

_____

Handle the slippery delivered infant firmly but gently, keeping the neck in _____ position to _____ the airway.

4

Workbook Activities

The following activities have been designed to help you. Your instructor may require you to complete some or all of these activities as a regular part of your OEC training program. You are encouraged to complete any activity that your instructor does not assign as a way to enhance your learning in the classroom.

Chapter Review

The following exercises provide an opportunity to refresh your knowledge of this chapter.

■ NOTES ■

Matching

Match each of the terms in the left column to the appropriate definition in the right column.

_____ **1.** Deceleration

_____ **2.** Kinetic energy

_____ **3.** Mechanism of injury

_____ **4.** Potential energy

_____ **5.** Blunt trauma

_____ **6.** Penetrating trauma

A. impact on the body by objects that cause injury without penetrating soft tissue or internal organs and cavities

B. product of mass, gravity, and height

C. injury caused by objects that pierce the surface of the body

D. how trauma occurs

E. energy of moving object

F. slowing

Multiple Choice

Read each item carefully, then select the best response.

_____ **1.** The following are concepts of energy typically associated with injury except:

A. potential energy.

B. thermal energy.

C. kinetic energy.

D. work.

_____ **2.** The energy of a moving object is called:

A. potential energy.

B. thermal energy.

C. kinetic energy.

D. work.

Mechanisms and Patterns of Injury

_____ **3.** Energy may be:

   A. created.

   B. destroyed.

   C. converted.

   D. all of the above

_____ **4.** The amount of kinetic energy that is converted to do work on the body dictates the _____ of the injury.

   A. location

   B. severity

   C. cause

   D. speed

_____ **5.** Potential energy is mostly associated with the energy of:

   A. falling objects.

   B. vehicle crashes.

   C. pedestrian vs. bicycle crashes.

   D. gunshot wounds.

_____ **6.** If a powerful force is exerted on the body, the rescuer should suspect shock (possibly severe) and:

   A. coma.

   B. heart attack.

   C. internal injuries.

   D. death.

_____ **7.** The three collisions in a frontal impact include all of the following except:

   A. person vs. stationary object.

   B. person vs. moving object.

   C. flying objects vs. people.

   D. internal organs vs. solid structures of the body.

_____ **8.** The mechanism of injury provides information about the severity of the collision and therefore has a(n) _____ effect on patient care.

    A. direct

    B. positive

    C. indirect

    D. negative

_____ **9.** Damage to the body caused by an external force is:

    A. negative force.

    B. trauma.

    C. energy.

    D. mass.

_____ **10.** In a motor vehicle crash, as the passenger's head hits the windshield, the brain continues to move forward until it strikes the inside of the skull resulting in a _____ injury.

    A. compression

    B. laceration

    C. lateral

    D. motion

_____ **11.** Your quick initial assessment of the patient and the evaluation of the _____ can help to direct lifesaving care and provide critical information to the hospital staff.

    A. scene

    B. index of suspicion

    C. mechanism of injury

    D. abdominal area

_____ **12.** A contusion to a patient's forehead along with a "star" pattern on the windshield suggests possible injury to the:

    A. nose.

    B. brain.

    C. face.

    D. heart.

_____ **13.** Significant mechanisms of injury include:

    A. moderate intrusions from a lateral impact.

    B. severe damage from the rear.

    C. collisions in which rotation is involved.

    D. all of the above

_____ **14.** The twisting type of fall that can cause a knee sprain or a spiral fracture of the tibia and fibula is an example of _____ force.

    A. bending

    B. compression

    C. rotational

    D. crushing

_____ **15.** A nontwisting fall forward could produce all of the following except a:

    A. sprained knee or ankle.

    B. ruptured Achilles' tendon.

    C. boot top fracture.

    D. fractured scapula.

_____ **16.** Hyperextension and stretching trauma would be most probable in:

   A. a twisting fall.

   B. a ski pole basket catching on a tree while the pole straps are on the skier's wrist.

   C. an abrupt collision-stopping motion.

   D. a bicyclist falling sideways.

_____ **17.** Signs of most injuries sustained from diving into water that is too shallow can be found by simply inspecting the _____ during extrication of the patient.

   A. head and neck

   B. chest

   C. hands

   D. torso

_____ **18.** A fall from more than _____ times the patient's height is considered to be significant.

   A. two

   B. three

   C. four

   D. five

_____ **19.** Factors that should be taken into account when evaluating a patient following a fall include:

   A. the height of the fall.

   B. the surface struck.

   C. the part of the body that hit first.

   D. all of the above

_____ **20.** Low-energy penetrating trauma may be caused accidentally by impalement or intentionally by a(n):

   A. knife.

   B. pair of scissors.

   C. ice pick.

   D. all of the above

Vocabulary www.OECzone.com vocab explorer

Define the following terms using the space provided.

   1. Newton's First Law of Motion:

   _____

   _____

   _____

   2. Distraction trauma:

   _____

   _____

   _____

5

3. Velocity:

_____

_____

_____

Fill-in

Read each item carefully, then complete the statement by filling in the missing word(s).

1. A skier catching an edge and falling to the ground is an example of _____ energy.

2. Hitting a lift tower at great speed could cause _____ trauma.

3. _____ occurs to the body when the body's tissues are exposed to energy levels beyond their tolerance.

4. The formula for calculating kinetic energy is _____.

5. Being pinned between a rock and a kayak in Class 5 water is a possible _____ trauma.

6. A(n) _____ force can cause a hyperextension type of injury.

7. Trauma caused by bullets, ice axes, ski poles, and other sharp objects is called _____.

True/False

If you believe the statement to be more true than false, write the letter "T" in the space provided. If you believe the statement to be more false than true, write the letter "F."

1. _____ Energy can be both created and destroyed.

2. _____ The energy of a moving object is called potential energy.

3. _____ Solid organs are more prone to rupture from force than are hollow organs.

4. _____ The cervical spine has little tolerance for lateral bending.

5. _____ The injury potential of a fall is related to the height from which the patient fell.

6. _____ Knowledge of the causes of accidents will not prevent them, but will help a rescuer in the emergency care of an injured person.

Short Answer

Complete this section with short written answers using the space provided.

1. Describe potential energy.

_____

_____

_____

2. List at least five causes where multiple and/or serious injuries should be suspected.

_____

_____

_____

_____

3. List the three factors to consider when evaluating a patient who has fallen.

_____

_____

_____

4. What actions of the patient and other aspects need to be considered at an accident scene to determine the mechanism of injury?

_____

_____

_____

5. List the five types of trauma caused by changes in speed or direction.

_____

_____

_____

_____

NOTES

5

Word Fun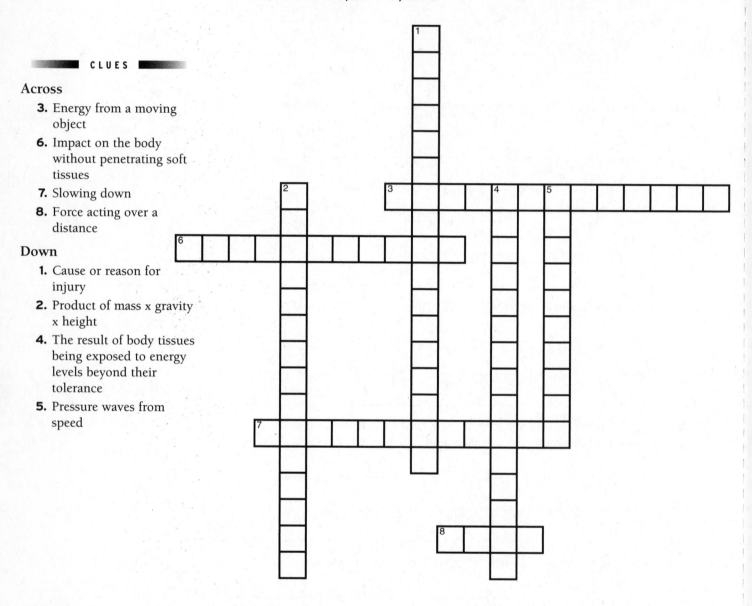

The following crossword puzzle is an activity provided to reinforce correct spelling and understanding of medical terminology associated with emergency care. Use the clues in the column to complete the puzzle.

■■■■ CLUES ■■■■

Across

3. Energy from a moving object

6. Impact on the body without penetrating soft tissues

7. Slowing down

8. Force acting over a distance

Down

1. Cause or reason for injury

2. Product of mass x gravity x height

4. The result of body tissues being exposed to energy levels beyond their tolerance

5. Pressure waves from speed

■■■■ NOTES ■■■■

Calls to the Scene

The following case scenarios provide an opportunity to explore the concerns associated with patient management. Read each scenario, then answer each question in detail.

1. While watching a giant slalom race, you observe a racer miss the gate at a tremendous rate of speed. He spins and swirls in a cloud of snow, striking his head on the left side two times. You ski over to him and find that he has collided with a horizontal, rigid, metal pipe and is doubled over on it. One ski released and the other is still on. You know that the injuries will be severe. Both legs are broken.

What kind of trauma should you suspect? Seeing the patient doubled over a pipe tells you that he may have sustained what kind of injury? The pipe that the skier struck has caused what kind of trauma to the pelvic area?

_____

_____

_____

_____

_____

_____

_____

_____

2. You are biking down a black diamond slope that is located beside a lift. You spot a person lying on the ground below the lift. Bystanders inform you that they saw the person fall from the lift. The lift is approximately 20' from the ground. Your patient, a 32-year-old man, was found lying on the ground with obvious deformity to his right lower leg. He is alert and oriented and tells you he slipped off the lift. Bleeding is controlled and his airway is intact.

How would you best manage this patient?

5

_____

_____

_____

_____

_____

_____

_____

_____

Workbook Activities

The following activities have been designed to help you. Your instructor may require you to complete some or all of these activities as a regular part of your OEC training program. You are encouraged to complete any activity that your instructor does not assign as a way to enhance your learning in the classroom.

Chapter Review

The following exercises provide an opportunity to refresh your knowledge of this chapter.

■ NOTES ■

Matching

Match each of the terms in the left column to the appropriate definition in the right column.

_____ **1.** Dermis

_____ **2.** Sweat glands

_____ **3.** Epidermis

_____ **4.** Mucous membranes

_____ **5.** Sebaceous glands

_____ **6.** Abrasion

_____ **7.** Laceration

_____ **8.** Hemothorax

_____ **9.** Penetrating wound

_____ **10.** Avulsion

_____ **11.** Evisceration

_____ **12.** Pneumothorax

A. embedded pole

B. cool the body by discharging a substance through the pores

C. tissue hanging as a flap from a wound

D. tough external layer forming a watertight covering for the body

E. knife cut

F. secrete a watery substance that lubricates the openings of the mouth and nose

G. inner layer of skin that contains the structures that give skin its characteristic appearance

H. air around lungs

I. produce oil, which waterproofs the skin and keeps it supple

J. blood collecting inside the chest

K. exposed intestines

L. skinned knee

Multiple Choice

Read each item carefully, then select the best response.

_____ **1.** The _____ is (are) our first line of defense against external forces.

   A. extremities

   B. hair

   C. skin

   D. lips

CHAPTER 19

Soft-Tissue Injuries

_____ **2.** The skin covering the _____ is quite thick.
   A. lips
   B. scalp
   C. ears
   D. eyelids

_____ **3.** As the cells on the surface of the skin are worn away, new cells form in the _____ layer.
   A. dermal
   B. germinal
   C. epidermal
   D. subcutaneous

_____ **4.** The hair follicles, sweat glands, and sebaceous glands are found in the:
   A. dermis.
   B. germinal layer.
   C. epidermis.
   D. subcutaneous layer.

_____ **5.** The skin regulates temperature in a cold environment by:
   A. secreting sweat through sweat glands.
   B. constricting the blood vessels.
   C. dilating the blood vessels.
   D. increasing the amount of heat that is radiated from the body's surface.

_____ **6.** Closed soft-tissue injuries are characterized by all of the following except:
   A. pain at the site of injury.
   B. swelling beneath the skin.
   C. damage of the protective layer of skin.
   D. a history of blunt trauma.

_____ **7.** A(n) _____ occurs whenever a large blood vessel is damaged and bleeds.
   A. contusion
   B. hematoma
   C. crushing injury
   D. avulsion

_____ **8.** A(n) _____ is usually associated with extensive tissue damage.

   A. contusion

   B. hematoma

   C. abrasion

   D. avulsion

_____ **9.** A hematoma can result from:

   A. a soft-tissue injury.

   B. a fracture.

   C. any injury to a large blood vessel.

   D. all of the above

_____ **10.** A(n) _____ occurs when a great amount of force is applied to the body for a long period of time.

   A. contusion

   B. hematoma

   C. crushing injury

   D. avulsion

_____ **11.** More extensive open injuries may involve significant internal organ damage and soft-tissue damage, which could lead to:

   A. compartment syndrome.

   B. contamination.

   C. hypovolemic shock.

   D. hemothorax.

_____ **12.** The "S" in ICES stands for:

   A. swelling.

   B. soft-tissue.

   C. splinting.

   D. shock.

_____ **13.** Open soft-tissue wounds include all of the following except:

   A. abrasions.

   B. contusions.

   C. lacerations.

   D. avulsions.

_____ **14.** An abrasion is:

   A. superficial.

   B. deep.

   C. full-thickness.

   D. none of the above

_____ **15.** A laceration may be:

   A. superficial.

   B. deep.

   C. jagged.

   D. all of the above

_____ **16.** Bleeding from avulsions can usually be controlled by:

   A. elevation.

   B. pressure dressings.

   C. tourniquets.

   D. pressure points.

_____ **17.** A laceration completely through the cheek and into the mouth will require a pressure dressing:

   A. on both sides.

   B. on the outside only.

   C. on the inside only.

   D. Dressings should not be used anywhere.

_____ **18.** Because shootings usually end up in court, it is important to factually and completely document the:

   A. circumstances surrounding any gunshot injury.

   B. patient's condition.

   C. treatment given.

   D. all of the above

_____ **19.** All open wounds are assumed to be _____ and present a risk of infection.

   A. contaminated

   B. life-threatening

   C. minimal

   D. extensive

_____ **20.** Before you begin caring for a patient with an open wound, you should:

   A. survey the scene.

   B. follow BSI precautions.

   C. be sure the patient has an open airway.

   D. all of the above

_____ **21.** Splinting an extremity even when there is no fracture can help:

   A. reduce pain.

   B. minimize damage to an already-injured extremity.

   C. make it easier to move the patient.

   D. all of the above

_____ **22.** On inhalation, pressure inside the chest cavity _____, allowing air to enter.

   A. increases

   B. decreases

   C. equalizes

   D. stabilizes

_____ **23.** Treatment for an abdominal evisceration includes:

   A. pushing the exposed organs back into the abdominal cavity.

   B. covering the organs with dry dressings.

   C. flexing the knees and legs to relieve pressure on the abdomen.

   D. applying moist, adherent dressings.

_____ **24.** An open neck injury may result in _____ if enough air is sucked into a blood vessel.

   A. hypovolemic shock

   B. tracheal deviation

   C. air embolism

   D. subcutaneous emphysema

5

_____25. Burns may result from:
   A. heat.
   B. toxic chemicals.
   C. electricity.
   D. all of the above

_____26. Factors in helping to determine the severity of a burn include:
   A. the depth of the burn.
   B. the extent of the burn.
   C. whether or not there are critical areas involved.
   D. all of the above

_____27. _____ burns involve only the epidermis.
   A. Full-thickness
   B. Second-degree
   C. Superficial
   D. Third-degree

_____28. _____ burns cause intense pain.
   A. First-degree
   B. Second-degree
   C. Superficial
   D. Third-degree

_____29. _____ burns may involve subcutaneous layers, muscle, bone, or internal organs.
   A. Superficial
   B. Partial-thickness
   C. Full-thickness
   D. Second-degree

_____30. With _____ burns, the area is dry and leathery and may appear white, dark brown, or even charred.
   A. first-degree
   B. second-degree
   C. partial-thickness
   D. third-degree

_____31. Significant airway burns may be associated with:
   A. singeing of the hair within the nostrils.
   B. hoarseness.
   C. hypoxia.
   D. all of the above

_____32. The most important consideration when dealing with electrical burns is:
   A. BSI precautions.
   B. scene safety.
   C. level of responsiveness.
   D. airway.

_____33. Treatment of electrical burns includes:
   A. maintaining the airway.
   B. monitoring the patient closely for respiratory or cardiac arrest.
   C. splinting any suspected injuries.
   D. all of the above

_____**34.** All of the following, except _____ , may be used as an occlusive dressing:
  A. gauze pads
  B. Vaseline gauze
  C. aluminum foil
  D. plastic

_____**35.** Using elastic bandages to secure dressings may result in _____ if the injury swells or if improperly applied.
  A. additional tissue damage
  B. loss of a limb
  C. impaired circulation
  D. all of the above

Labeling www.OECzone.com anatomy review

Label the following diagrams with the correct terms.

1. The Skin

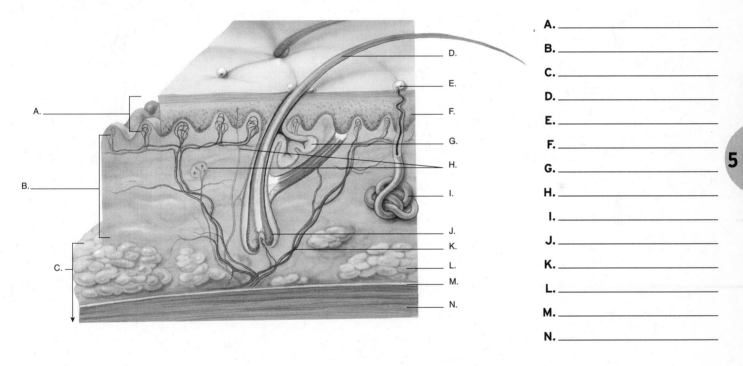

A. _____

B. _____

C. _____

D. _____

E. _____

F. _____

G. _____

H. _____

I. _____

J. _____

K. _____

L. _____

M. _____

N. _____

5

2. The Rule of Nines

A. _____

B. _____

C. _____

D. _____

E. _____

F. _____

G. _____

H. _____

A. _____

B. _____

C. _____

D. _____

E. _____

F. _____

G. _____

H. _____

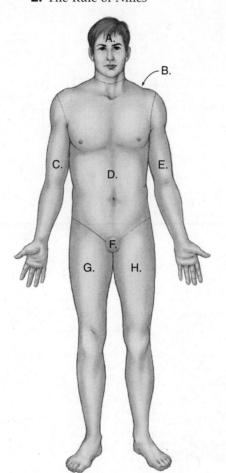

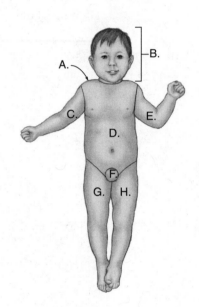

Vocabulary

Define the following terms using the space provided.

1. Partial-thickness burn:

_____

_____

_____

2. Closed injury:

_____

_____

_____

3. Evisceration:

_____

_____

_____

4. Compartment syndrome:

_____

_____

_____

5. Contamination:

_____

_____

_____

Fill-in

Read each item carefully, then complete the statement by filling in the missing word(s).

1. Mucous membranes are _____.

2. A person will sweat in an effort to _____ the body.

3. Nerve endings are located in the _____.

4. Below the dermis lies the _____ tissue.

5. In cold weather, skin blood vessels will _____.

6. The skin protects the body by keeping _____ out and

_____ in.

7. Because nerve endings are present, injury to the _____ may be painful.

8. A major function of the skin is regulating body _____.

9. The external layer of skin is the _____ and the inner layer is the

_____.

10. When the vessels of the skin dilate, heat is _____ from the body.

True/False

If you believe the statement to be more true than false, write the letter "T" in the space provided. If you believe the statement to be more false than true, write the letter "F."

1. _____ Partial-thickness burns involve the epidermis and some portion of the dermis.

2. _____ Blisters are commonly seen with superficial burns.

3. _____ Severe burns are usually a combination of superficial, partial-thickness, and full-thickness burns.

4. _____ The Rule of Nines allows you to estimate the percentage of body surface area that has been burned.

5. _____ Two factors, depth and extent, are critical in assessing the severity of a burn.

6. _____ Your first responsibility with a burn patient is to stop the burning process.

7. _____ Burned areas should be immersed in cool water for up to 30 minutes.

8. _____ Electrical burns are always more severe than the external signs indicate.

9. _____ The universal dressing is ideal for covering large open wounds.

10. _____ Occlusive dressings are usually made of Vaseline gauze, aluminum foil, or plastic.

11. _____ Gauze pads prevent air and liquids from entering or exiting the wound.

12. _____ Elastic bandages can be used to secure dressings.

13. _____ Soft roller bandages are slightly elastic and the layers adhere somewhat to one another.

14. _____ Ecchymosis is associated with open wounds.

15. _____ A laceration is considered a closed wound.

Short Answer

Complete this section with short written answers using the space provided.

1. List the three major classifications of depth of burns.

_____

_____

_____

2. List the three general classifications of soft-tissue injuries.

_____

_____

_____

3. Define the acronym ICES.

I: _____

C: _____

E: _____

S: _____

4. Describe the classifications of a critical burn for an infant or child.

_____

_____

_____

5. What treatment should be used with a patient burned by a dry chemical?

_____

_____

_____

5

6. Why are electrical burns particularly dangerous to a patient?

_____

_____

_____

7. Describe a sucking chest wound.

_____

_____

_____

8. List the three primary functions of dressings and bandages.

_____

_____

_____

9. List the four types of open soft-tissue injuries.

_____

_____

_____

_____

10. List the five factors used to determine the severity of a burn.

_____

_____

_____

_____

_____

■ CLUES ■

Across

4. Displacement of organs outside the body

6. Lining of body cavities and passages with contact to outside

7. Torn completely loose or hanging as a flap

8. Presence of infective organisms

9. Inner layer of skin

10. Bruise

11. Blood collected in soft tissues

Down

1. Discoloration associated with closed injury

2. Injury from sharp, pointed object

3. Assigns percentages to burns

5. Scraping wound

Word Fun www.OECzone.com vocab explorer

The following crossword puzzle is an activity provided to reinforce correct spelling and understanding of medical terminology associated with emergency care.
Use the clues in the column to complete the puzzle.

Calls to the Scene

The following case scenarios provide an opportunity to explore the concerns associated with patient management. Read each scenario, then answer each question in detail.

1. You are sitting in the aid room when one of the kitchen crew comes in holding his arm. He says that he has spilled the contents of the French fry cooker on his arm and on his body. His arm and hand have large blisters and are very red. Upon examination, it is clear that he has also been saturated in the groin area. His genitals are also blistered and red.

   How would you classify these burns? What emergency care would you recommend?

   _____

   _____

   _____

   _____

   _____

   _____

   _____

   _____

5

2. You are called to the scene of a 25-year-old snowboarder who has fallen after a jump. He states that he "got a lot of air" but landed on his right side. After landing, a skier following too closely ran over his outstretched right arm. He denies injury to his head, neck, or back. Your exam reveals an enlarging, discolored area on his right calf, but no pain over the tibia or fibula. He has a 3" laceration over the right elbow with moderate bleeding.

   Describe the emergency care of his injuries. What complications would you anticipate?

   _____

   _____

   _____

   _____

   _____

_____

_____

_____

3. You are called to the lower level of the main lodge where you find a maintenance worker unconscious in front of an open electrical service panel. A witness states that there was a large flash before he collapsed. He is lying on his side, and you observe a small burn on his palm.

What is your first concern as you approach the patient? What equipment or other needs would you communicate to the base? Describe the steps of assessment and emergency care.

You have started CPR and are notified that EMS is 20 minutes away. The patient does not seem to be responding. How long will you continue CPR?

_____

_____

_____

_____

_____

_____

_____

_____

_____

_____

Skill Drills

www.OECzone.com
video clips

Skill Drill 19-1: Controlling Bleeding from a Soft-Tissue Injury
Test your knowledge of this skill drill by filling in the correct words in the photo captions.

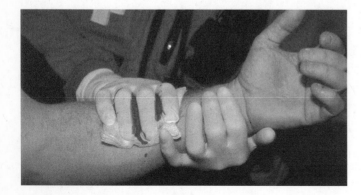

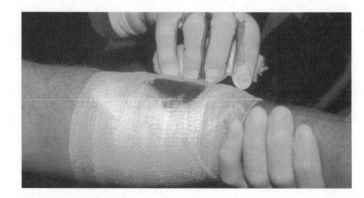

1. Apply _____ _____ with a _____ bandage.

2. Maintain pressure with a _____ bandage.

(continued)

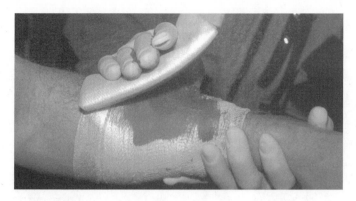

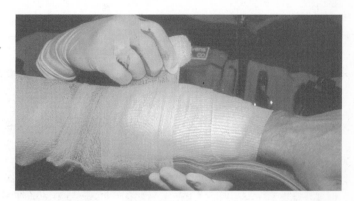

3. If bleeding continues, apply a second _____ and _____ bandage over the first, and apply pressure to the corresponding arterial pressure point.

4. _____ the extremity.

Skill Drill 19-2: Sealing a Sucking Chest Wound
Test your knowledge of this skill drill by filling in the correct words in the photo captions.

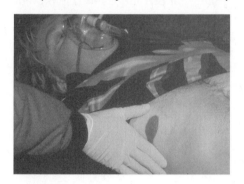

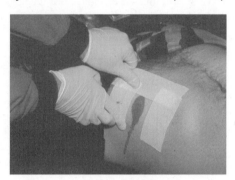

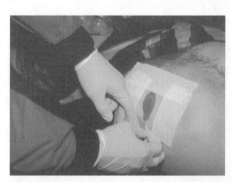

1. Keep the patient _____ and give _____ .

2. Seal the wound with a(n) _____ dressing.

3. Follow _____ _____ regarding sealing or _____ _____ the dressing's fourth side.

Skill Drill 19-3: Stabilizing an Impaled Object
Test your knowledge of this skill drill by filling in the correct words in the photo captions.

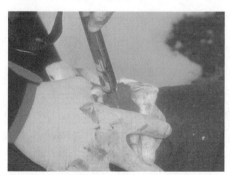

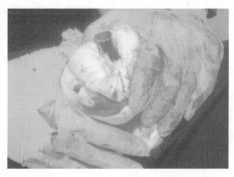

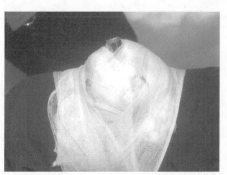

1. Do not attempt to _____ or _____ the object.

2. Control _____ and _____ the object in place using _____ _____, _____, and/or _____ .

3. Add _____ _____ to stabilize and protect the impaled object during transport.

5

Skill Drill 19-4: Caring for Burns
Test your knowledge of this skill drill by placing the photos below in the correct order. Number the first step with a "1," the second step with a "2," etc.

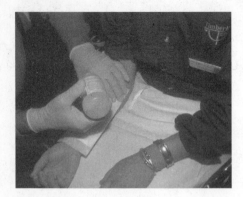

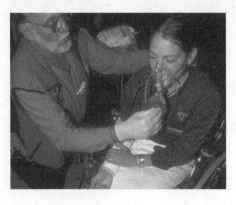

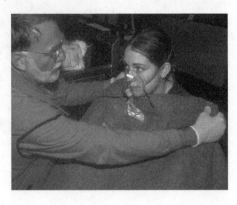

_____
Prepare for transport.
Treat for shock if needed.

_____
Give supplemental oxygen and continue to assess the airway.
Estimate the severity of the burn, then cover the area with a dry, sterile dressing or clean sheet.
Assess and treat the patient for any other injuries.

_____
Follow BSI precautions to help prevent infection.
Remove the patient from the burning area; extinguish or remove hot clothing and jewelry as needed.
If the wound(s) is still burning or hot, immerse the hot area in cool, sterile water, or cover with a wet, cool dressing.

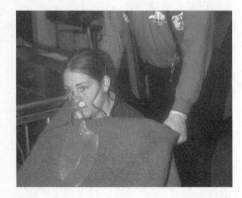

_____
Cover the patient with blankets to prevent loss of body heat.
Transport promptly.

Notes

Workbook Activities

The following activities have been designed to help you. Your instructor may require you to complete some or all of these activities as a regular part of your OEC training program. You are encouraged to complete any activity that your instructor does not assign as a way to enhance your learning in the classroom.

Chapter Review

The following exercises provide an opportunity to refresh your knowledge of this chapter.

NOTES

Matching

Match each of the terms in the left column to the appropriate definition in the right column.

_____ 1. Cornea	**A.** membrane that covers the exposed surface of the eye
_____ 2. Iris	**B.** focuses light
_____ 3. Lens	**C.** muscle behind the cornea
_____ 4. Pupil	**D.** transparent tissue in front of the pupil and iris
_____ 5. Sclera	**E.** circular opening in the iris
_____ 6. Orbit	**F.** the eyeball
_____ 7. Conjunctiva	**G.** eye socket
_____ 8. Globe	**H.** the light-sensitive area of the eye where images are projected
_____ 9. Lacrimal glands	**I.** tear glands
_____ 10. Retina	**J.** white portion of the eye

Multiple Choice

Read each item carefully, then select the best response.

_____ 1. The conjunctiva covers the:

    A. outer surface of the eyelids.

    B. exposed surface of the eye.

    C. lens.

    D. iris.

_____ 2. The purpose of the _____, an extremely tough, fibrous tissue, is to help maintain the eye's globular shape.

    A. cornea

    B. lens

    C. retina

    D. sclera

Eye Injuries

_____ **3.** The _____ allows light to enter the eye.

    A. cornea

    B. lens

    C. retina

    D. sclera

_____ **4.** The circular muscle that adjusts the size of the opening behind the cornea to regulate the amount of light that enters the eye is called the:

    A. iris.

    B. lens.

    C. retina.

    D. sclera.

_____ **5.** In a normal, uninjured eye, the pupils:

    A. are round.

    B. are equal in size.

    C. react equally when exposed to light.

    D. all of the above

_____ **6.** Important signs and symptoms to record include all of the following except:

    A. how the injury occurred.

    B. any changes in vision.

    C. any history of color blindness.

    D. the use of any eye medications.

_____ **7.** The delicate tissues of the eye can be burned by _____, often causing permanent damage.

    A. chemicals

    B. heat

    C. light rays

    D. all of the above

_____ **8.** To care for thermal burns of the eyes and eyelids, you should:

    A. cover both eyes with a sterile dressing moistened with sterile saline.

    B. apply eye shields over the dressing.

    C. transport promptly.

    D. all of the above

_____ **9.** Retinal injuries that are caused by exposure to extremes of light are generally not _____ but may result in permanent damage to vision.

    A. deep

    B. painful

    C. lacerated

    D. none of the above

_____ **10.** Superficial burns of the eyes can result from:

    A. light from prolonged exposure to a sunlamp.

    B. reflected light from a bright snow-covered area.

    C. ultraviolet rays from an arc welding unit.

    D. all of the above

_____ **11.** Lacerations of the eyelids may cause heavy bleeding that can usually be controlled by:

    A. firm pressure.

    B. gentle pressure.

    C. pressure dressings.

    D. flushing the eyes.

_____ **12.** If there is a laceration of the globe itself, you should apply:

    A. firm pressure.

    B. gentle pressure.

    C. no pressure.

    D. pressure dressings.

_____ **13.** Which of the following guidelines should not be included as treatment of penetrating injuries of the eye?

    A. Do not exert any pressure on or manipulate the globe.

    B. If part of the eyeball is exposed, gently apply a moist, sterile dressing to prevent drying.

    C. Cover the injured eye with a protective metal eye shield or sterile dressing.

    D. Gently replace the eyeball if it is displaced out of its socket.

_____ **14.** A "black eye" is a result of:

    A. bleeding into tissue around the orbit.

    B. a fracture of the orbit.

    C. a torn retina.

    D. none of the above

_____ **15.** Bleeding into the anterior chamber of the eye that obscures part or all of the iris is called:

    A. hematemesis.

    B. hyphema.

    C. hyphoma.

    D. hemoptysis.

_____ **16.** Fracture of the orbit, particularly of the bones that form its floor and support of the globe, is known as a:

A. blowout fracture.

B. retinal detachment.

C. hyphema.

D. black eye.

_____ **17.** Eye findings that should alert you to the possibility of a head injury include:

A. one pupil larger than the other.

B. bleeding under the conjunctiva.

C. protrusion or bulging of one eye.

D. all of the above

_____ **18.** Which of the following situations is the only time that contact lenses should be removed in the field?

A. blowout fracture

B. retinal detachment

C. chemical burn

D. broken or torn contact lens

Labeling www.OECzone anatomy review

Label the following diagram with the correct terms.

1. The major components of the eye.

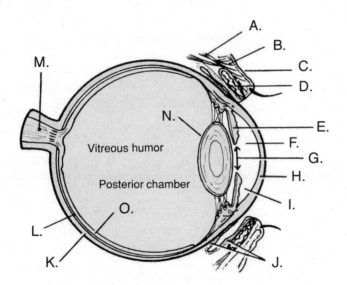

A. _____

B. _____

C. _____

D. _____

E. _____

F. _____

G. _____

H. _____

I. _____

J. _____

K. _____

L. _____

M. _____

N. _____

O. _____

5

Vocabulary

Define the following terms using the space provided.

1. Blowout fracture:

_____

_____

_____

2. Hyphema:

_____

_____

_____

3. Conjunctivitis:

_____

_____

_____

Fill-in

Read each item carefully, then complete the statement by filling in the missing word(s).

1. The glands that produce fluids to keep the eye moist are called _____

_____.

2. A cranial nerve that transmits visual information to the brain is called an

_____ _____.

3. The eye works like a _____, with the iris and pupil making

adjustments to light and the retina acting like _____.

4. Never remove contact lenses from an injured eye unless the injury is a

_____ _____.

5. The _____ is composed of the adjacent bones of the face and skull.

6. When performing an examination, you are looking for specific _____
or conditions that may suggest the nature of the problem.

7. Large objects are prevented from penetrating the eye by the protective

_____ that surrounds it.

8. _____ is inflammation and redness of the conjunctiva.

True/False

If you believe the statement to be more true than false, write the letter "T" in the space provided. If you believe the statement to be more false than true, write the letter "F."

1. _____ Objects impaled in the eye should be removed before applying a dressing.

2. _____ Vitreous humor can be replaced.

3. _____ Aqueous humor can be replaced.

4. _____ Lacrimal glands help keep the eye dry.

5. _____ Contact lenses should always be removed in the field.

6. _____ Foreign objects stuck to the cornea should be removed prior to transport.

7. _____ Bleeding soon after irritation or injury can result in a bright yellow conjunctiva.

8. _____ In a normal, uninjured eye, the entire circle of the iris is visible.

9. _____ If a small foreign object is lying on the surface of the patient's eye, you should use a dextrose solution to gently irrigate the eye.

Short Answer

Complete this section with short written answers using the space provided.

1. Describe a retinal detachment.

_____

_____

_____

2. List the three guidelines for treating penetrating eye injuries.

_____

_____

_____

3. List assessment findings in the eye that may indicate head injury.

_____

_____

_____

5

Word Fun

The following crossword puzzle is an activity provided to reinforce correct spelling and understanding of medical terminology associated with emergency care. Use the clues in the column to complete the puzzle.

■■■■ CLUES ■■■

Across

2. White portion of the eye
5. Membrane that lines eyelids and surface of eye
6. Eye socket
7. Bleeding into anterior chamber of the eye
8. Transmits visual sensations to the brain
9. Muscle regulating light into the eye

Down

1. Break in the bones of the orbit
3. Tear producer
4. Transparent tissue in front of the pupil

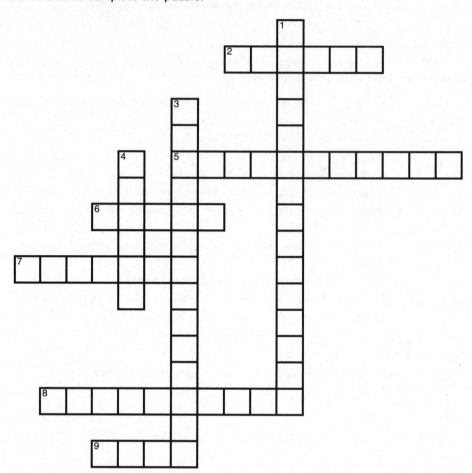

■■■■ NOTES ■■■

Calls to the Scene

The following case scenarios provide an opportunity to explore the concerns associated with patient management. Read each scenario, then answer each question in detail.

1. You are dispatched to a 12-year-old boy who has skied into a tree and hit his face. The impact has resulted in a branch through his goggles that has impaled his right eye. The patient is alert and very upset. His mother is hysterical.

   How would you best manage this patient?

   _____

   _____

   _____

   _____

   _____

   _____

_____

_____

_____

2. You are called to the park's cafeteria kitchen. A 32-year-old man had dry dish detergent splashed into his eyes. Coworkers have tried brushing the powder off his face and pouring water into his eyes, but he is still unable to see and is in severe pain.

How would you best manage this patient?

_____

_____

_____

_____

_____

_____

_____

3. You are dispatched to a skier collision where a 15-year-old boy wearing sunglasses crashed into a stationary skier. He is sitting, holding his broken sunglasses, complaining of double vision, and presents with swelling and bruising around his right orbit.

How would you best manage this patient?

_____

_____

_____

_____

_____

_____

_____

5

Skill Drills

Skill Drill 20-1: Removing a Foreign Object from Under the Upper Eyelid
Test your knowledge of skill drills by filling in the correct words in the photo captions.

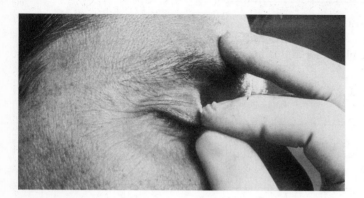

1. Have the patient look _____ , grasp the
_____ _____, and gently pull
the lid away from the eye.

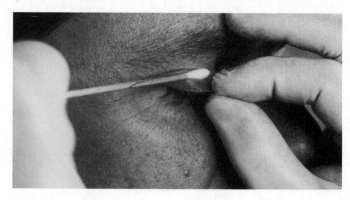

2. Place a _____ _____ on the
upper lid, ½" from the lashes.

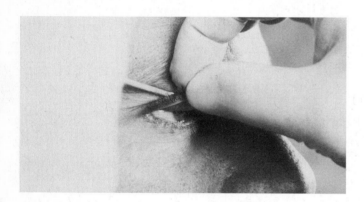

3. Pull the lid _____ and _____,
folding it back over the applicator.

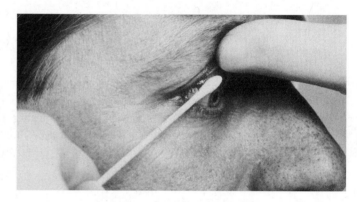

4. Gently remove the foreign object with a
_____, _____ applicator.

Skill Drill 20-2: Stabilizing a Foreign Object Impaled in the Eye
Test your knowledge of skill drills by filling in the correct words in the photo captions.

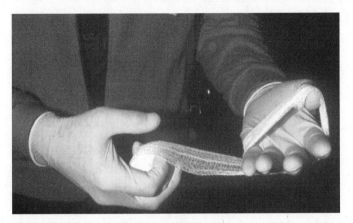

1. To prepare a doughnut ring, wrap a _____ _____ roll around your fingers and thumb _____ or _____ times. Adjust the diameter by _____ your fingers.

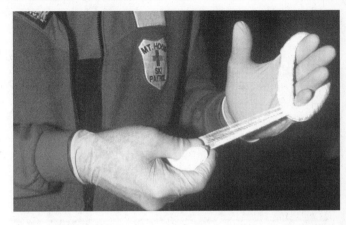

2. Wrap the remainder of the roll, . . .

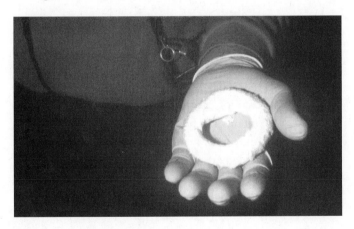

3. . . . working around the ring.

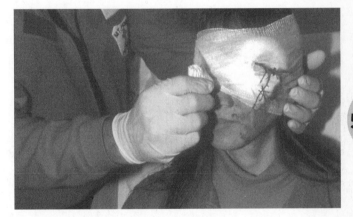

4. Place the dressing over the _____ to hold the impaled object in place, then _____ it with a _____ dressing.

Workbook Activities

The following activities have been designed to help you. Your instructor may require you to complete some or all of these activities as a regular part of your OEC training program. You are encouraged to complete any activity that your instructor does not assign as a way to enhance your learning in the classroom.

Chapter Review

The following exercises provide an opportunity to refresh your knowledge of this chapter.

■ NOTES ■

Matching

Match each of the terms in the left column to the appropriate definition in the right column.

_____ **1.** Cranium   **A.** upper jaw

_____ **2.** Occiput   **B.** posterior cranium

_____ **3.** Pinna   **C.** contains the brain

_____ **4.** Zygomas   **D.** pull/tear away

_____ **5.** Mandible   **E.** visible part of ear

_____ **6.** Avulse   **F.** cheekbones

_____ **7.** Maxilla   **G.** lower jawbone

Multiple Choice

Read each item carefully, then select the best response.

_____ **1.** As a rescuer, your objective is to:
  A. prevent further injury.
  B. manage any acute airway problems.
  C. control bleeding.
  D. all of the above

_____ **2.** The head is divided into two parts: the cranium and the:
  A. brain.
  B. face.
  C. skull.
  D. medulla oblongata.

_____ **3.** The brain connects to the spinal cord through a large opening at the base of the skull known as the:
  A. eustachian tube.
  B. spinous process.
  C. foramen magnum.
  D. vertebral foramina.

Face and Throat Injuries

_____ **4.** Approximately _____ of the nose is composed of bone. The
remainder is composed of cartilage.

    A. nine tenths

    B. two thirds

    C. three fourths

    D. one third

_____ **5.** Motion of the mandible occurs at the:

    A. temporomandibular joint.

    B. mastoid process.

    C. chin.

    D. mandibular angle.

_____ **6.** The _____ may be found on either side of the trachea, along with
the jugular veins and several nerves.

    A. hypothalamus

    B. subclavian arteries

    C. cricoid cartilage

    D. carotid arteries

_____ **7.** The _____ connects the cricoid cartilage and thyroid cartilage.

    A. larynx

    B. cricoid membrane

    C. cricothyroid membrane

    D. thyroid membrane

_____ **8.** Upper airway obstructions caused by facial injuries may be due to:

    A. heavy bleeding.

    B. loosened teeth or dentures.

    C. soft-tissue swelling.

    D. all of the above

_____ 9. If you find portions of avulsed skin that have become separated, you should:

A. wrap the skin in a moist, sterile dressing, place it in a plastic bag, and transport it with the patient.

B. place the skin in a plastic "biohazard" bag and dispose of properly.

C. place the skin in a plastic bag filled with ice and arrange for transport to the emergency department.

D. leave it at the scene to be disposed of later.

_____ 10. The nasal cavity is divided into two chambers by the:

A. frontal sinus.

B. middle turbinate.

C. zygoma.

D. nasal septum.

_____ 11. You may be able to control bleeding from the nose by:

A. applying a sterile dressing.

B. pinching the nostrils together.

C. putting the patient in a supine position.

D. having the patient hold ice in his or her mouth.

_____ 12. The middle ear is connected to the nasal cavity by the:

A. frontal sinus.

B. zygomatic process.

C. eustachian tube.

D. superior trachea.

_____ 13. A basilar skull fracture may present with:

A. leakage of cerebrospinal fluid from the ears and nose.

B. distended neck veins.

C. Battle's sign.

D. periorbital ecchymosis.

_____ 14. Signs of a possible facial fracture include:

A. bleeding in the mouth.

B. absent or loose teeth.

C. loose and/or moveable bone fragments.

D. all of the above

_____ 15. The presence of air in the soft tissues of the neck that produces a crackling sensation is called:

A. the "Rice Krispy" effect.

B. a pneumothorax.

C. rales.

D. subcutaneous emphysema.

_____ 16. Most bleeding from the neck can be controlled by:

A. direct pressure.

B. a pressure point.

C. elevation.

D. a tourniquet.

Labeling www.OECzone.com anatomy review

Label the following diagrams with the correct terms.

1. Face/Skull

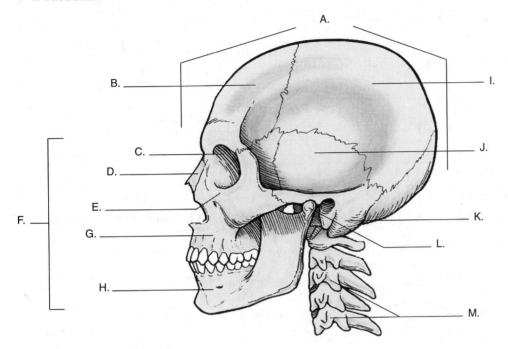

A. _____

B. _____

C. _____

D. _____

E. _____

F. _____

G. _____

H. _____

I. _____

J. _____

K. _____

L. _____

M. _____

Vocabulary www.OECzone.com vocab explorer

Define the following terms using the space provided.

1. Air embolism:

_____

_____

_____

2. Hematoma:

_____

_____

_____

3. Sternocleidomastoid muscle:

_____

_____

_____

NOTES

5

4. Subcutaneous emphysema:

_____

_____

_____

5. Temporomandibular joint (TMJ):

_____

_____

_____

Fill-in

Read each item carefully, then complete the statement by filling in the missing word(s).

1. Pulsations in the neck are felt in the _____ vessels.

2. The _____ vertebrae are in the neck.

3. The _____ lobes of the cranium are located on the lateral portion of the head.

4. The _____ is located in the anterior portion of the neck.

5. The rings of the trachea are made of _____.

6. The Adam's apple is more prominent in _____ than in _____.

7. The _____ _____ is a large opening at the base of the skull.

8. The _____ is the upper part of the jaw.

9. The _____ lobes lie laterally between the temporal and occipital lobes.

10. The _____ connects the larynx with the main air passage.

True/False

If you believe the statement to be more true than false, write the letter "T" in the space provided. If you believe the statement to be more false than true, write the letter "F."

1. _____ Injuries to the face often lead to airway problems.

2. _____ Care for facial injuries begins with BSI precautions and the ABCs.

3. _____ Exposed eye or brain injuries are covered with a dry dressing.

4. _____ Clear fluid in the outer ear is normal.

5. _____ Any crushing injury of the upper part of the neck likely involves the larynx or the trachea.

6. _____ Soft-tissue injuries to the face are common.

7. _____ Epistaxis is another word for nosebleed.

Short Answer

Complete this section with short written answers using the space provided.

1. Describe bleeding control methods for facial injuries.

_____

_____

_____

2. Describe bleeding control methods for lacerations to veins or arteries in the neck.

_____

_____

_____

Word Fun www.OECzone.com vocab explorer

The following crossword puzzle is a good way to review correct spelling and meaning of medical terminology associated with emergency care. Use the clues in the column to complete the puzzle.

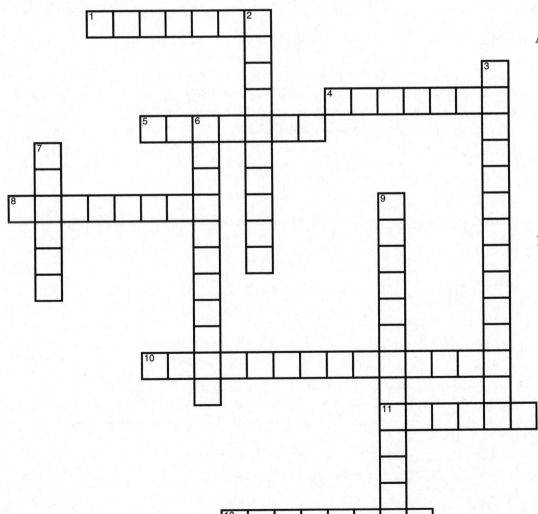

Across

1. Posterior portion of the skull

4. Upper jawbone

5. Skull

8. Lower jawbone

10. Connects the middle ear to the nasal cavity

11. To pull or tear away

12. Blood accumulated in soft tissue

Down

2. Layers of bones in the nasal cavity

3. Bony mass about 1" posterior to the ear

6. Air in the veins

7. Fleshy bulge anterior to the ear canal

9. Large opening in the base of the skull

5

Calls to the Scene

The following case scenarios provide an opportunity to explore the concerns associated with patient management. Read each scenario, then answer each question in detail.

1. You are called to a local school playground for a 7-year-old girl complaining of moderate epistaxis. She has no history and her mother has been called. The child is sitting in the nurse's office holding her face over a trash can.

   How would you best manage this patient?

   _____

   _____

   _____

   _____

   _____

   _____

   _____

   _____

2. You are dispatched to a 37-year-old man with a large laceration to the right side of his neck. Bleeding is dark and heavy. He is alert, but weak.

   How would you best manage this patient?

   _____

   _____

   _____

   _____

   _____

   _____

   _____

   _____

   _____

3. You are at the lumberyard where a 25-year-old man had his ear cut completely off with a saw. Bleeding is controlled with direct pressure. He is alert and oriented. How would you best manage this patient?

_____

_____

_____

_____

_____

_____

_____

_____

_____

Skill Drills www.OECzone.com video clips

Test your knowledge of skill drills by filling in the correct words in the photo captions.

Skill Drill 21-1: Controlling Bleeding from a Neck Injury

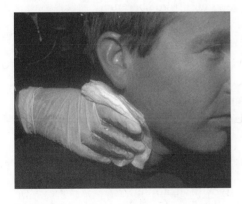 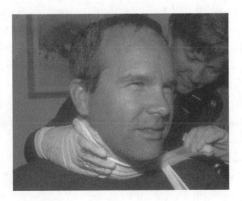 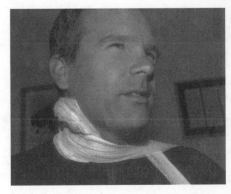

1. Apply _____ _____ to control bleeding.

2. Use a _____ _____ to secure a dressing in place.

3. Wrap the bandage around and under the patient's _____.

5

Workbook Activities

The following activities have been designed to help you. Your instructor may require you to complete some or all of these activities as a regular part of your OEC training program. You are encouraged to complete any activity that your instructor does not assign as a way to enhance your learning in the classroom.

Chapter Review

The following exercises provide an opportunity to refresh your knowledge of this chapter.

■ **NOTES** ■

Matching

Match each of the terms in the left column to the appropriate definition in the right column.

_____ **1.** Thoracic cage

_____ **2.** Diaphragm

_____ **3.** Exhalation

_____ **4.** Inhalation

_____ **5.** Aorta

_____ **6.** Closed chest injury

_____ **7.** Hemoptysis

_____ **8.** Pericardium

_____ **9.** Open chest injury

_____ **10.** Tachypnea

_____ **11.** Dyspnea

_____ **12.** Pneumothorax

_____ **13.** Hemothorax

A. chest rises

B. chest

C. chest falls

D. separates chest from abdomen

E. major artery in the chest

F. penetrating wound

G. rapid respirations

H. generally caused by blunt trauma

I. coughing up blood

J. sac around the heart

K. air enters chest hole, causing lung collapse

L. blood collects in pleural space, compressing lung

M. difficulty with breathing

Multiple Choice

Read each item carefully, then select the best response.

_____ **1.** Air is supplied to the lungs via the:

    A. esophagus.

    B. trachea.

    C. nares.

    D. oropharnyx.

Chest Injuries

_____ 2. The _____ separates the thoracic cavity from the abdominal cavity.
    A. diaphragm
    B. mediastinum
    C. xyphoid process
    D. inferior border of the ribs

_____ 3. Which of the following does not occur during inhalation?
    A. The intercostal muscles contract, elevating the rib cage.
    B. The diaphragm contracts.
    C. The pressure inside the chest increases.
    D. Air enters through the nose and mouth.

_____ 4. Blunt trauma to the chest may:
    A. bruise the lungs and heart.
    B. fracture whole areas of the chest wall.
    C. damage the aorta.
    D. all of the above

_____ 5. Symptoms of chest injury include:
    A. cyanosis around the lips or fingertips.
    B. rapid, weak pulse.
    C. hemoptysis.
    D. pain at the site of injury.

_____ 6. Common causes of dyspnea include:
    A. airway obstruction.
    B. lung compression.
    C. damage to the chest wall.
    D. all of the above

_____ 7. _____ occurs when one segment of the chest wall moves opposite the remainder of the chest.
    A. Flail segment
    B. Paradoxical motion
    C. Pneumothorax
    D. Hemoptysis

_____ **8.** The principle reason for concern about a patient who has a chest injury is:

    A. hemoptysis.

    B. cyanosis.

    C. loss of oxygen-storing capabilities.

    D. a rapid, weak pulse and low blood pressure.

_____ **9.** A _____ results when an injury allows air to enter through a hole in the chest wall or the surface of the lung as the patient attempts to breathe, causing the lung on that side to collapse.

    A. tension pneumothorax

    B. hemothorax

    C. hemopneumothorax

    D. pneumothorax

_____ **10.** A sucking chest wound should be treated:

    A. after assessing ABCs.

    B. after confirming mental status.

    C. clear and maintain airway, immediately cover the wound with a gloved hand, then an occlusive dressing.

    D. by using a stack of gauze dressings.

_____ **11.** Which of the following statements about a spontaneous pneumothorax is true?

    A. It presents with a sudden sharp chest pain.

    B. It presents with increasing difficulty breathing.

    C. It should be treated the same as a traumatic pneumothorax.

    D. all of the above

_____ **12.** What occurs as a pneumothorax develops tension?

    A. Air gradually increases the pressure in the chest.

    B. The affected lung completely collapses.

    C. Blood is prevented from returning through the venae cavae to the heart.

    D. all of the above

_____ **13.** Common signs and symptoms of tension pneumothorax include:

    A. increasing respiratory distress.

    B. distended neck veins.

    C. tracheal deviation away from the injured site.

    D. all of the above

_____ **14.** A hemothorax results from blood collecting in the pleural space from bleeding in the:

    A. rib cage.

    B. lung.

    C. great vessel.

    D. all of the above

_____ **15.** A fractured rib that penetrates into the pleural space may lacerate the surface of the lung, causing a:

    A. tension pneumothorax.

    B. hemothorax.

    C. hemopneumothorax.

    D. all of the above

_____ **16.** In what is called paradoxical movement, the detached portion of the chest wall:

A. moves opposite of normal.

B. moves out instead of in during inhalation.

C. moves in instead of out during expiration.

D. all of the above

_____ **17.** Traumatic asphyxia occurs when:

A. the lung is bruised.

B. three or more adjacent ribs are fractured in two or more places.

C. the chest is suddenly and severely compressed.

D. all of the above

_____ **18.** Traumatic asphyxia results in a very characteristic appearance, including:

A. distended neck veins.

B. cyanosis in the face and neck.

C. hemorrhage into the sclera of the eye.

D. all of the above

_____ **19.** Signs and symptoms of a pericardial tamponade include:

A. low blood pressure.

B. a weak pulse.

C. muffled heart tones.

D. all of the above

_____ **20.** Large blood vessels in the chest that can result in massive hemorrhaging include all of the following except the:

A. pulmonary arteries.

B. femoral arteries.

C. aorta.

D. four main pulmonary veins.

Labeling `www.OECzone.com anatomy review`

Label the following diagrams with the correct terms.

1. Anterior Aspect of the Chest

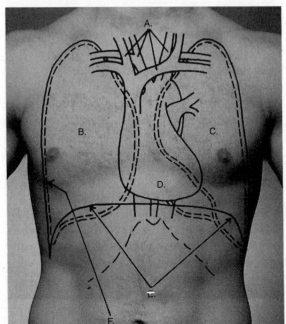

A. _____

B. _____

C. _____

D. _____

E. _____

F. _____

2. The Ribs

A. _____

B. _____

C. _____

D. _____

E. _____

F. _____

G. _____

Vocabulary

Define the following terms using the space provided.

1. Flail chest:

_____

_____

_____

2. Paradoxical motion:

_____

_____

_____

3. Pericardial tamponade:

_____

_____

_____

4. Spontaneous pneumothorax:

_____

_____

_____

NOTES

5. Sucking chest wound:

_____

_____

_____

6. Tension pneumothorax:

_____

_____

_____

Fill-in

Read each item carefully, then complete the statement by filling in the missing word.

1. The esophagus is located in the _____ of the chest.

2. During inhalation, the pressure in the chest _____.

3. In the anterior chest, ribs connect to the _____.

4. The trachea divides into the right and left main stem _____.

5. The _____ nerves supply the diaphragm.

6. Contents of the chest are protected by the _____.

7. The chest extends from the lower end of the neck to the _____.

8. _____ line the area between the lungs and chest wall.

9. A great vessel located in the chest is the _____.

10. During inhalation, the diaphragm _____.

True/False

If you believe the statement to be more true than false, write the letter "T" in the space provided. If you believe the statement to be more false than true, write the letter "F."

1. _____ Dyspnea is difficulty with breathing.

2. _____ Tachypnea is slow respirations.

3. _____ Distended neck veins may be a sign of a tension pneumothorax.

4. _____ Rib fractures are common in children.

5. _____ Decreased pulse pressure is related to spontaneous pneumothorax.

6. _____ Laceration of the large blood vessels in the chest can cause minimal hemorrhage.

7. _____ The thoracic cage extends from the lower end of the neck to the umbilicus.

8. _____ Patients with spinal cord injuries at C3 or above can lose their ability to breathe entirely.

9. _____ Almost one third of people who are killed immediately in car crashes die as a result of traumatic rupture of the aorta.

Short Answer

Complete this section with short written answers using the space provided.

1. List the signs and symptoms associated with a chest injury.

_____

_____

_____

2. Describe the two methods for sealing a sucking chest wound.

_____

_____

_____

3. Describe the method(s) for immobilizing a flail chest wall segment.

_____

_____

_____

4. Define traumatic asphyxia and describe its signs.

_____

_____

_____

Word Fun

www.OECzone.com
vocab explorer

The following crossword puzzle is an activity provided to reinforce correct spelling and understanding of medical terminology associated with emergency care. Use the clues in the column to complete the puzzle.

CLUES

Across

1. Blood in the pleural cavity
5. Opposite movement from normal
7. Rapid breathing
8. Fractured ribs that become detached from the rib cage
9. Buildup of blood in sac around the heart
11. Air in the pleural cavity

Down

2. Spitting or coughing up blood
3. Accumulation of air in the pleural cavity, causing pressure in the cavity to rise
4. Bruise of the lung
6. One-way valve allowing air to leave
10. Difficulty breathing

5

Calls to the Scene

The following case scenarios provide an opportunity to explore the concerns associated with patient management. Read each scenario, then answer each question in detail.

1. You are dispatched to a skier/tree collision. Your patient, a 67-year-old man, is unresponsive and has a very weak pulse and decreasing respirations as you move him from the tree well. Once you have him immobilized on the long backboard, he becomes apneic and pulseless.

   How would you best manage this patient?

   _____

   _____

   _____

   _____

   _____

   _____

   _____

   _____

   _____

   _____

2. Your patient, a 22-year-old man, is complaining of a sudden onset of right-sided chest pain with a sudden onset of difficulty breathing. He tells you he was out running when it started.

   How would you best manage this patient?

   _____

   _____

   _____

   _____

   _____

   _____

   _____

   _____

   _____

   _____

3. You are dispatched to a local climbing site where a 27-year-old man was crushed by a piece of heavy rock. Fellow climbers pulled the rock off the patient. He presents with distended neck veins, cyanosis, and bloodshot eyes.

How would you best manage this patient?

_____

_____

_____

_____

_____

_____

_____

_____

_____

5

Workbook Activities

The following activities have been designed to help you. Your instructor may require you to complete some or all of these activities as a regular part of your OEC training program. You are encouraged to complete any activity that your instructor does not assign as a way to enhance your learning in the classroom.

Chapter Review

The following exercises provide an opportunity to refresh your knowledge of this chapter.

NOTES

Matching

Match each of the terms in the left column to the appropriate definition in the right column.

_____ 1. Hollow organs	**A.** blood in urine
_____ 2. Solid organs	**B.** organs outside of the body
_____ 3. Peritonitis	**C.** abdominal lining inflammation
_____ 4. Genitourinary system	**D.** kidneys, liver, spleen
_____ 5. Filtering system	**E.** kidneys
_____ 6. Evisceration	**F.** abdomen
_____ 7. Hematuria	**G.** stomach, bladder, ureters
_____ 8. Peritoneal cavity	**H.** controls reproductive functions and the waste discharge system

Multiple Choice

Read each item carefully, then select the best response.

_____ 1. The abdomen contains several organs that make up the:

　　A. digestive system.

　　B. urinary system.

　　C. genitourinary system.

　　D. all of the above

_____ 2. Hollow organs of the abdomen include the:

　　A. stomach.

　　B. ureters.

　　C. bladder.

　　D. all of the above

C H A P T E R 2

Abdomen and Genitalia Injuries

_____ **3.** Solid organs of the abdomen include all of the following except the:
  A. liver.
  B. spleen.
  C. gallbladder.
  D. pancreas.

_____ **4.** The first signs of peritonitis include:
  A. severe abdominal pain.
  B. tenderness.
  C. muscular spasm.
  D. all of the above

_____ **5.** Late signs of peritonitis may include:
  A. a soft abdomen.
  B. nausea.
  C. normal bowel sounds.
  D. all of the above

_____ **6.** _____ takes place in the solid organs.
  A. Digestion
  B. Excretion
  C. Energy production
  D. all of the above

_____ **7.** Because solid organs have a rich supply of blood, any injury can result in major:
  A. hemorrhaging.
  B. damage.
  C. pain.
  D. guarding.

_____ **8.** A patient who has abdominal bleeding may experience all of the following except:

    A. pain or tenderness.

    B. rigidity.

    C. urticaria.

    D. distention.

_____ **9.** The major soft-tissue landmark(s) is (are) the _____, which overlie(s) the fourth lumbar vertebra.

    A. iliac crests

    B. umbilicus

    C. pubic symphysis

    D. anterior iliac spines

_____ **10.** The abdomen is divided into four:

    A. quadrants.

    B. planes.

    C. sections.

    D. angles.

_____ **11.** Injuries to the abdomen may involve:

    A. hollow organs.

    B. open injuries.

    C. solid organs.

    D. all of the above

_____ **12.** Open abdominal injuries are also known as:

    A. blunt injuries.

    B. eviscerations.

    C. penetrating injuries.

    D. peritoneal injuries.

_____ **13.** Closed abdominal injuries may result from:

    A. a stab wound.

    B. seat belt injury.

    C. a gunshot wound.

    D. all of the above

_____ **14.** The major complaint of patients with abdominal injury is:

    A. pain.

    B. tachycardia.

    C. rigidity.

    D. swelling.

_____ **15.** The most common sign of significant abdominal injury is:

    A. pain.

    B. tachycardia.

    C. rigidity.

    D. distention.

_____ **16.** Late signs of abdominal injury include all of the following except:

    A. distention.

    B. increased blood pressure.

    C. rigidity.

    D. shallow respirations.

_____ **17.** Your primary concern when dealing with an unresponsive patient with an open abdominal injury is:

   A. covering the wound with a moist dressing.

   B. maintaining the airway.

   C. controlling the bleeding.

   D. monitoring vital signs.

_____ **18.** A patient with blunt abdominal trauma may present with:

   A. severe bruises on the abdominal wall.

   B. laceration of the liver or spleen.

   C. rupture of the intestine.

   D. all of the above

_____ **19.** It is imperative that a patient who has received severe blunt abdominal trauma be:

   A. log rolled onto a backboard.

   B. transported rapidly.

   C. given oxygen.

   D. all of the above

_____ **20.** Patients with penetrating abdominal injuries often complain of:

   A. pain.

   B. nausea.

   C. vomiting.

   D. all of the above

_____ **21.** When caring for a patient with a penetrating abdominal injury, you should assume that the object has:

   A. penetrated the peritoneum.

   B. entered the abdominal cavity.

   C. possibly injured one or more organs.

   D. all of the above

_____ **22.** When treating a patient with an evisceration, you should:

   A. attempt to replace the abdominal contents.

   B. cover the protruding organs with a dry, sterile dressing.

   C. cover the protruding organs with moist, adherent dressings.

   D. cover the protruding contents with moist, sterile gauze compresses.

_____ **23.** The solid organs of the urinary system include the:

   A. kidneys.

   B. ureters.

   C. bladder.

   D. urethra.

_____ **24.** All of the male genitalia lie outside the pelvic cavity with the exception of the:

   A. urethra, bladder, and penis.

   B. penis and urethra.

   C. seminal vesicles, prostate, and parts of the urethra.

   D. testes, penis, and prostate.

5

_____25. Suspect kidney damage if the patient has a history or physical evidence of:

   A. an abrasion, laceration, or contusion in the flank.

   B. a penetrating wound in the region of the lower rib cage or the upper abdomen.

   C. fractures on either side of the lower rib cage.

   D. all of the above

_____26. Signs of injury to the kidney may include:

   A. bruises or lacerations on the overlying skin.

   B. shock.

   C. hematuria.

   D. all of the above

_____27. Suspect a possible injury of the urinary bladder in all of the following findings except:

   A. bruising to the left upper quadrant.

   B. blood at the urethral opening.

   C. blood at the tip of the penis or a stain on the patient's underwear.

   D. physical signs of trauma on the lower abdomen, pelvis, or perineum.

_____28. When treating a patient with an amputation of the penile shaft, your top priority is:

   A. locating the amputated part.

   B. controlling bleeding.

   C. keeping the remaining tissue dry.

   D. delaying transport until bleeding is controlled.

_____29. Treatment of injuries involving the external male genitalia includes:

   A. making the patient as comfortable as possible.

   B. using sterile, moist compresses to cover areas that have been stripped of skin.

   C. applying direct pressure with dry, sterile gauze dressings to control bleeding.

   D. all of the above

Labeling

www.OECzone.com anatomy review

Label the following diagrams with the correct terms.

1. Hollow Organs

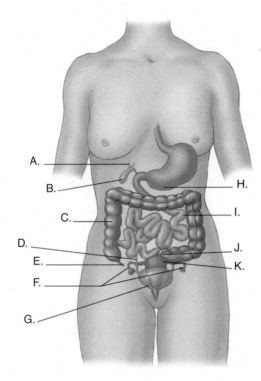

A. _____

B. _____

C. _____

D. _____

E. _____

F. _____

G. _____

H. _____

I. _____

J. _____

K. _____

2. Solid Organs

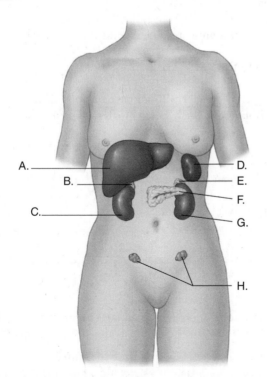

A. _____

B. _____

C. _____

D. _____

E. _____

F. _____

G. _____

H. _____

5

Vocabulary

Define the following terms using the space provided.

1. Closed abdominal injury:

_____

_____

_____

2. Open abdominal injury:

_____

_____

_____

3. Guarding:

_____

_____

_____

Fill-in

Read each item carefully, then complete the statement by filling in the missing word.

1. Severe bleeding may occur with injury to _____ organs.

2. The _____ system is responsible for filtering waste.

3. Kidneys are located in the _____ space.

4. Injuries to the kidneys or bladder will not have obvious _____, but there are usually more subtle clues such as lower rib pain or a possible pelvic fracture.

5. When ruptured, the organs of the abdominal cavity can spill their contents into the peritoneal cavity, causing an intense inflammatory reaction called _____.

6. Blood within the peritoneal cavity does not provoke a(n) _____ and may not cause pain or tenderness.

7. Closed abdominal injuries are also known as _____.

True/False

If you believe the statement to be more true than false, write the letter "T" in the space provided. If you believe the statement to be more false than true, write the letter "F."

1. _____ Hollow organs will bleed profusely if injured.

2. _____ The most common sign of an abdominal injury is an elevated heart rate.

3. _____ Patients with abdominal injuries should be kept supine with the head elevated.

4. _____ Peritoneal irritation is in response to a hollow organ injury.

5. _____ Eviscerated organs should be covered with a dry dressing.

6. _____ Injuries to the kidneys usually occur in isolation.

Short Answer

Complete this section with short written answers using the space provided.

1. List the hollow organs of the abdomen and urinary system.

_____

_____

_____

2. List the solid organs of the abdomen and urinary system.

_____

_____

_____

3. List the signs and symptoms of an abdominal injury.

_____

_____

_____

4. List the steps to care for a penetrating abdominal injury.

_____

_____

_____

5. List the steps to care for an open abdominal wound with exposed organs.

_____

_____

_____

6. List the major history or physical findings associated with possible kidney damage.

_____

_____

_____

5

Word Fun

The following crossword puzzle is an activity provided to reinforce correct spelling and understanding of medical terminology associated with emergency care. Use the clues in the column to complete the puzzle.

CLUES

Across

4. Contracting of muscle to protect

5. Stomach, small intestines, bladder

7. Displacement of organs outside of the abdomen

8. Inflammation of the abdominal lining

Down

1. Liver, spleen, pancreas

2. Abdominal cavity

3. Penetrating wound of the belly

6. Blood in the urine

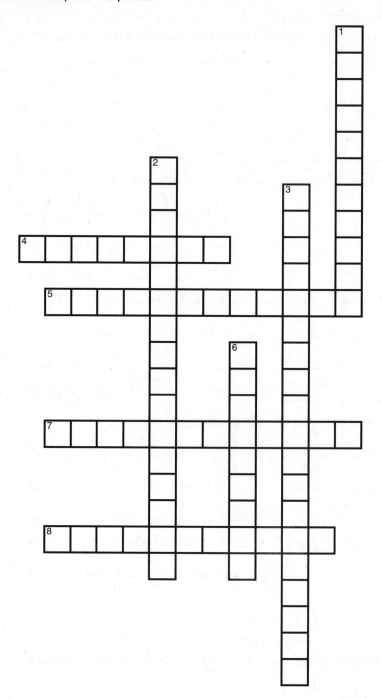

Calls to the Scene

The following case scenarios provide an opportunity to explore the concerns associated with patient management. Read each scenario, then answer each question in detail.

1. You are dispatched to a gladed trail where you find a 26-year-old man. He has several superficial lacerations to his arms, and a tree branch is impaled in his right upper quadrant. He is lying supine on the snow. He is alert, and bystanders tell you that this incident occurred about 5 minutes ago.

   How would you best manage this patient?

   _____

   _____

   _____

   _____

   _____

   _____

   _____

   _____

   _____

   _____

2. A 35-year-old woman loses control while skiing and falls on her left side onto an exposed runner of a moveable snow gun. Upon arrival, you find no altered level of responsiveness. The skier's initial vital signs indicate a pulse of 92 and respirations of 16. Her abdomen on the left side is tender on palpation and is beginning to become rigid. A second set of vital signs taken 5 minutes after the first set reveals a pulse of 110 and respirations of 24.

   How would you best manage this patient?

   _____

   _____

   _____

   _____

   _____

   _____

   _____

   _____

5

3. A 35-year-old man was hiking through some ranch property and fell onto a barbed wire fence. He has a bowel evisceration and is in extreme pain. His hiking partner tells you that there was no trauma involved; he slipped and fell from a standing position onto the wire, tearing open his abdomen in the process. He lowered himself to the ground before passing out. He is voice responsive and tachycardic. His rate of breathing is 24 breaths/min and deep.

How would you best manage this patient?

_____

_____

_____

_____

_____

_____

_____

_____

_____

Notes

5

Workbook Activities

The following activities have been designed to help you. Your instructor may require you to complete some or all of these activities as a regular part of your OEC training program. You are encouraged to complete any activity that your instructor does not assign as a way to enhance your learning in the classroom.

Chapter Review

The following exercises provide an opportunity to refresh your knowledge of this chapter.

NOTES

Matching

Match each of the terms in the left column to the appropriate definition in the right column.

_____ **1.** Striated

_____ **2.** Tendons

_____ **3.** Smooth

_____ **4.** Joint

_____ **5.** Ligaments

_____ **6.** Closed fracture

_____ **7.** Point tenderness

_____ **8.** Displaced fracture

_____ **9.** Articular cartilage

_____ **10.** Open fracture

_____ **11.** Traction

A. Any injury that makes the limb appear to be in an unnatural position

B. Any fracture in which the skin has not been broken

C. A thin layer of cartilage, covering the articular surface of bones in synovial joints

D. Involuntary muscle

E. Any break in the bone in which the overlying skin has been damaged as well

F. Hold joints together

G. Skeletal muscle

H. The act of exerting a pulling force on a structure

I. Where two bones contact

J. Attach muscle to bone

K. Tenderness sharply located at the site of an injury

Multiple Choice

Read each item carefully, then select the best response.

_____ **1.** Blood in the urine is known as a:

   A. hematuria.

   B. hemoptysis.

   C. hematocrit.

   D. hemoglobin.

Principles of Musculoskeletal Injuries

_____ **2.** Smooth muscle is found in the:

  A. back.

  B. blood vessels.

  C. heart.

  D. all of the above

_____ **3.** The bones in the skeleton produce _____ in the bone marrow.

  A. red blood cells

  B. minerals

  C. electrolytes

  D. white blood cells

_____ **4.** _____ are held together in a tough fibrous structure known as a capsule.

  A. Tendons

  B. Joints

  C. Ligaments

  D. Bones

_____ **5.** Joints are bathed and lubricated by _____ fluid.

  A. cartilaginous

  B. articular

  C. synovial

  D. cerebrospinal

_____ **6.** A _____ is a disruption of a joint in which the bone ends are no longer in contact.

  A. torn ligament

  B. dislocation

  C. fracture dislocation

  D. sprain

_____ **7.** A _____ is a joint injury in which there is some partial or temporary dislocation of the bone ends and partial stretching or tearing of the supporting ligaments.

  A. dislocation

  B. strain

  C. sprain

  D. torn ligament

_____ **8.** A _____ is a stretching or tearing of the muscle.

  A. strain

  B. sprain

  C. torn ligament

  D. split

_____ **9.** The zone of injury includes the:

  A. adjacent nerves.

  B. adjacent blood vessels.

  C. surrounding soft tissue.

  D. all of the above

_____ **10.** A(n) _____ fractures the bone at the point of impact.

  A. direct blow

  B. indirect force

  C. twisting force

  D. high-energy injury

_____ **11.** A(n) _____ may cause a fracture or dislocation at a distant point.

  A. direct blow

  B. indirect force

  C. twisting force

  D. high-energy injury

_____ **12.** When caring for patients who have fallen, you must identify the _____ and the mechanism of injury so that you will not overlook associated injuries.

  A. site of injury

  B. height of fall

  C. point of contact

  D. twisting forces

_____ **13.** _____ produce severe damage to the skeleton, surrounding soft tissues, and vital internal organs.

  A. Direct blows

  B. Indirect forces

  C. Twisting forces

  D. High-energy injuries

_____ **14.** Regardless of the extent and severity of the damage to the skin, you should treat any injury that breaks the skin as a possible:

  A. closed fracture.

  B. open fracture.

  C. nondisplaced fracture.

  D. displaced fracture.

_____ **15.** A(n) _____ is also known as a hairline fracture.

    A. closed fracture

    B. open fracture

    C. nondisplaced fracture

    D. displaced fracture

_____ **16.** A(n) _____ produces actual deformity, or distortion, of the limb by shortening, rotating, or angulating it.

    A. closed fracture

    B. open fracture

    C. nondisplaced fracture

    D. displaced fracture

_____ **17.** When examining an injured extremity, you should compare the injured limb to:

    A. the opposite uninjured limb.

    B. one of your limbs or one of your partner's limbs.

    C. an injury chart.

    D. none of the above

_____ **18.** _____ is the most reliable indicator of an underlying fracture.

    A. Crepitus

    B. Deformity

    C. Point tenderness

    D. Absence of distal pulse

_____ **19.** A(n) _____ is a fracture that occurs in a growth section of a child's bone, which may prematurely stop growth if not properly treated.

    A. greenstick fracture

    B. comminuted fracture

    C. pathologic fracture

    D. epiphyseal fracture

_____ **20.** A(n) _____ is an incomplete fracture that passes only partway through the shaft of a bone but may still cause severe angulation.

    A. greenstick fracture

    B. comminuted fracture

    C. pathologic fracture

    D. epiphyseal fracture

_____ **21.** A(n) _____ is a fracture of a weakened or diseased bone, seen in patients with osteoporosis or cancer.

    A. greenstick fracture

    B. comminuted fracture

    C. pathologic fracture

    D. epiphyseal fracture

_____ **22.** A(n) _____ is a fracture in which the bone is broken into two or more fragments.

    A. greenstick fracture

    B. comminuted fracture

    C. pathologic fracture

    D. epiphyseal fracture

5

_____23. Rapid swelling usually indicates _____ from a fracture site and is typically followed by severe pain.

A. bleeding

B. laceration

C. locked joint

D. compartment syndrome

_____24. Fractures are almost always associated with _____ of the surrounding soft tissue.

A. laceration

B. crepitus

C. ecchymosis

D. swelling

_____25. Assessment of patients with musculoskeletal injuries must include:

A. initial assessment followed by a focused physical exam.

B. evaluation of neurovascular function.

C. applying oxygen as needed.

D. all of the above

_____26. Always check neurovascular function:

A. after any manipulation of the limb.

B. before applying a splint.

C. after applying a splint.

D. all of the above

_____27. Splinting will help to prevent:

A. excessive bleeding of the tissues at the injury site caused by broken bone ends.

B. laceration of the skin by broken bone ends.

C. increased pain from movement of bone ends.

D. all of the above

_____28. In-line _____ is the act of exerting a pulling force on a body structure in the direction of its normal alignment.

A. stabilization

B. immobilization

C. traction

D. direction

_____29. Basic types of splints include:

A. rigid.

B. formable.

C. traction.

D. all of the above

_____30. Do not use traction splints for any of the following conditions except:

    A. injuries of the pelvis.

    B. an isolated femur fracture.

    C. partial amputation or avulsions with bone separation.

    D. lower leg or ankle injury.

_____ 31. Hazards associated with improper application of splints include:

    A. compression of nerves, tissues, and blood vessels.

    B. delay in transport of a patient with a life-threatening injury.

    C. reduction of distal circulation if the splint is too tight.

    D. all of the above

Labeling www.OECzone anatomy review

Label the following diagram with the correct terms.

1. The Human Skeleton

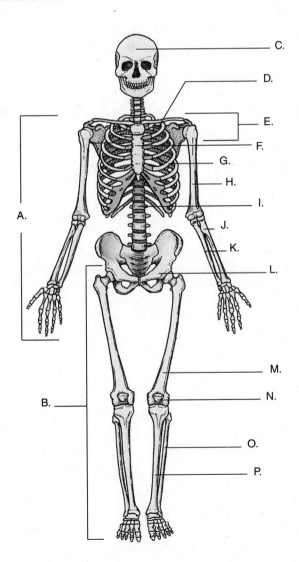

A. _____

B. _____

C. _____

D. _____

E. _____

F. _____

G. _____

H. _____

I. _____

J. _____

K. _____

L. _____

M. _____

N. _____

O. _____

P. _____

5

Vocabulary

Define the following terms using the space provided.

1. Traction:

_____

_____

_____

2. Dislocation:

_____

_____

_____

3. Nondisplaced fracture:

_____

_____

_____

4. Sling:

_____

_____

_____

5. Swathe:

_____

_____

_____

Fill-in

Read each item carefully, then complete the statement by filling in the missing word(s).

1. Atrophy is the _____ of muscle tissue.

2. Bone marrow produces _____ blood cells.

3. The knee and elbow are _____ joints.

4. Always carefully assess the _____ to try to determine the amount of kinetic energy that an injured limb has absorbed.

5. Penetrating injury should alert you to the possibility of a(n) _____.

6. The _____ is the longest and largest bone in the body.

7. A grating or grinding sensation known as _____ can be felt and sometimes even heard when fractured bone ends rub together.

8. A dislocated joint sometimes will spontaneously _____, or return to its normal position.

9. If you suspect that a patient has compartment syndrome, splint the affected limb, keeping it at the level of the heart, and provide immediate transport out of the outdoor environment, frequently checking _____.

10. Describe the types of injuries and additional supplies that are most appropriate with each splint listed below.

Quick splint _____

Cardboard splint _____

Wire, ladder splint _____

Malleable metal splint _____

Air splint _____

Vacuum splint _____

Sling and swathe _____

Hare traction splint _____

Sager or Kendrick traction splint _____

Thomas (modified) splint _____

True/False

If you believe the statement to be more true than false, write the letter "T" in the space provided. If you believe the statement to be more false than true, write the letter "F."

1. _____ All extremity injuries should be splinted before moving a patient unless the patient's life is in immediate danger.

2. _____ Splinting reduces pain and prevents the motion of bone fragments.

3. _____ You should use traction to reduce a fracture and force all bone fragments back into alignment.

4. _____ When applying traction, the direction of pull is always along the axis of the limb.

5. _____ Cover wounds with a dry, sterile dressing before applying a splint.

6. _____ When splinting a fracture, you should be careful to immobilize only the joint above the injury site.

7. _____ One of the steps of the neurologic examination is to palpate the pulse distal to the point of injury.

8. _____ Assessment of neurovascular function should be repeated every 5 to 10 minutes until the patient arrives at definitive care.

9. _____ A patient's ability to sense light touch in the fingers and toes distal to the injury site is a good indication that the nerve supply is intact.

Short Answer

Complete this section with short written answers using the space provided.

1. List the four types of forces that may cause injury to a limb.

_____

_____

_____

_____

2. List five of the signs associated with a possible fracture.

_____

_____

_____

_____

_____

3. List the four items to check when assessing neurovascular function.

_____

_____

_____

_____

4. List the general principles of splinting.

_____

_____

_____

5. What are the three goals of in-line traction?

_____

_____

_____

5

■ CLUES ■

Across

3. Exerting a pulling force

5. Major lower extremity nerve

6. Hand position for splinting

7. Elevation of pressure within fibrous tissues

8. Blood in urine

11. Collarbone

12. Joint between the two pubic bones

13. Forearm bone on small finger side

14. Striated, attached to bones

Down

1. Part of the scapula that joins with the humerus

2. Broken bone with overlying skin injured

4. Bone fragments are separated

9. Discoloration from bleeding under skin

10. Grating sound of bone ends

Word Fun

The following crossword puzzle is an activity provided to reinforce correct spelling and understanding of medical terminology associated with emergency care. Use the clues in the column to complete the puzzle.

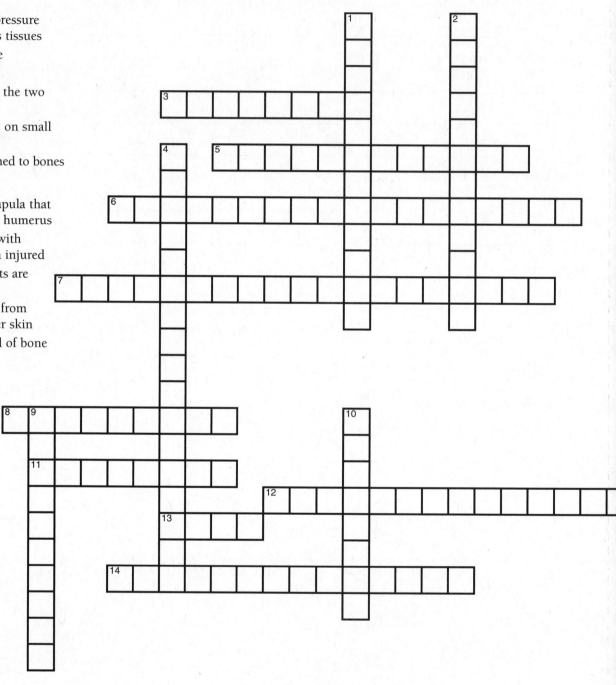

Calls to the Scene

The following case scenarios provide an opportunity to explore the concerns associated with patient management. Read each scenario, then answer each question in detail.

1. You are dispatched to a summer construction site for a 27-year-old man complaining of severe thoracic pain posteriorly. Coworkers tell you he was hit in the upper back by the bucket of a backhoe. He is alert and oriented and closer inspection reveals bruising and deformity over the left scapula with pain and crepitus on palpation.

   How would you best manage this patient?

   _____

   _____

   _____

   _____

   _____

   _____

   _____

   _____

   _____

2. You are called to a local park where an 11-year-old girl fell off the parallel bars onto her right elbow. She is cradling the arm to her chest. She has obvious swelling and deformity in the area. She has good pulse, motor, and sensation at the wrist. ABCs are normal.

   How would you best manage this patient?

   _____

   _____

   _____

   _____

   _____

   _____

   _____

   _____

5

3. A skier hits a snow-making machine that is off the edge of the trail. He is found lying on his side with the injured leg under him, supported by the upper leg and the snow. He has pain about 4" above the knee. As long as the leg is not moved, the patient remains calm. He resists any attempt to straighten the knee.

How would you best manage this patient?

_____

_____

_____

_____

_____

_____

_____

_____

_____

Skill Drills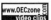

Skill Drill 24-1: Assessing Pulse, Motor and Sensory Functions
Test your knowledge of this skill drill by filling in the correct words in the photo captions.

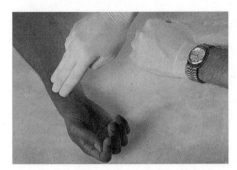

1. Palpate the _____ pulse in the upper extremity.

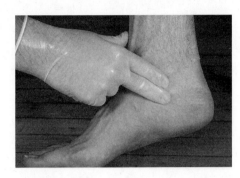

2. Palpate the _____ _____ pulse in the lower extremity. Remember to palpate the _____ _____ pulse as well.

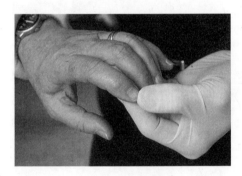

3. Assess capillary refill by blanching a fingernail or _____.

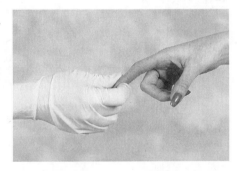

4. Assess sensation on the flesh near the _____ of the _____ finger and thumb, and the _____ _____ as well.

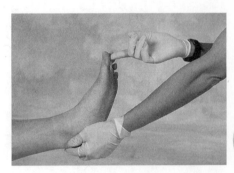

5. On the foot, first check sensation on the flesh near the _____ of the _____ _____.

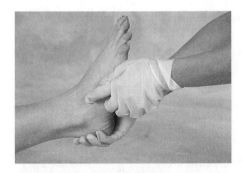

6. Also check foot sensation on the _____ _____.

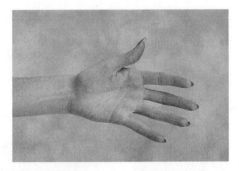

7. Evaluate motor function by asking the patient to _____ the hand. (Perform motor tests only if the hand or foot is not _____. _____ a test if it causes pain.)

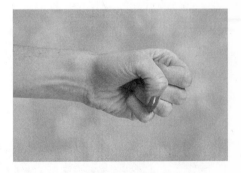

8. Also ask the patient to _____ _____ _____.

(continued)

5

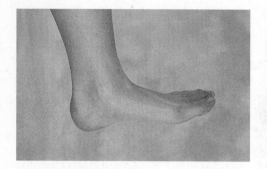
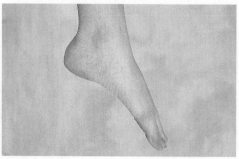

9. To evaluate motor function in the foot, ask the patient to _____ the foot.

10. Also have the patient _____ the foot and _____ the toes.

Skill Drill 24-2: Caring for Musculoskeletal Injuries
Test your knowledge of this skill drill by filling in the correct words in the photo captions.

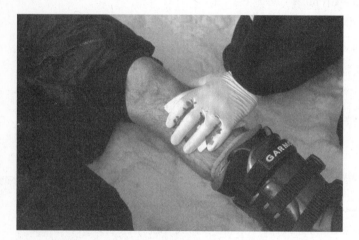

1. Cover open wounds with a _____, _____ dressing, and _____ _____ to control bleeding. Assess _____ CMS functions.

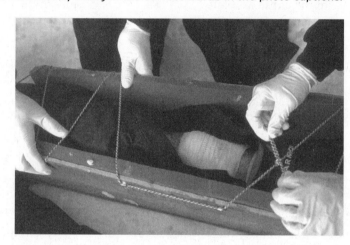

2. Apply a _____ splint.

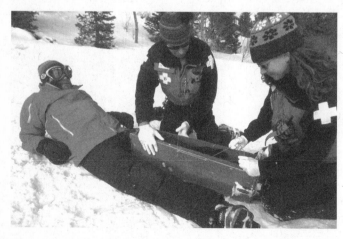

3. _____ the extremity and the patient for transport.

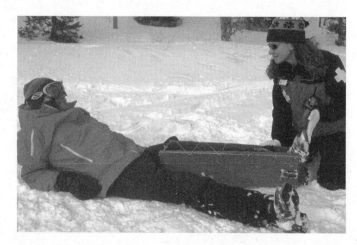

4. Assess distal _____ functions and _____ the patient for transport.

Skill Drill 24-3: Applying a Quick Splint
Test your knowledge of this skill drill by filling in the correct words in the photo captions.

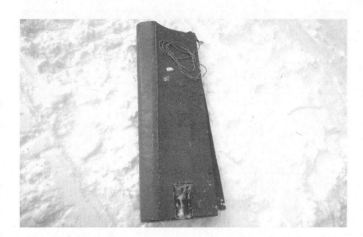

1. Open the quick splint _____ next to the patient's injured _____ .

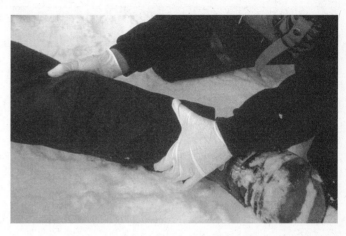

2. Grasp the booted foot with one hand, using slight _____ traction, and place the other hand just below the _____ or under the lower thigh to _____ the extremity.

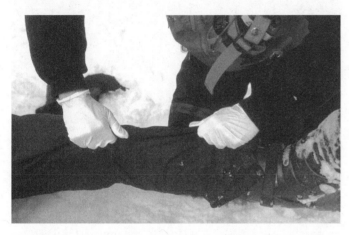

3. The "_____ lift" is another useful method for lifting and supporting the injured extremity.

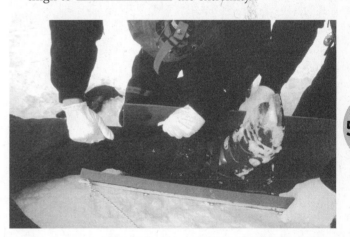

4. Have a second rescuer _____ the splint underneath the leg while you gently _____ the injured extremity into the splint.

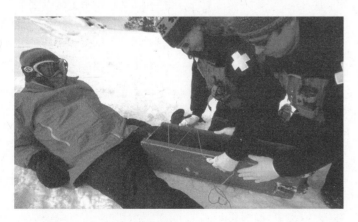

5. The second rescuer then _____ up the sides of the splint like a clamshell and secures the splint _____ firmly.

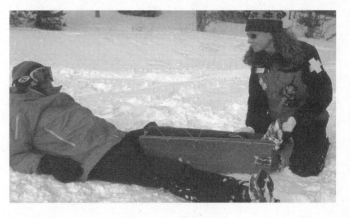

6. Reassess _____ function.

5

Skill Drill 24-4: Applying a Sling and Swathe
Test your knowledge of this skill drill by filling in the correct words in the photo captions.

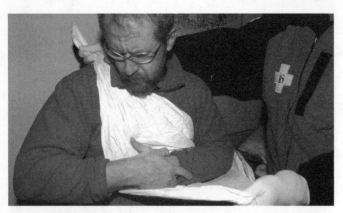

1. Bend the patient's elbow to just under a _____ angle and lay a _____ bandage on the chest wall under the injured arm. The injured forearm lays across the _____.

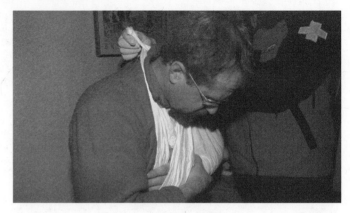

2. Tie the two ends together at the _____ of the neck. Bring the apex _____ and pin it to the _____ of the sling, or tie a knot in the apex.

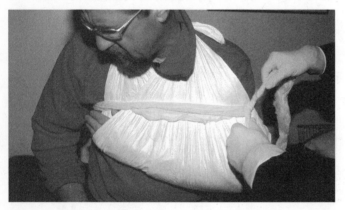

3. Wrap a _____ around the patient's chest, include the _____ _____ on the injured side, and tie it snugly under the _____ armpit.

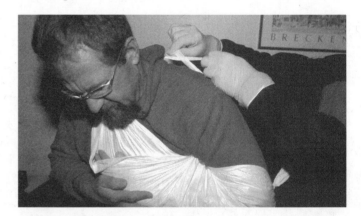

4. To avoid pressure on an injured shoulder or fractured clavicle, bring the lower corner of the sling under the near _____. Tie it to the opposite corner behind the patient's _____.

Skill Drill 24-5: Forming and Applying a Blanket Roll Splint
Test your knowledge of this skill drill by filling in the correct words in the photo captions.

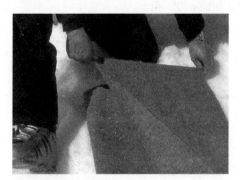

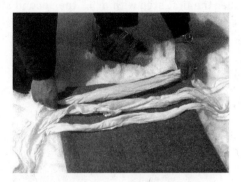

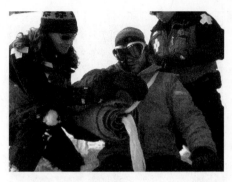

1. Fold a blanket _____ in thirds.

2. Lay _____ across the blanket. Tie knots in the two ends of one cravat(s) for _____ purposes later.

3. Position the _____ blanket snugly and in the _____ angle of the dislocated shoulder.

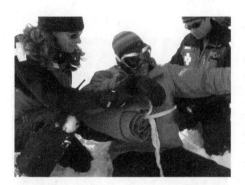

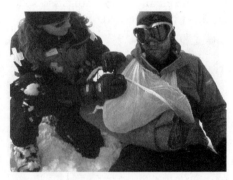

4. Securely _____ the cravats around the _____ and _____.

5. Secure the injured arm with a _____ and _____.

5

Skill Drill 24-6: Initial Application of All Traction Splints
Test your knowledge of this skill drill by placing the photos below in the correct order.
Number the first step with a "1," the second step with a "2," etc.

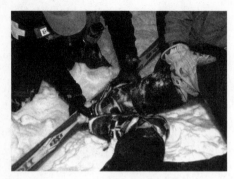

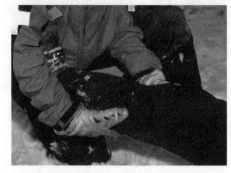

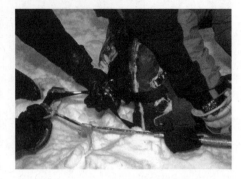

_____

After the fracture has been stabilized, another rescuer(s) removes the ski or snowboard and assesses the CMS status of the extremity.

_____

The first rescuer firmly grasps the injured leg below the knee and realigns the fracture by manual, longitudinal (axial) traction. The boot can be removed and CMS status assessed at this time as needed.

_____

The leg is placed in the splint, secured to the upper thigh, and mechanical traction is evenly substituted for manual traction.

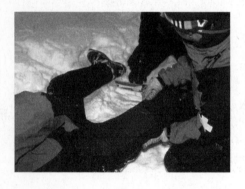

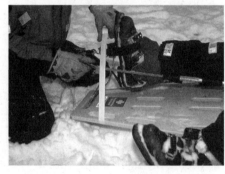

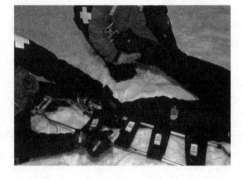

_____

One rescuer manually stabilizes the fracture site.

_____

Log roll the patient onto his or her uninjured side and place the patient on a long backboard. Secure the splint to the backboard to prevent movement.

_____

The second rescuer sizes and prepares the splint. The ankle hitch should be applied at this time and can be used to maintain manual traction.

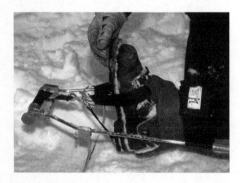

_____

Reassess the CMS status of the injured extremity after all the straps have been applied.

Skill Drill 24-7: Applying a Sager Traction Splint

Test your knowledge of this skill drill by placing the photos below in the correct order.
Number the first step with a "1," the second step with a "2," etc.

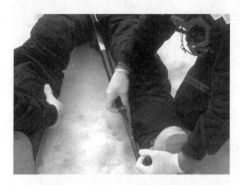

_____

Estimate the proper length of the splint by placing it next to the uninjured limb.

Fit the ankle pads to the ankle.

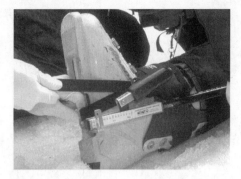

_____

Tighten the ankle harness just above the malleoli.

Snug the cable ring against the bottom of the foot.

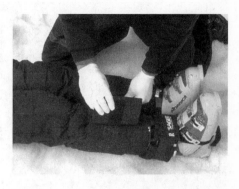

_____

Secure the splint with elasticized cravats.

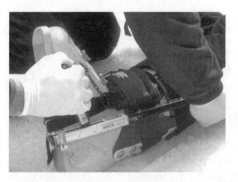

_____

Extend the splint's inner shaft to apply traction of about 10% of body weight.

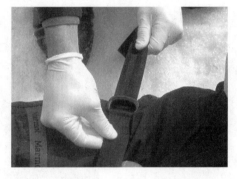

_____

Place the splint at the inner thigh, apply the thigh strap at the upper thigh, and secure snugly.

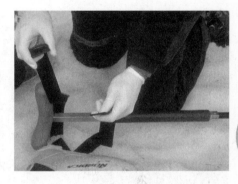

_____

Adjust the thigh strap so that it lies anteriorly when secured.

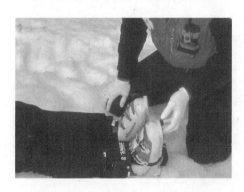

_____

Check circulation, motor, and sensory functions.

Secure the patient to a long backboard.

5

Skill Drill 24-8: Boot Removal
Test your knowledge of this skill drill by filling in the correct words in the photo captions.

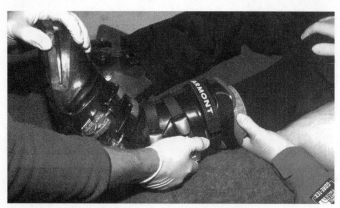

1. Stabilize the _____ leg and the
   _____.

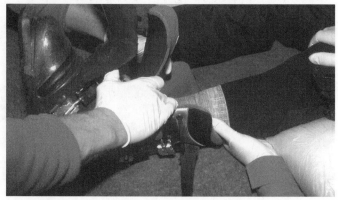

2. While maintaining _____ stabilization,
   spread the boot shell, pulling the _____ out
   or opening a rear entry boot as wide as possible.
   _____ all devices and provide
   _____ to the assisting rescuer.

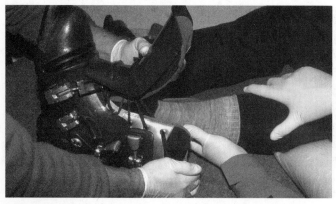

3. With the boot shell held open and the leg stabilized,
   apply _____ to the boot. Firmly and
   smoothly _____ and _____ the
   boot off the foot, while using your _____ as
   counterpressure against the boot toe.

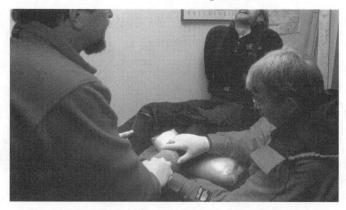

4. Monitor the patient for indications of excessive
   _____ or _____. Stop or modify
   the procedure as appropriate.

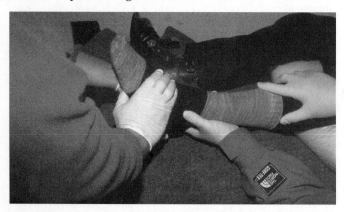

5. Assess distal _____ and _____
   function, swelling, _____, or bruising
   (remove clothing).

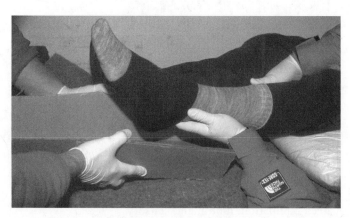

6. Prepare to _____ the lower extremity.

Notes

Workbook Activities

The following activities have been designed to help you. Your instructor may require you to complete some or all of these activities as a regular part of your OEC training program. You are encouraged to complete any activity that your instructor does not assign as a way to enhance your learning in the classroom.

Chapter Review

The following exercises provide an opportunity to refresh your knowledge of this chapter.

▬ **N O T E S** ▬

Matching

Match each of the terms in the left column to the appropriate definition in the right column.

_____ **1.** Compression   **A.** Hitting a lift tower at great speed

_____ **2.** Glenoid fossa   **B.** Larger of the two lower leg bones

_____ **3.** Tibia   **C.** Supporting bone of the upper arm

_____ **4.** Humerus   **D.** Reduce or eliminate motion

_____ **5.** Stabilization   **E.** Part of the scapula

Match the symptom with the bone or joint:

_____ **6.** Knee   **F.** injury just above the boot

_____ **7.** Pelvic   **G.** limb shortened and externally rotated

_____ **8.** Hip   **H.** blood in urine

_____ **9.** Femur   **I.** tender over the malleoli

_____ **10.** Ankle   **J.** sound of "pop"

_____ **11.** Tibia   **K.** leg externally rotated

Multiple Choice

Read each item carefully, then select the best response.

_____ **1.** Fractures of the clavicle are best treated using a:

     A. sling and swathe.

     B. blanket roll in the armpit.

     C. traction splint.

     D. cardboard splint.

Assessment and Care of Bone and Joint Injuries

_____ **2.** A patient with a dislocated shoulder will usually be most comfortable when transported in a toboggan in which of the following positions?

A. the supine position

B. the prone position

C. the fetal position, injured side up

D. a sitting position, supported from behind

_____ **3.** The position of the knee when it is strongest and most stable is:

A. slightly flexed.

B. fully extended.

C. fully flexed.

D. hyperextended.

_____ **4.** The knee ligament that is most frequently injured by skiers is the:

A. anterior cruciate.

B. lateral collateral.

C. medial collateral.

D. posterior cruciate.

_____ **5.** Downward pressure followed by inward pressure on the iliac crests is a test for injury to the:

A. spine.

B. femur.

C. abdomen.

D. pelvis.

_____ **6.** A patient with a suspected knee sprain should be encouraged to consult an orthopaedic surgeon if symptoms do not subside in:

A. 3 to 4 days.

B. 1 week.

C. 24 hours.

D. 2 weeks.

_____ **7.** Signs and symptoms of a dislocated joint include:

    A. marked deformity.

    B. tenderness on palpation.

    C. locked joint.

    D. all of the above

_____ **8.** Signs and symptoms of sprains include all of the following except:

    A. point tenderness.

    B. Pain prevents the patient from moving or using the limb normally.

    C. marked deformity.

    D. instability of the joint is indicated by increased motion.

_____ **9.** Signs and symptoms associated with hip dislocation include:

    A. severe pain in the hip.

    B. lateral and posterior aspects of the hip region will be tender on palpation.

    C. you may be able to palpate the femoral head deep within the muscles of the buttock.

    D. all of the above

_____ **10.** There is always a significant amount of blood loss, as much as _____ mL, after a fracture of the shaft of the femur.

    A. 250 to 500

    B. 100 to 250

    C. 1,500 to 2,000

    D. 100 to 1,500

_____ **11.** The knee is especially susceptible to _____ injuries, which occur when abnormal bending or twisting forces are applied to the joint.

    A. tendon

    B. ligament

    C. dislocation

    D. fracture-dislocation

_____ **12.** Signs and symptoms of knee ligament injury include:

    A. swelling.

    B. point tenderness.

    C. joint effusion.

    D. all of the above

_____ **13.** Because of local tenderness and swelling, it is easy to confuse a nondisplaced or minimally displaced fracture about the knee with a:

    A. tendon injury.

    B. ligament injury.

    C. dislocation.

    D. fracture-dislocation.

_____ 14. Fracture of the tibia and fibula are often associated with _____ as a result of the distorted positions of the limb following injury.

   A. vascular injury.

   B. muscular injury

   C. tendon injury

   D. ligament injury

_____ 15. A boot top fracture affects the:

   A. fibula and/or tibia.

   B. ulna and/or radius.

   C. ilium and/or ischium.

   D. patella and/or femur.

_____ 16. A pelvic fracture can injure the:

   A. spleen.

   B. liver.

   C. pancreas.

   D. bladder.

_____ 17. Stretching and tearing of the joint capsule and ligaments without bone-end displacement is called a:

   A. strain.

   B. hernia.

   C. fracture.

   D. sprain.

_____ 18. Femur fractures immediately above the knee should be splinted with a:

   A. traction splint.

   B. backboard.

   C. fixation splint extending ankle to groin.

   D. fixation splint extending just below to just above the knee.

_____ 19. If you suspect a lower leg fracture, you need to consider all except which of the following?

   A. Support the injured area as you move the limb.

   B. Make sure the splint is cardboard.

   C. Extend the splint to past the knee and ankle.

   D. Pad the hollows and secure the splint snugly.

5

A. _____

B. _____

C. _____

D. _____

E. _____

F. _____

G. _____

H. _____

I. _____

J. _____

K. _____

L. _____

M. _____

N. _____

O. _____

P. _____

Q. _____

R. _____

S. _____

T. _____

U. _____

V. _____

Labeling

Label the following diagrams with the correct terms.

1. Anatomy of the Knee

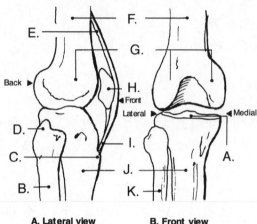

A. Lateral view   B. Front view

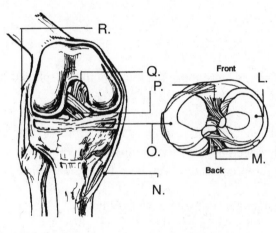

C. Front view   D. Top view

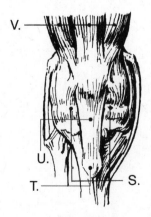

E. Front view

Vocabulary

Define the following terms using the space provided.

1. Acromioclavicular (A/C) joint:

_____

_____

_____

2. Colles fracture:

_____

_____

_____

3. Sciatic nerve:

_____

_____

_____

4. Glenohumeral joint:

_____

_____

_____

5. Supracondylar fracture of the humerus:

_____

_____

_____

6. Retroperitoneal space:

_____

_____

_____

5

Fill-in

Read each item carefully, then complete the statement by filling in the missing word.

1. When providing emergency care to a patient with an injured upper extremity, be

   sure to remove rings, bracelets, and other jewelry before _____ occurs

   and before you splint the extremity.

2. Fractures of the _____ occur infrequently because the bone is well
   protected by major large muscles.

3. In patients with elbow injuries, if you find _____ and _____ in
   the hand, splint the injury in the position in which you find it.

4. Fractures of the pelvis most often result from _____ in the form of a
   heavy blow.

5. _____ are the most common injury in skiing.

6. The term hip fracture refers to a fracture of the _____.

True/False

If you believe the statement to be more true than false, write the letter "T" in the space provided. If you believe the statement to be more false than true, write the letter "F."

1. _____ A dislocation occurs only at a joint; a fracture can occur anywhere along the bone.

2. _____ The best splint to use is a fixation splint.

3. _____ The muscles attached to the femur are small and weak.

4. _____ A fracture of the femoral shaft can be associated with extensive blood loss even if the fracture is closed.

5. _____ If exposed bone ends retract into the wound during alignment and splinting, they should immediately be reexposed.

6. _____ An open angulated fracture must be aligned before a splint can be applied.

7. _____ A sling and swathe immobilizes upper extremity injuries by using the chest wall as part of the splint.

8. _____ With fracture-dislocation injuries, the rescuer should monitor the distal extremity for nerve and circulation supply.

9. _____ Traction splints are designed to increase heat and muscle spasms of the injured limb, thereby delaying shock.

10. _____ A traction splint is indicated for all femur fractures.

Short Answer

Complete this section with short written answers using the space provided.

1. When the splinting process for lower extremities is completed, what must be reassessed and why?

_____

_____

_____

2. List three symptoms of a pelvic fracture.

_____

_____

_____

3. In what position is a fracture or dislocation generally best treated and transported?

_____

_____

_____

4. Describe the possible injury that could occur if the patient falls with the arm in an adducted position.

_____

_____

_____

5. Describe the possible injury that could occur if the patient falls with the arm in an abducted position.

_____

_____

_____

6. Describe the difference between posterior and anterior shoulder dislocation.

_____

_____

Word Fun

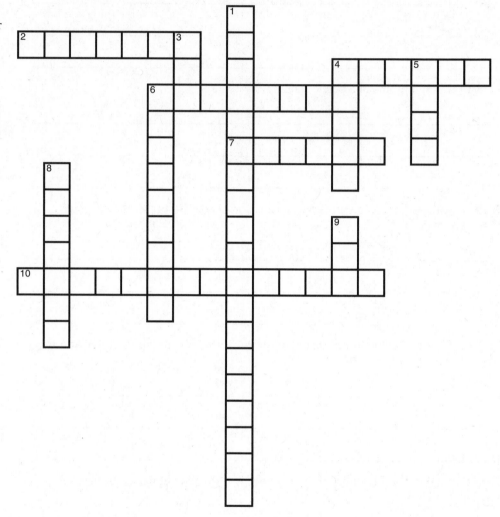

The following crossword puzzle is an activity provided to reinforce correct spelling and understanding of medical terminology associated with emergency care. Use the clues in the column to complete the puzzle.

CLUES

Across

2. Shoulder blade
4. Smaller bone in the lower leg
6. Collarbone
7. Lower arm bone on the thumb side of the forearm
10. Fracture to the lower end of the tibia and/or fibula

Down

1. Fractures of the distal radius
3. Anterior cruciate ligaments
4. Thigh bone
5. Lower arm bone on the small finger side of the forearm
6. Heel bone
8. Supporting bone of the upper arm
9. Posterior cruciate ligaments

Calls to the Scene

The following case scenarios provide an opportunity to explore the concerns associated with patient management. Read each scenario, then answer each question in detail.

1. A skier traveling very fast through the trees loses control while trying to avoid a collision with a blue spruce. The skier crashes into the tree and dislocates her right shoulder. The skier is in a supine position with her right arm above her head. During assessment she will not allow you to bring the arm to near-normal position.

   How would you manage this patient?

   _____

   _____

   _____

   _____

   _____

   _____

   _____

   _____

   _____

   _____

   _____

2. You come upon a skier in his mid-20s who, while telemarking, went into a twisting fall as he crossed a section of ice on the advanced slope. His fall carried him into some rocks where he sustained an open fracture at boot top with deformity and exposed bone. His pulse is 100 beats/min, and his respirations are 24 breaths/min.

   How would you manage this patient?

   _____

   _____

   _____

   _____

   _____

_____

_____

_____

_____

_____

3. A 20-year-old woman, skiing for the first time, catches an inside edge and falls off the T-bar lift. The patient complains of severe pain in her right lower leg. She says she can move her toes. Her pulse is 100 beats/min, and her respirations are 20 breaths/min.

How would you manage this patient?

_____

_____

_____

_____

_____

_____

_____

_____

_____

_____

Skill Drills

Skill Drill 25-1: Splinting the Hand and Wrist
Test your knowledge of this skill drill by filling in the correct words in the photo captions.

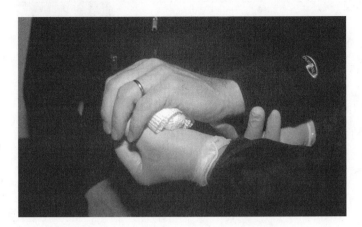

1. Move the hand into the _____ _____ _____. Place a soft _____ _____ in the _____.

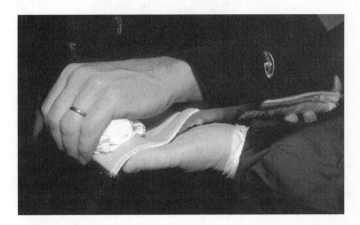

2. Apply a padded _____ _____ on the palmar side with _____ exposed.

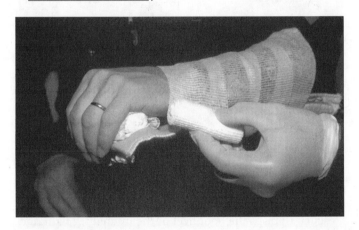

3. Secure the splint with a _____ _____.

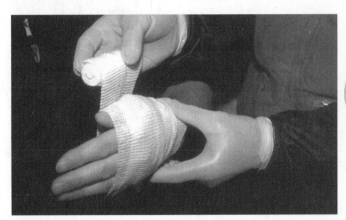

4. Stabilize a _____ ulnar collateral ligament sprain to the _____ with a _____ _____.

Skill Drill 25-2: Realignment of Angulated, Rotated, Fractured Tibia/Fibula with Application of a Quick Splint

Test your knowledge of this skill drill by placing the photos below in the correct order. Number the first step with a "1," the second step with a "2", etc.

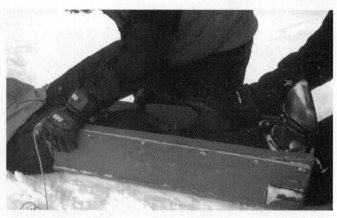

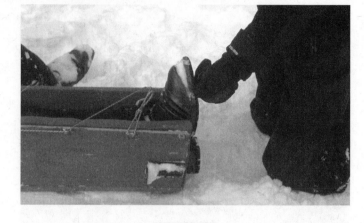

Rescuer 2 closes the splint and secures the straps, while rescuer 1 removes his or her upper hand.

_____

Rescuer 1 slides his or her hand out from around the heel, and then checks CMS in the foot.

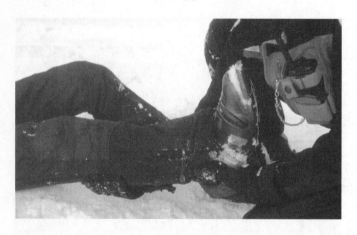

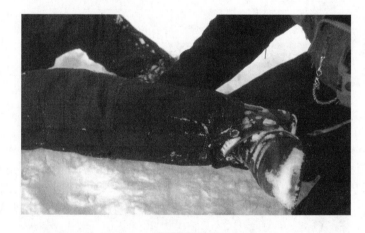

When the splint is ready, rescuer 1 applies gentle longitudinal traction, and with both hands, lifts, straightens, and derotates the deformed tibia all in one continuous motion.

_____

Rescuer 1 grasps the boot heel of the injured leg with one hand, while the other hand is placed under the calf just below the knee.

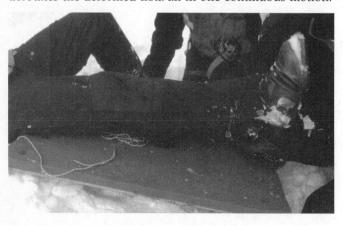

Rescuer 2 slides the splint under the leg from medial and below, then rescuer 1 lowers the leg into the splint.

Notes

Workbook Activities

The following activities have been designed to help you. Your instructor may require you to complete some or all of these activities as a regular part of your OEC training program. You are encouraged to complete any activity that your instructor does not assign as a way to enhance your learning in the classroom.

Chapter Review

The following exercises provide an opportunity to refresh your knowledge of this chapter.

NOTES

Matching

Match each of the terms in the left column to the appropriate definition in the right column.

_____ 1. Cerebellum

_____ 2. Brain stem

_____ 3. Somatic nervous system

_____ 4. Autonomic nervous system

_____ 5. Spinal column

_____ 6. Central nervous system

_____ 7. Cerebral edema

_____ 8. Connecting nerves

_____ 9. Intervertebral disk

_____ 10. Meninges

A. consists of 33 bones

B. swelling of the brain

C. the brain and spinal cord

D. controls movement

E. the part of the central nervous system that controls virtually all the functions that are absolutely necessary for life

F. three distinct layers of tissue that surround and protect the brain and spinal cord within the skull and spinal cord

G. the part of the nervous system that regulates involuntary functions

H. the part of the nervous system that regulates voluntary activities

I. located in the brain and spinal cord, these connect the motor and sensory nerves

J. cushion that lies between the vertebrae

Multiple Choice

Read each item carefully, then select the best response.

_____ 1. The nervous system includes:

A. the brain.

B. the spinal cord.

C. billions of nerve fibers.

D. all of the above

Head and Spine Injuries

_____ **2.** The nervous system is divided into two parts: the central nervous system and the:

A. autonomic nervous system.

B. peripheral nervous system.

C. sympathetic nervous system.

D. somatic nervous system.

_____ **3.** The brain is divided into three major areas: the cerebrum, the cerebellum, and the:

A. foramen magnum.

B. meninges.

C. brain stem.

D. spinal column.

_____ **4.** Injury to the head and neck may indicate injury to the:

A. thoracic spine.

B. lumbar spine.

C. cervical spine.

D. sacral spine.

_____ **5.** The _____ is composed of three layers of tissue that surround the brain and spinal cord within the skull and spinal canal.

A. meninges

B. dura mater

C. pia mater

D. arachnoid space

_____ **6.** The skull is divided into two large structures: the cranium and the:

A. occiput.

B. face.

C. parietal.

D. foramen magnum.

_____ **7.** Peripheral nerves include:

   A. connecting nerves.

   B. sensory nerves.

   C. motor nerves.

   D. all of the above

_____ **8.** The brain and spinal cord float in cerebrospinal fluid (CSF), which:

   A. acts as a shock absorber.

   B. bathes them.

   C. buffers them from injury.

   D. all of the above

_____ **9.** The autonomic nervous system is composed of two parts: the sympathetic nervous system and the:

   A. peripheral nervous system.

   B. central nervous system.

   C. parasympathetic nervous system.

   D. somatic nervous system.

_____ **10.** The most prominent and most easily palpable spinous process is at the _____ cervical vertebra at the base of the neck.

   A. 7th

   B. 6th

   C. 5th

   D. 4th

_____ **11.** When identifying the mechanism of injury of an unresponsive patient, _____ may have helpful information.

   A. first responders

   B. family members

   C. bystanders

   D. all of the above

_____ **12.** Emergency medical care of a patient with a possible spinal injury begins with:

   A. opening the airway.

   B. determining level of consciousness.

   C. scene safety.

   D. taking BSI precautions.

_____ **13.** The _____ is a tunnel running the length of the spine, which encloses and protects the spinal cord.

   A. foramen magnum

   B. spinal canal

   C. foramen foramina

   D. meninges

_____ **14.** Once the head and neck are manually stabilized, you should assess:

   A. pulse.

   B. motor function.

   C. sensation.

   D. all of the above

_____ **15.** You must maintain manual stabilization of the head until the:

    A. patient's head and torso are in line.

    B. patient is secured to a backboard with the head immobilized.

    C. rigid cervical collar is in place.

    D. patient arrives at the hospital.

_____ **16.** The ideal procedure for moving a patient from the ground to the backboard is the:

    A. four-person log roll.

    B. lateral slide.

    C. four-person lift.

    D. push and pull maneuver.

_____ **17.** You can almost always control bleeding from a scalp laceration by:

    A. direct pressure.

    B. elevation.

    C. pressure point.

    D. tourniquet.

_____ **18.** Exceptions to using a short spinal extrication device include all of the following except if:

    A. you or the patient is in danger.

    B. the patient is conscious and complaining of lumbar pain.

    C. you need to gain immediate access to other patients.

    D. the patient's injuries justify immediate removal.

_____ **19.** Applying excessive pressure to an open wound with a skull fracture could:

    A. increase intracranial pressure.

    B. push bone fragments into the brain.

    C. increase the size of the soft-tissue injury.

    D. all of the above

_____ **20.** A _____ is a temporary loss or alteration of a part or all of the brain's abilities to function, without actual physical damage to the brain.

    A. contusion

    B. concussion

    C. hematoma

    D. subdural hematoma

_____ **21.** Symptoms of a concussion include:

    A. dizziness.

    B. weakness.

    C. visual changes.

    D. all of the above

_____ **22.** Intracranial bleeding outside of the dura and under the skull is known as a(n):

    A. concussion.

    B. intracerebral hemorrhage.

    C. subdural hematoma.

    D. epidural hematoma.

5

_____23. The difference in signs and symptoms of traumatic vs. nontraumatic brain injuries is the:

A. lack of altered mental status.

B. lack of mechanism of injury.

C. lack of swelling.

D. increase in blood pressure.

_____24. _____ is the most reliable sign of a closed brain injury.

A. Vomiting

B. Decreased level of responsiveness

C. Seizures

D. Numbness and tingling in the extremities

_____25. _____ is one of the most common, and one of the most serious, complications of a brain injury.

A. Cyanosis

B. Hypoxia

C. Vomiting

D. Cerebral edema

_____26. Common causes of brain injuries include all of the following except:

A. direct blows.

B. motor vehicle crashes.

C. seizure activity.

D. sports injuries.

_____27. Assessment of mental status is accomplished through the use of the mnemonic:

A. SAMPLE.

B. OPQRST.

C. AVPU.

D. AEIOU-TIPS.

_____28. Unequal pupil size may indicate:

A. increased intracranial pressure.

B. a congenital problem.

C. damage to the nerves that control dilation and constriction.

D. all of the above

_____29. Patients with brain injuries often have injuries to the _____ as well.

A. face

B. torso

C. cervical spine

D. extremities

_____30. Proper order of treatment for traumatic head injuries includes:

A. scene safety, airway, LOR with c-spine control, breathing, circulation.

B. LOR with c-spine control, airway, breathing, circulation.

C. LOR, airway, breathing, circulation, c-spine.

D. BSI, ABCs, LOR, c-spine control.

_____31. A cervical collar should be applied to a patient with a possible spinal injury based on the:

A. mechanism of injury.

B. history.

C. signs and symptoms.

D. all of the above

_____**32.** Helmets should be removed in all of the following cases except:

A. cardiac arrest.

B. when the helmet allows for excessive movement.

C. when there are no impending airway or breathing problems.

D. when a shield cannot be removed.

_____**33.** Your best choice of action for a child involved in a motor vehicle crash and found in a car seat is to:

A. immobilize the child in the car seat.

B. rule out spinal injury and place the child with a parent.

C. pad sides of car seat but leave space to allow for lateral movement.

D. move the child to a pediatric immobilization device.

Labeling www.OECzone anatomy review

Label the following diagrams with the correct terms.

1. The Brain

A. _____
B. _____
C. _____
D. _____
E. _____
F. _____
G. _____
H. _____
I. _____

2. The Connecting Nerves in the Spinal Cord

A. _____
B. _____
C. _____
D. _____

3. The Spinal Column

A. _____

B. _____

C. _____

D. _____

E. _____

A.

B.

C.

D.

E.

Vocabulary

Define the following terms using the space provided.

1. Retrograde amnesia:

_____

_____

_____

2. Anterograde (posttraumatic) amnesia:

_____

_____

_____

3. Closed brain injury:

_____

_____

_____

4. Eyes-forward position:

_____

_____

_____

5. Open brain injury:

_____

_____

_____

Fill-in

Read each item carefully, then complete the statement by filling in the missing word(s).

1. The _____ nerves carry information to the muscles.

2. The dura mater, arachnoid, and pia mater are layers of _____ within the skull and spinal canal.

3. The brain and spinal cord are part of the _____ nervous system.

4. Within the peripheral nervous system, there are _____ pairs of spinal nerves.

5. The _____ nerves pass through holes in the skull and transmit sensations directly to the brain.

6. Vertebrae are separated by cushions called _____.

7. The skull has two large structures of bone, the _____ and the

_____.

8. The _____ produces cerebrospinal fluid (CSF).

9. The _____ nervous system reacts to stress.

10. The _____ nervous system causes the body to relax.

True/False

If you believe the statement to be more true than false, write the letter "T" in the space provided. If you believe the statement to be more false than true, write the letter "F."

1. _____ A distracted spine has been moved along its length.

2. _____ If a sensory nerve in the reflex arc detects an irritating stimulus, it will bypass the motor nerve and send a message directly to the brain.

3. _____ Voluntary activities are those actions we perform unconsciously.

4. _____ The autonomic nervous system is composed of the sympathetic nervous system and the parasympathetic nervous system.

5. _____ The parasympathetic nervous system reacts to stress with the fight-or-flight response whenever it is confronted with a threatening situation.

6. _____ All patients with suspected head and/or spine injuries should have their head realigned to an in-line neutral position.

7. _____ When assessing a patient for possible spine injury, you should begin with a focused history and physical exam.

Short Answer

Complete this section with short written answers using the space provided.

1. List the five basic questions to ask a conscious patient when conducting an assessment of a head or head and spine injury.

_____

_____

_____

_____

_____

2. List the reasons for not placing the head/spine injury patient's head into a neutral in-line position.

_____

_____

_____

3. List the three major types of brain injuries.

_____

_____

_____

4. List at least five signs and symptoms of a brain injury.

_____

_____

_____

_____

_____

5. List the three general principles for treating a brain injury.

_____

_____

_____

6. List the six questions to ask yourself when deciding whether or not to remove a helmet.

_____

_____

_____

_____

_____

_____

5

■ CLUES ■

Across

5. Swelling of the brain
6. Inability to remember after the event
8. Controls primary life functions
9. Cushion between vertebrae
10. Layers of tissues surrounding the brain
11. Cerebral trauma without broken skin

Down

1. Inability to remember the event
2. Coordinates body movement
3. Voluntary part of CNS
4. Join motor and sensory nerves
7. Pulling the spine along its length

Word Fun

The following crossword puzzle is an activity provided to reinforce correct spelling and understanding of medical terminology associated with emergency care. Use the clues in the column to complete the puzzle.

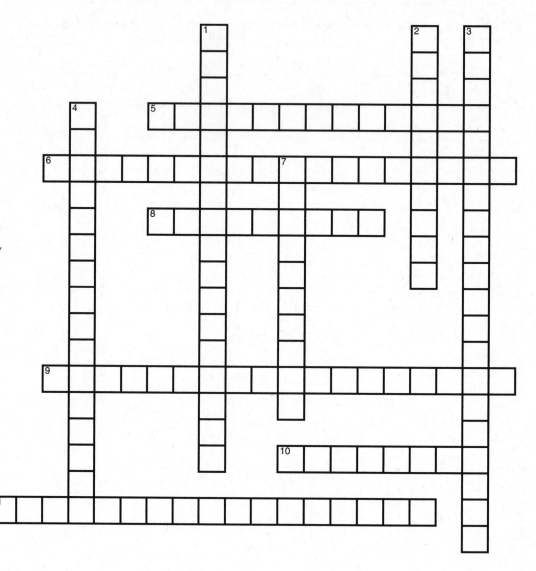

Calls to the Scene

The following case scenarios provide an opportunity to explore the concerns associated with patient management. Read each scenario, then answer each question in detail.

1. A 22-year-old man falls forward in a "head plant" while aggressively skiing an expert mogul slope. You quickly ski over to him. Although he appears stunned, he is fully responsive and exhibits no altered level of responsiveness. He tells you he felt a sharp pain in his neck when he hit the slope. He also said that he attempted to move but laid back down when he felt a tingly sensation in his upper back. Your initial assessment reveals a pulse of 110 beats/min and respirations of 20 breaths/min.

   How would you best manage this patient?

   _____

   _____

   _____

   _____

   _____

   _____

   _____

   _____

   _____

   _____

2. You are called to the scene of a baseball game where a 10-year-old boy was accidentally hit with a baseball bat on the left side of his head. He has a depression in the left temporal region and severe vomiting. He is responsive to pain and bleeding is minimal.

   How would you best manage this patient?

   _____

   _____

   _____

   _____

   _____

   _____

   _____

   _____

5

3. During a freestyle contest, a 14-year-old boy, while performing a double daffy jump, is thrown backward and lands on his upper back. The patient is unresponsive initially. He regains consciousness but has no recollection of his jump. He complains of pain in the upper thoracic spine and lower neck areas and has good movement and sensation in all extremities. Vital signs are within normal ranges.

How would you best manage this patient?

_____

_____

_____

_____

_____

_____

_____

_____

_____

_____

Skill Drills

Skill Drill 26-1: Performing Manual In-Line Stabilization
Test your knowledge of this skill drill by filling in the correct words in the photo captions.

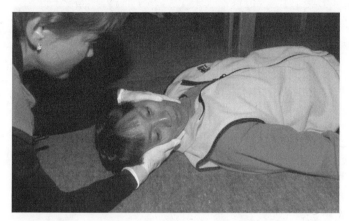

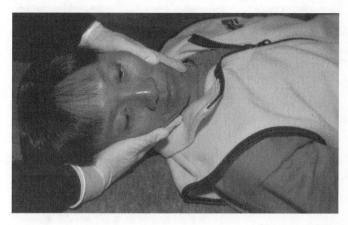

1. Kneel at the head of the patient and place your hands firmly around the _____ of the _____ on either _____.

2. Support the lower jaw with your _____ and _____ fingers, and the head with your _____.

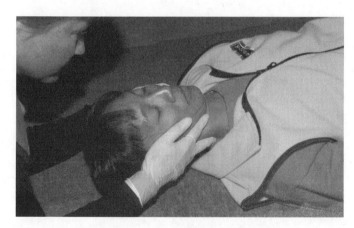

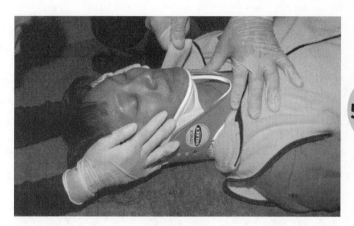

3. Gently _____ the head into a _____, _____ position, aligned with the torso. Do not _____ the head or neck excessively.

4. Continue to _____ the head manually while your partner places a rigid _____ _____ around the neck. Maintain _____ _____ until you have the patient secured to a backboard.

5

Skill Drill 26-2: Immobilizing a Patient to a Long Backboard

Test your knowledge of this skill drill by placing the photos below in the correct order. Number the first step with a "1," the second step with a "2," etc. Also, fill in the correct words in the photo captions.

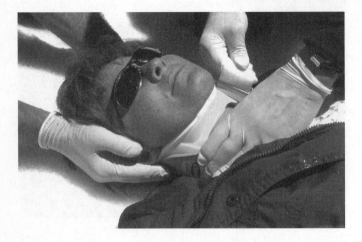

_____

Apply a_____ _____.

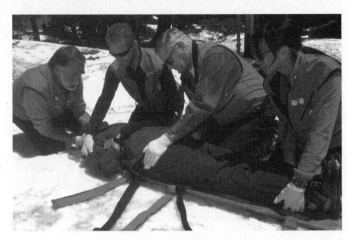

_____

_____ the patient on the board.

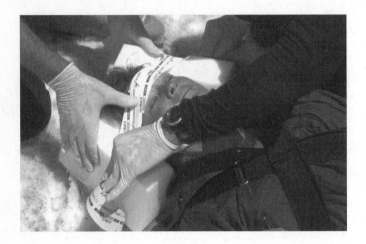

_____

Place _____ across the patient's forehead.

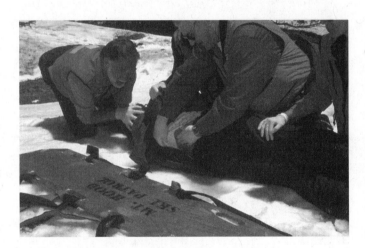

_____

On command, rescuers _____ the patient toward themselves, quickly examine the _____, slide the backboard under the patient, and roll the patient onto the board.

(continued)

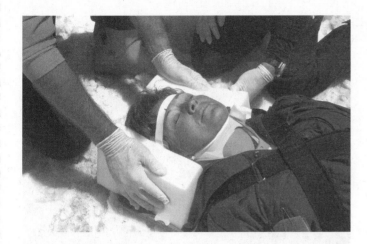

_____

Begin to secure the patient's head using a commercial immobilization device, _____ _____, and/or _____ _____.

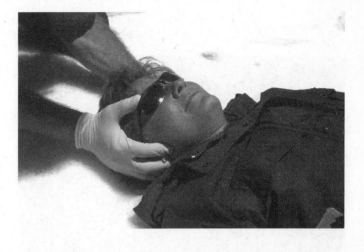

_____

Apply and maintain _____ _____.
Assess _____ _____ in all extremities.

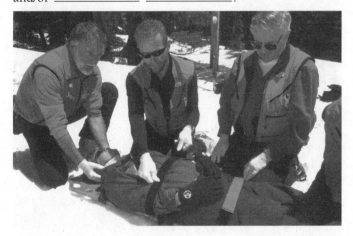

_____

Secure the _____, _____, and _____.

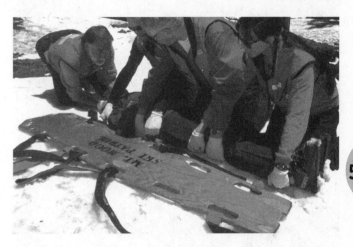

_____

Rescuers _____ on one side of the patient and place _____ on the far side of the patient.

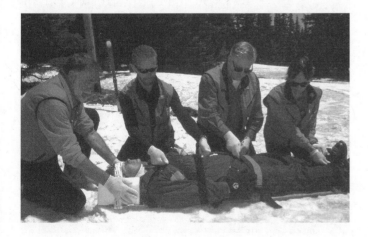

_____

Check all _____ and readjust as needed.
Reassess _____ _____ in all extremities.

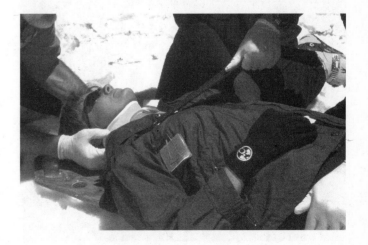

_____

Secure the _____ _____ first.

5

Skill Drill 26-3: Immobilizing a Patient Found in a Standing Position
Test your knowledge of this skill drill by filling in the correct words in the photo captions.

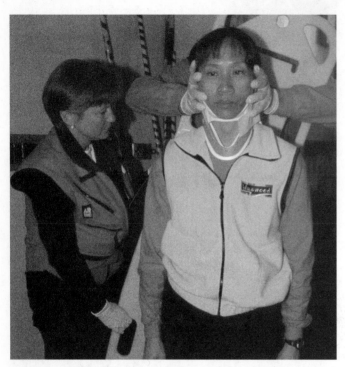

1. After _____ stabilizing the head and neck, apply a _____ _____. Position the board _____ the patient.

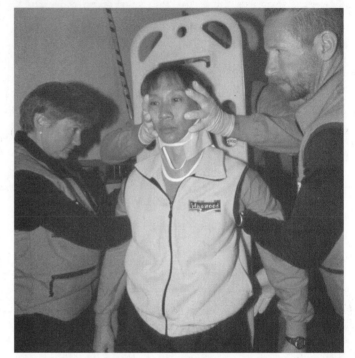

2. Position rescuers at _____ and _____ the patient. Side rescuers reach under patient's _____ and grasp _____ at or slightly above _____ level.

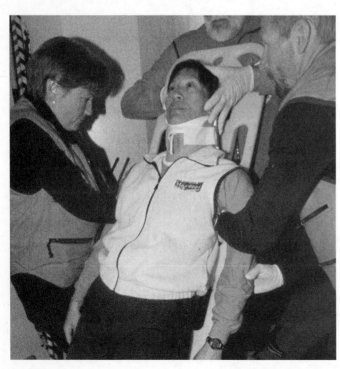

3. Prepare to lower the patient. Rescuers on the sides should be _____ the rescuer at the head and _____ for his or her _____.

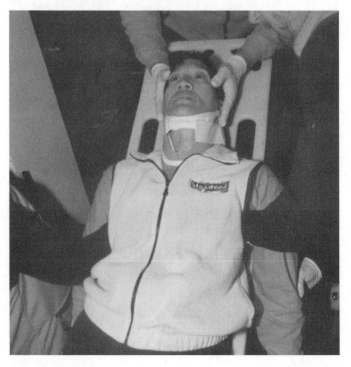

4. On command, _____ the backboard to the ground.

Skill Drill 26-4: Application of a Cervical Collar

Test your knowledge of this skill drill by filling in the correct words in the photo captions.

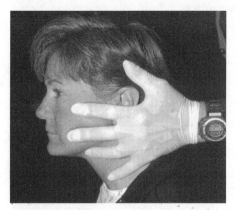

1. Apply _____ stabilization.

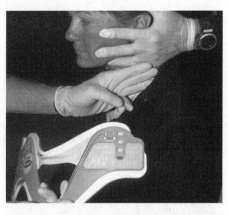

2. Measure the proper _____ _____.

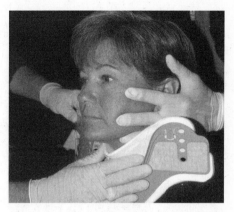

3. Place the _____ _____ first.

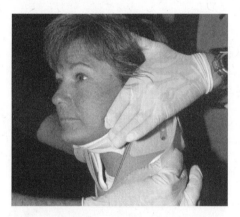

4. _____ the collar around the neck and _____ the collar.

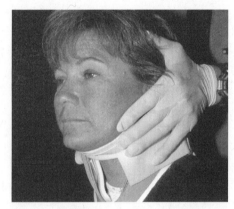

5. Ensure proper _____ and maintain _____, _____ stabilization.

5

Skill Drill 26-5: Removing a Helmet
Test your knowledge of this skill drill by placing the photos below in the correct order. Number the first step with a "1," the second step with a "2," etc. Also, fill in the correct words in the photo captions.

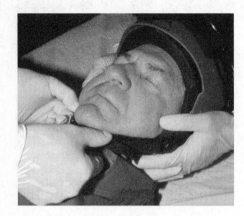

_____

Prevent head movement by placing your _____ on either side of the helmet and fingers on the _____ _____ . Have another rescuer _____ the strap.

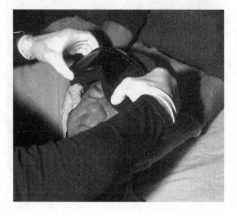

_____

Kneel down at the patient's head with another _____ at one side. Open the face shield to assess _____ and _____ . Remove _____ or goggles if present.

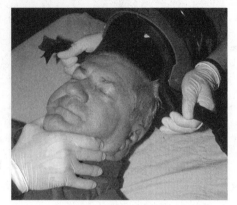

_____

Have another rescuer slide his or her hand from the _____ of the patient's head and cervical spine to the _____ of the head to prevent it from snapping back.

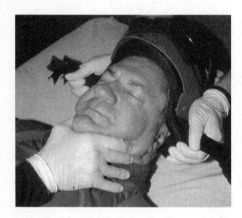

_____

Gently slip the helmet about _____ off, then stop.

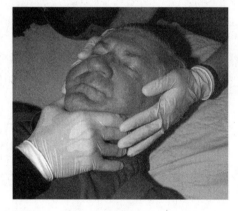

_____

Remove the helmet and _____ the cervical spine. Apply a _____ _____ and secure the patient to a _____ _____ . _____ as needed to prevent neck flexion or extension.

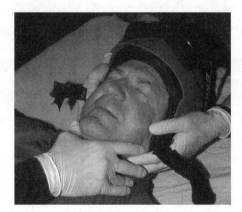

_____

Have another rescuer place one hand at the _____ of the _____ _____ and the other at the _____ of the head and cervical spine.

Notes

Workbook Activities

The following activities have been designed to help you. Your instructor may require you to complete some or all of these activities as a regular part of your OEC training program. You are encouraged to complete any activity that your instructor does not assign as a way to enhance your learning in the classroom.

Chapter Review

The following exercises provide an opportunity to refresh your knowledge of this chapter.

■ NOTES ■

Matching

Match each of the terms in the left column to the appropriate definition in the right column.

_____ 1. Extremity lift   **A.** separates into two or four pieces

_____ 2. Flexible stretcher   **B.** tubular framed stretcher with rigid fabric stretched across it

_____ 3. Stair chair   **C.** used for patients without a spinal injury who are supine

_____ 4. Basket stretcher   **D.** specifically designed stretcher that can be rolled along the ground

_____ 5. Scoop stretcher   **E.** used to carry patients across uneven terrain

_____ 6. Backboard   **F.** used for patients who are found lying supine with no suspected spinal injury

_____ 7. Direct ground lift   **G.** can be folded or rolled up

_____ 8. Portable stretcher   **H.** used to carry patients up and down stairs

_____ 9. Wheeled ambulance stretcher   **I.** spine board or longboard

Multiple Choice

Read each item carefully, then select the best response.

_____ 1. _____ safety depends on the use of proper lifting techniques and maintaining a proper hold when lifting or carrying a patient.

    A. Your

    B. Your team's

    C. The patient's

    D. all of the above

Rescue Techniques: Lifts and Loads

_____ 2. You should perform an urgent move:

    A. if a patient has an altered level of consciousness.

    B. if a patient has inadequate ventilation or shock.

    C. in extreme weather conditions.

    D. all of the above

_____ 3. The _____ is the mechanical weight-bearing base of the spinal column and the fused central posterior section of the pelvic girdle.

    A. coccyx

    B. sacrum

    C. lumbar region

    D. thorax

_____ 4. You may injure your back if you lift with your:

    A. back curved.

    B. back straight, but bent significantly forward at the hips.

    C. back straight, but arms extended away from the body.

    D. all of the above

_____ 5. When lifting, you should:

    A. spread your legs shoulder width apart.

    B. never lift a patient while reaching any significant distance in front of your torso.

    C. keep the weight that you are lifting as close to your body as possible.

    D. all of the above

_____ 6. When lifting a patient to a cot, be sure:

    A. to flex at the hips.

    B. to bend at the knees.

    C. that you do not hyperextend your back.

    D. all of the above

_____ **7.** A backboard is a device that provides support to patients who you suspect have:

   A. hip injuries.

   B. pelvic injuries.

   C. spinal injuries.

   D. all of the above

_____ **8.** The team leader should do all of the following except _____ before any lifting is initiated.

   A. give a command of execution

   B. indicate where each team member is to be located

   C. rapidly describe the sequence of steps that will be performed

   D. give a brief overview of the stages

_____ **9.** To move a patient that weighs more than 250 lb will require special:

   A. techniques.

   B. equipment.

   C. resources.

   D. all of the above

_____ **10.** When carrying a patient in a stair chair, always remember to:

   A. keep your back in a locked-in position.

   B. flex at the hips, not at the waist.

   C. keep the patient's weight and your arms as close to your body as possible.

   D. all of the above

_____ **11.** When you use a body drag to move a patient, you should:

   A. make sure your back is locked and straight.

   B. avoid any twisting so that the vertebrae remain in normal alignment.

   C. avoid hyperextending.

   D. all of above

_____ **12.** When pulling a patient, you should do all of the following, except:

   A. extend your arms no more than about 15" to 20".

   B. reposition your feet so that the force of pull will be balanced equally.

   C. when you can pull no farther, lean forward another 15" to 20".

   D. pull the patient by slowly flexing your arms.

_____ **13.** When log rolling a patient, you should:

   A. kneel as close to the patient's side as possible.

   B. lean solely from the hips.

   C. use your shoulder muscles to help with the roll.

   D. all of the above

_____ **14.** If the weight you are pulling is lower than your waist, you should pull from:

   A. the waist.

   B. a kneeling position.

   C. the shoulder.

   D. a squatting position.

_____ **15.** Situations in which you should use an emergency move include those in which:

    A. there is the presence of fire, explosives, or hazardous materials.

    B. you are unable to protect the patient from other hazards.

    C. you are unable to gain access to others in a vehicle who need lifesaving care.

    D. all of the above

_____ **16.** You should use a one-person technique to move a patient only:

    A. if a potentially life-threatening danger exists and you are alone.

    B. because of the pressing nature of the danger.

    C. if your partner is moving a second patient.

    D. all of the above

_____ **17.** You can move a patient on his or her back along the floor or ground by using all of the following methods except:

    A. pulling on the patient's clothing in the neck and shoulder area.

    B. placing the patient on a blanket, coat, or other item that can be pulled.

    C. pulling the patient by the legs if they are the most accessible part.

    D. placing your arms under the patient's shoulders and through the armpits, while grasping the patient's arms, dragging the patient backward.

_____ **18.** An urgent move may be necessary for moving a patient with:

    A. an altered level of consciousness.

    B. inadequate ventilation.

    C. shock.

    D. all of the above

_____ **19.** In which of the following situations should you use the rapid extrication technique?

    A. The vehicle on the scene is unsafe.

    B. The patient's condition cannot be properly assessed before being removed from the car.

    C. The patient blocks access to another seriously injured patient.

    D. all of the above

_____ **20.** Before you attempt any move, the team leader must be sure that:

    A. there are enough personnel and that the proper equipment is available.

    B. any obstacles have been identified or removed.

    C. the procedure and path to be followed have been clearly identified and discussed.

    D. all of the above

_____ **21.** To avoid the strain of unnecessary lifting and carrying, you should use _____ or assist an able patient to the cot whenever possible.

    A. the direct ground lift

    B. the extremity lift

    C. the draw sheet method

    D. a scoop stretcher

6

_____22. To move a patient from the ground or the floor onto the cot, you should:

   A. lift and carry the patient to the nearby prepared cot using a direct body carry.

   B. use a scoop stretcher.

   C. use a log roll or long-axis drag to place the patient onto a backboard, and then lift and carry the backboard to the cot.

   D. all of the above

_____23. The _____ is the most uncomfortable of all the various devices; however, it provides excellent support and immobilization.

   A. portable stretcher

   B. flexible stretcher

   C. wooden backboard

   D. scoop stretcher

_____24. If _____ are used, you must follow infection control procedures before you can reuse the backboards.

   A. plastic backboards

   B. wooden backboards

   C. metal backboards

   D. all of the above

_____25. You should use a rigid _____, often called a Stokes litter, to carry a patient across uneven terrain from a remote location that is inaccessible by ambulance or other vehicle.

   A. basket stretcher

   B. scoop stretcher

   C. molded backboard

   D. flotation device

_____26. Basket stretchers can be used:

   A. for technical rope rescues and some water rescues.

   B. to carry a patient across fields on an all-terrain vehicle.

   C. to carry a patient on a toboggan.

   D. all of the above

_____27. Every time you have to move a patient, you must take special care that _____ are (is) not injured.

   A. you

   B. your team

   C. the patient

   D. all of the above

_____28. Certain patient conditions, such as _____, call for special lifting and moving techniques.

   A. head or spinal injury

   B. shock

   C. pregnancy

   D. all of the above

Vocabulary

Define the following terms using the space provided.

1. Jams and pretzels:

_____

_____

_____

2. Log roll:

_____

_____

_____

3. Bridge lift:

_____

_____

_____

4. Power lift:

_____

_____

_____

5. Emergency move:

_____

_____

_____

6

Fill-in

Read each item carefully, then complete the statement by filling in the missing word.

1. To avoid injury to you, the patient, or your partners, you will have to learn how to

   lift and carry the patient properly, using proper _____ and a power grip.

2. The key rule of lifting is to always keep the back in a straight, _____
   position and to lift without twisting.

3. The safest and most powerful way to lift, lifting by extending the properly placed

   flexed legs, is called a _____.

4. The arm and hand have their greatest lifting strength when facing

   _____ up.

5. Be sure to pick up and carry the backboard with your back in the

   _____ position.

6. You should not attempt to lift a patient who weighs more than _____
   lb with fewer than four rescuers, regardless of individual strength.

7. During a body drag where you and your partner are on each side of the patient,
   you will have to alter the usual pulling technique to prevent pulling

   _____ and producing adverse lateral leverage against your lower back.

8. Be careful that you do not push or pull from a(n) _____ position.

9. Remember to always consider whether there is an option that will cause

   _____ _____ to you and the other rescuers.

10. The manual support and immobilization that you provide when using the rapid

    extrication technique produce a greater risk of _____.

11. The _____ is used for patients with no suspected spinal injury who

    are found lying supine on the ground.

12. The _____ may be especially helpful when the patient is in a very
    narrow space or there is not enough room for the patient and a team of rescuers
    to stand side by side.

13. A _____ may be a useful device to transfer a patient.

True/False

If you believe the statement to be more true than false, write the letter "T" in the space provided. If you believe the statement to be more false than true, write the letter "F."

1. _____ Patient packaging and handling are technical skills you will learn and perfect through practice and training.

2. _____ A portable stretcher is typically a lightweight folding device that does not have the undercarriage and wheels of a true ambulance stretcher.

3. _____ The term "power lift" refers to a posture that is safe and helpful for rescuers when they are lifting.

4. _____ If you find that lifting a patient is a strain, try to move to the ambulance as quickly as possible to minimize the possibility of back injury.

5. _____ The use of adjunct devices and equipment, such as sheets and blankets, may make the job of lifting and moving a patient more difficult.

6. _____ One-person techniques for moving patients should only be used when immediate patient movement is necessary due to a life-threatening hazard and only one rescuer is available.

7. _____ A scoop stretcher may be used alone for a standard immobilization of a patient with a spinal injury.

8. _____ When carrying a patient down stairs or on an incline, make sure the stretcher is carried with the head end first.

9. _____ The rapid extrication technique is the preferred technique to use on all sitting patients with possible spinal injuries.

10. _____ It is unprofessional for you to discuss and plan a lift at the scene in front of the patient.

Short Answer

Complete this section with short written answers using the space provided.

1. List the one-rescuer drags, carries, and lifts.

_____

_____

_____

2. List the situations in which the rapid extrication technique is used.

_____

_____

_____

3. List the guidelines to safely lift a patient onto a device.

_____

_____

_____

_____

_____

6

4. Describe the key rule of lifting.

_____

_____

_____

5. Describe the general positioning guidelines for loading a patient into a toboggan.

_____

_____

_____

Word Fun www.OECzone.com vocab explorer

The following crossword puzzle is an activity provided to reinforce correct spelling and understanding of medical terminology associated with emergency care. Use the clues in the column to complete the puzzle.

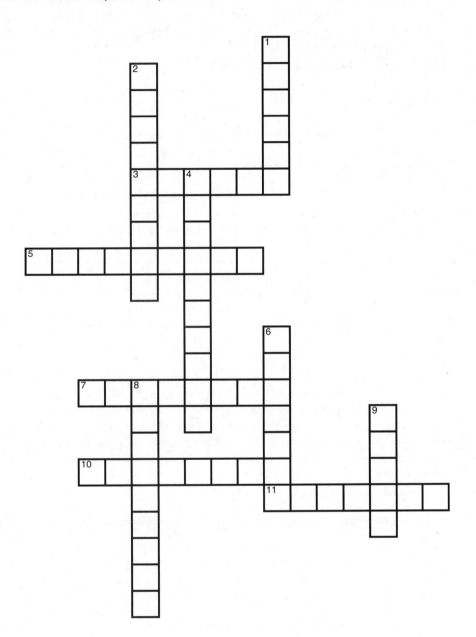

◼◼◼◼ C L U E S ◼◼◼◼

Across

3. Stretcher used with technical rescues, particularly when water is involved

5. Safest way to lift

7. Stretcher that becomes rigid when secured around patient

10. Tubular framed stretcher with fabric across

11. Four-rescuer carry with one at the head, one at the foot, and one on each side

Down

1. A ground lift used with patients with no suspected spinal injury

2. Used to support a patient with a hip, pelvic, or spine injury

4. Folding device for moving seated patients up or down floors

6. Stretcher designed to roll along the ground

8. Using the patient's limbs to lift

9. Stretcher that can be split into two or four sections

6

Calls to the Scene

The following case scenarios provide an opportunity to explore the concerns associated with patient management. Read each scenario, then answer each question in detail.

1. You are dispatched to a site for a 26-year-old man who fell into a ravine. He is approximately 35' down a rocky ledge. He is alert with an unstable pelvis and weak radial pulses. You have all the help you need from the rescue crew and the volunteer fire department.

   How would you best manage this patient?

   _____

   _____

   _____

   _____

   _____

   _____

   _____

   _____

2. You are working at a head-on snowmobile/snowcat crash where you have a patient in critical condition. As your partner works with the driver in the snowcat, you assess the driver of the snowmobile. He is a 58-year-old man with weak radial pulses and a respiratory rate of 4 breaths/min. No other help has arrived on the scene and your partner is equally busy with his patient. You cannot effectively ventilate the patient where he is seated. More rescuers are en route to your location.

   How would you best manage this patient?

   _____

   _____

   _____

   _____

   _____

   _____

   _____

   _____

3. You are working a mountain bike race and see a mountain bike crash. The patient, a 34-year-old female, is lying face down, responds to pain, and has absent radial pulses. She is breathing shallowly at a rate of 10 breaths/min. Race officials have called for backup assistance.

How would you best manage this patient?

_____

_____

_____

_____

_____

_____

_____

_____

Skill Drills

Skill Drill 27-1: Log Roll

Test your knowledge of this skill drill by placing the photos below in the correct order. Number the first step with a "1," the second step with a "2," etc.

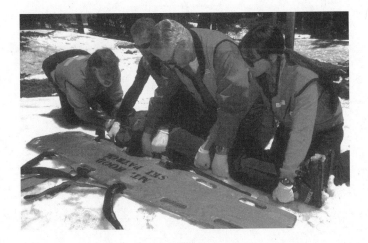

_____

Position sufficient rescuers on the side of the patient, kneeling as close to the patient's side as possible. Position hands on the far side, taking body mass into consideration. Keep your back straight and lean solely from the hips. Overlap hands if possible.

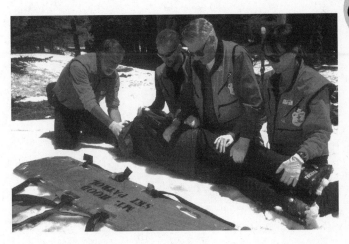

_____

Roll the patient as a unit toward the rescuers on command from the leader (at the head), keeping the body in line and while monitoring vital signs. The patient's arm may be alongside the body or elevated, depending on local protocols.

(continued)

6

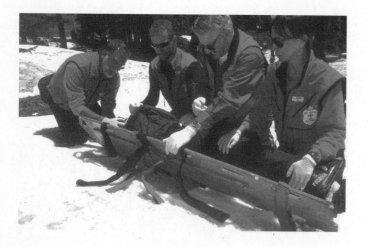

When using a backboard, bring the device as close as practical to the patient's back.

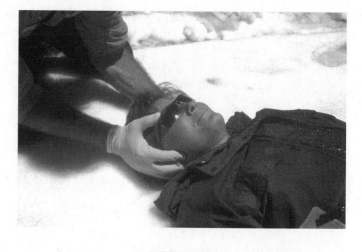

Manually stabilize the head and neck.

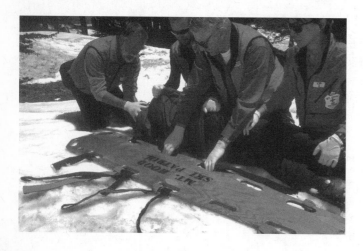

Place the backboard, blanket, or stretcher alongside the patient and underneath as far as possible without excessive movement.

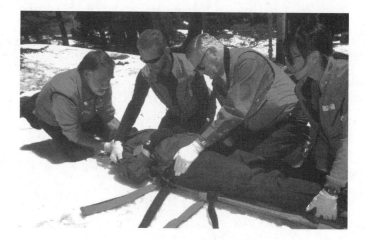

Roll the patient onto the device on command from the leader, keeping the body in line.

Skill Drill 27-2: Performing the Power Lift
Test your knowledge of this skill drill by filling in the correct words in the photo captions.

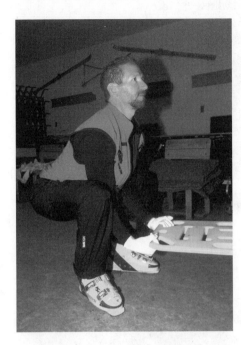

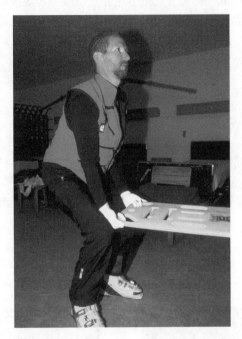

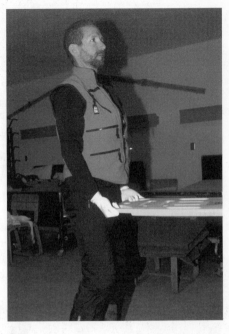

1. Lock your back into a(n) _____, slightly inward curve. _____ and bend your legs. Grasp the backboard, palms up and just in front of you. _____ and _____ the weight between your arms.

2. Position your feet, _____ the object, and _____ weight.

3. _____ your legs and lift, keeping your back locked in.

6

Skill Drill 27-3: The Bridge Lift

Test your knowledge of this skill drill by placing the photos below in the correct order. Number the first step with a "1," the second step with a "2," etc.

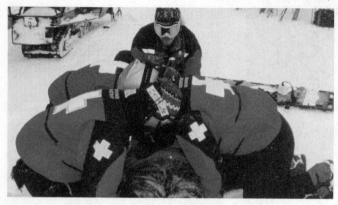

_____

Position the rescuers and have them form a bridge over the patient, head-to-shoulder or shoulder-to-shoulder. All rescuers must use the same configuration.

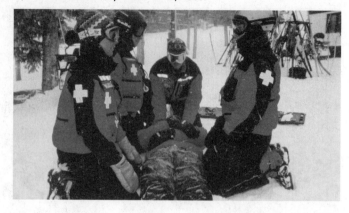

_____

With five rescuers, the first rescuer is at the head, rescuers 2 and 3 are at one side, and rescuers 4 and 5 are at the other side.

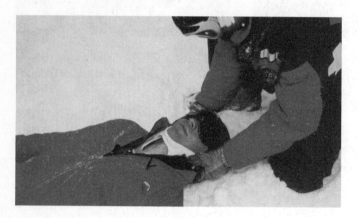

_____

Manually stabilize the head and neck.

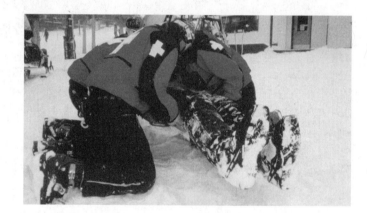

_____

Position hands underneath the patient to lift at points of body mass and ensure the rescuer's commitment and distribution across the bridge. Lift the patient just enough to place a backboard underneath.

Skill Drill 27-4: Direct Ground Lift
Test your knowledge of this skill drill by filling in the correct words in the photo captions.

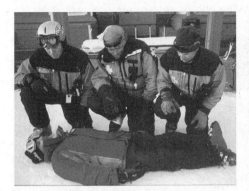

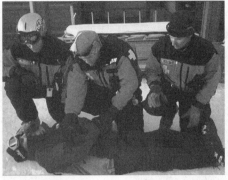

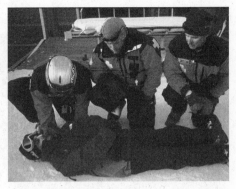

1. Line up on one side of the patient with rescuer 1 at the patient's _____, rescuer 2 at the patient's _____, and rescuer 3 at the patient's _____. All rescuers kneel on one knee, preferably the same knee.

2. The patient's arms should be placed on his or her _____, if possible.

3. Rescuer 1 then places the other arm under the patient's _____.

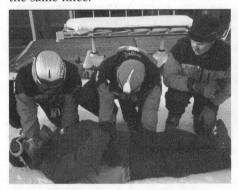

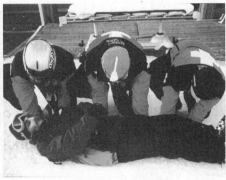

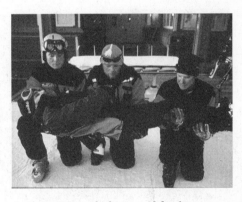

4. Rescuer 2 places both arms under the patient's _____ _____ and _____.

5. Rescuer 3 places both arms under the patient's _____.

6. On command, the team lifts the patient up to _____ _____ as each rescuer _____ an arm on his or her knee.

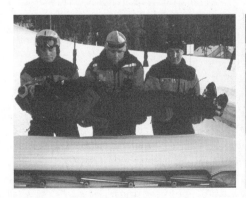

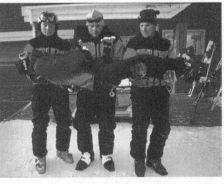

7. As a team and on _____, each rescuer _____ the patient in toward his or her chest. Again on _____, the team stands and carries the patient to the carrying or transportation device.

8. The steps are _____ to lower the patient onto the carrying or transportation device.

6

■ NOTES ■

Skill Drill 27-6: Lifting a Patient into a Toboggan or other Transportation Device

Test your knowledge of this skill drill by placing the photos below in the correct order. Number the first step with a "1," the second step with a "2," etc.

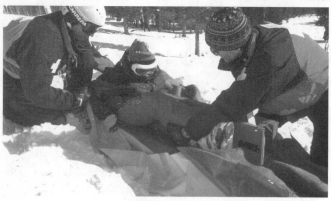

_____

Ensure that the patient clears the side of the device.

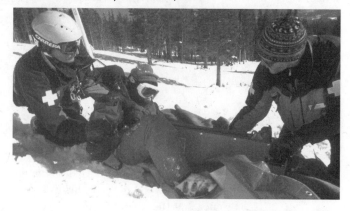

_____

Ensure all rescuers are in appropriate position.

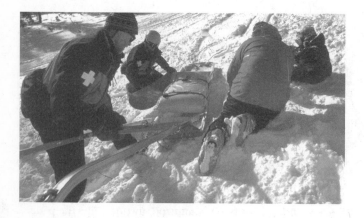

_____

Position the toboggan and all of the other equipment.

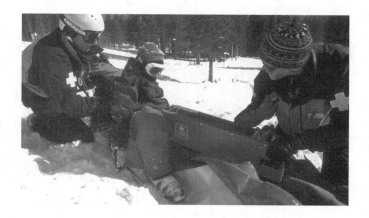

_____

Perform the lift smoothly without compromising the injury.

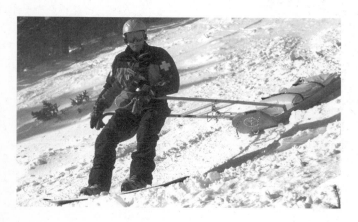

_____

Assess the factors:
   a. Position of the patient in the toboggan
   b. Nature and extent of the injury
   c. Patient responsive/unresponsive
   d. Patient mobility—ability to assist
   e. Number of people able to assist
   f. Terrain (steep or flat)
   g. Conditions (hard/soft; poor footing)
   h. Type of transportation device (with/without basket; height of edges)

Notes

6

Workbook Activities

The following activities have been designed to help you. Your instructor may require you to complete some or all of these activities as a regular part of your OEC training program. You are encouraged to complete any activity that your instructor does not assign as a way to enhance your learning in the classroom.

Chapter Review

The following exercises provide an opportunity to refresh your knowledge of this chapter.

■ NOTES ■

Matching

Match each of the priority terms in the right column to the appropriate triage injury in the left column.

_____ **1.** A middle-aged woman who is screaming hysterically. She has a large lump on her forehead and a fractured wrist. Her respirations and capillary refill are normal; she tells you that she hurt her head and wrist when the gondola fell.

_____ **2.** A middle-aged man who is lying in the gondola wreckage, unresponsive, breathing normally, frowning, and spontaneously moving all four extremities. His capillary refill time is 1 second.

_____ **3.** An elderly man with an obvious crushed chest. He has no detectable pulse and is not breathing.

_____ **4.** A young woman who is lying quietly. Her skin is pale, cold, and clammy, her pulse is fast, her respirations are rapid and shallow, and her capillary refill time is delayed. She complains weakly of abdominal pain.

_____ **5.** An obnoxious, middle-aged man who is yelling, cursing, and threatening to sue the ski area. He does not appear to be hurt.

_____ **6.** A young man who is lying quietly on his side, complaining of pain in the back between the shoulder blades. He says that he cannot move his legs. His breathing and capillary refill time seem normal.

Priority Terms
A. Red
B. Yellow
C. Green
D. Black

Triage

_____ **7.** An elderly woman who appears basically healthy and vigorous for her age. She is in respiratory distress and is complaining of chest pain. A brief inspection of the site of pain discloses a flail segment of her chest wall.

_____ **8.** A middle-aged woman who seems calm and does not appear to be injured.

Multiple Choice

Read each item carefully, then select the best response.

_____ **1.** The _____ defines the average amount of time that elapses before a patient with serious or multiple injuries starts to deteriorate rapidly.

    A. assessment period

    B. Golden Hour

    C. transportation period

    D. recovery period

_____ **2.** Patients with upper airway obstruction or chest wounds with respiratory distress fit into which triage priority color code?

    A. Red

    B. Yellow

    C. Green

    D. Black

_____ **3.** Patients with closed fractures or minor burns fit into which triage priority color code?

    A. Red

    B. Yellow

    C. Green

    D. Black

_____ **4.** Patients with cardiac arrest or obvious lethal injuries fit into which triage priority color code?

A. Red

B. Yellow

C. Green

D. Black

_____ **5.** Patients with progressing head injuries or major bleeding fit into which triage priority color code?

A. Red

B. Yellow

C. Green

D. Black

_____ **6.** Patients with localized soft-tissue injuries or closed fractures fit into which triage priority color code?

A. Red

B. Yellow

C. Green

D. Black

_____ **7.** Patients with injuries that are not a risk to life and may be able to wait for several hours before transport fit into which triage color code?

A. Red

B. Yellow

C. Green

D. Black

_____ **8.** Patients whose vital signs are absent fit into which triage color code?

A. Red

B. Yellow

C. Green

D. Black

_____ **9.** In the initial assessment process you ask, "Are you okay?" What do you say in triage assessment?

A. Are you okay?

B. Get up and walk.

C. May I help you?

D. It's time to move.

_____ **10.** During triage assessment, how long do you spend with each patient until you have seen them all?

A. 2 to 3 minutes per patient

B. 1 minute per patient

C. 45 seconds per patient

D. 15 to 30 seconds per patient

_____ **11.** Which of the following correctly states the highest to lowest priority for treating a single patient?

A. severe head injury, back injury, fractured leg

B. major multiple fractures, cardiac arrest, uncontrolled bleeding

C. fractured hip, severe shock, open abdominal wound

D. burns, diabetic coma, breathing difficulty

_____ **12.** What is the purpose of triage?

   A. to decide who will live or die

   B. to sort patients for treatment and transport

   C. to assign the proper rescuer to each patient

   D. to determine the injuries of each patient

_____ **13.** In a situation with multiple patients, which of the following injuries would have the highest priority for emergency care?

   A. dislocated shoulder

   B. open fracture

   C. decapitation

   D. breathing difficulty

_____ **14.** Safety of _____ must be your most important concern.

   A. you and your team

   B. the other responders

   C. the public

   D. all of the above

_____ **15.** When dealing with multiple patients, you should locate and rapidly _____ each patient.

   A. treat

   B. triage

   C. transport

   D. extricate

For the remainder of the multiple-choice section, the following answers are to be applied:

   A. First priority (red)

   B. Second priority (yellow)

   C. Third priority (green)

   D. Fourth priority (black)

Classify the following emergencies according to triage priority:

16. Shock _____

17. Major or multiple bone or joint injuries _____

18. Cardiac arrest _____

19. Minor fractures _____

20. Decreased level of consciousness _____

21. Obvious death _____

22. Airway and breathing difficulties _____

23. Burns without airway problems _____

24. Major open brain trauma _____

25. Minor soft-tissue injuries _____

Vocabulary

www.OECzone
vocab explorer

Define the following terms using the space provided.

   1. Mass-casualty incident:

   _____

   _____

   _____

6

2. Extrication:

_____

_____

_____

3. Secondary triage:

_____

_____

_____

4. Triage:

_____

_____

_____

5. Golden Hour:

_____

_____

_____

Fill-in

Fill in the blanks on the following table comparing triage assessment with standard assessment.

Initial Assessment	Triage Assessment (START)
1. Form general impression of the patients; Assess Mental Status	1.
2.	2. Respirations – open airway, tag
3. B-Assess Breathing – Provide rescue breathing, oxygen	3.
4. C-Assess Circulation – Take pulse, control external bleeding, evaluate skin color, temperature, and condition	4.

True/False

If you believe the statement to be more true than false, write the letter "T" in the space provided. If you believe the statement to be more false than true, write the letter "F."

1. _____ A person with altered mental status should be tagged with yellow ribbon.

2. _____ A person with no respirations should be tagged with a black ribbon.

3. _____ For every half hour after the first hour, the patient's chances of survival are cut in half.

4. _____ Highest priority triage patients have injuries to their nervous and skeletal systems.

5. _____ The yellow triage category includes those who appear able to wait for 45 minutes or longer before being transported to a hospital.

6. _____ In a triage situation, it is perfectly acceptable to ask those who can walk to do so without checking them first.

7. _____ In a patient with multiple injuries, triage refers to the proper order in which to treat each injury.

8. _____ Doing the greatest good for the greatest number is the principle behind triage.

Short Answer

Complete this section with short written answers using the space provided.

1. In the outdoor triage situation, which patients are provided the highest priority of care?

_____

_____

_____

2. Explain the steps and decisions used in the START triage plan.

_____

_____

_____

3. Explain the purpose of secondary triage.

_____

_____

_____

4. Identify situations that might require a variation in the standard triage process, ie, assigning a higher priority than the injury might otherwise warrant.

_____

_____

_____

6

Across

2. Simple triage and rapid treatment system of primary triage
5. Patients whose treatment and transportation can be delayed until last
6. Amount of time before a patient deteriorates rapidly
7. Used to rapidly identify a patient's priority for treatment and transport
8. Removal from a trapped area
9. Process of sorting patients by severity of injury

Down

1. Large-scale emergency situation involving more than one patient
3. In-depth assessment of patient's triage category
4. Patients whose treatment and transportation can be temporarily delayed

Word Fun www.OECzone.com vocab explorer

The following crossword puzzle is an activity provided to reinforce correct spelling and understanding of medical terminology associated with emergency care. Use the clues in the column to complete the puzzle.

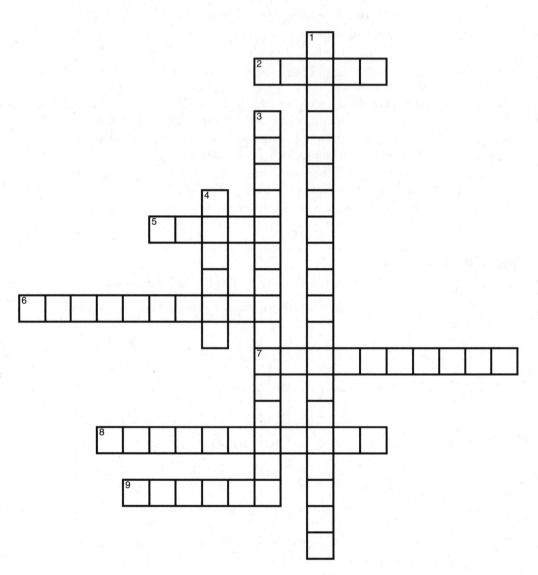

Calls to the Scene

The following case scenarios provide an opportunity to explore the concerns associated with patient management. Read each scenario, then answer each question in detail.

1. There is a small avalanche in which five skiers are found alive and breathing.

   #1 is unresponsive and has a crushed chest.

   #2 is responsive and has a dislocated hip and a scalp laceration.

   #3 is unresponsive with a bruise on his head.

   #4 is responsive and has a broken jaw, facial abrasions, and a broken clavicle.

   #5 is responsive and has a broken wrist.

   Three patrollers and two toboggans are available. How should you proceed with the injured skiers and in what order?

   _____

   _____

   _____

   _____

   _____

   _____

   _____

   _____

   _____

   _____

2. In the late afternoon on a warm spring day, a deck attached to the base lodge collapses. Twenty guests fall 15' to the ground. Your initial triage reveals that one person is pulseless and apneic, ten people are "walking wounded," six have serious injuries, and three have life-threatening injuries. Five minutes after the incident, two other rescuers join you at the site.

   Please include the answers to the following questions in your response.

   What BSI precautions are appropriate in this circumstance?

   Is oxygen administration appropriate?

   Explain the emergency care steps you would take in the order you would take them in handling this situation.

   What common problems and complications might develop?

   Describe the transportation decisions you would make.

   What documentation is needed for this situation and why?

   _____

   _____

6

_____

_____

_____

_____

_____

_____

_____

_____

_____

_____

3. You witness a multi-vehicle crash and pull over. You encounter three patients: a 4-year-old boy with bilateral femur fractures and absent radial pulse, a 27-year-old woman with a laceration to the head and a humerus fracture, and a 42-year-old man who is apneic and pulseless with an open skull fracture.

How should you triage these patients?

_____

_____

_____

_____

_____

_____

_____

_____

_____

_____

Notes

Workbook Activities

The following activities have been designed to help you. Your instructor may require you to complete some or all of these activities as a regular part of your OEC training program. You are encouraged to complete any activity that your instructor does not assign as a way to enhance your learning in the classroom.

Chapter Review

The following exercises provide an opportunity to refresh your knowledge of this chapter.

NOTES

Matching

Match each of the terms in the left column to the appropriate definition in the right column.

_____ **1.** Incident command system

_____ **2.** Casualty collection area

_____ **3.** Disaster

_____ **4.** Rehabilitation area

_____ **5.** Transportation area

_____ **6.** Treatment officer

A. area where patients can receive further triage and medical care

B. individual who is in charge of and directs EMS personnel at the treatment area

C. provides protection and treatment to firefighters and other personnel working at an emergency

D. area where ambulances and crews are organized

E. widespread event that disrupts community resources and functions

F. an organizational system to help control, direct, and coordinate emergency responders and resources; known more generally as an incident management system (IMS)

Multiple Choice

Read each item carefully, then select the best response.

_____ **1.** Functions normally centered at the command post include:

A. information.

B. safety.

C. liaison with other agencies and groups who are responding.

D. all of the above

Mass-Casualty Incident Management

_____ **2.** In extended operations, the typical incident command structure may have multiple sectors including:

A. operations.

B. planning.

C. logistics.

D. all of the above

_____ **3.** The _____ is a holding area for arriving ambulances and crews until they can be assigned a particular task.

A. staging area

B. treatment area

C. transportation area

D. rehabilitation area

_____ **4.** The _____ provides protection and treatment to firefighters and other personnel working at the emergency scene.

A. staging area

B. treatment area

C. transportation area

D. rehabilitation area

_____ **5.** The _____ is where ambulances and crews are organized to transport patients from the treatment area to local hospitals.

A. staging area

B. treatment area

C. transportation area

D. rehabilitation area

_____ **6.** As patients are loaded into the ambulance, the transport officer logs:

A. each patient's mass-casualty tag number.

B. each patient's overall condition.

C. the hospital to which they will be taken.

D. all of the above

_____ **7.** The _____ is where a more thorough assessment is made and on-scene treatment is begun while transport is being arranged.

    A. staging area

    B. treatment area

    C. transportation area

    D. rehabilitation area

_____ **8.** Examples of mass-casualty incidents include:

    A. airplane crashes.

    B. earthquakes.

    C. railroad crashes.

    D. all of the above

Vocabulary www.OECzone.com vocab explorer

Define the following terms using the space provided.

1. Command post:

_____

_____

_____

2. Casualty collection area:

_____

_____

_____

3. Triage officer:

_____

_____

_____

4. Incident commander:

_____

_____

_____

Fill-in

Read each item carefully, then complete the statement by filling in the missing word(s).

1. The _____ is more effective when used to organize large numbers of personnel at complex incidents such as hazardous materials spills and mass-casualty incidents.

2. The incident commander usually remains at a _____, the designated field command center.

3. The _____ is responsible for protecting all personnel and any victims of the incident.

4. A _____ is a widespread event that disrupts functions and resources of a community and threatens lives and property.

5. _____ is the sorting of patients based on the severity of their conditions to establish priorities for care based on available resources.

True/False

If you believe the statement to be more true than false, write the letter "T" in the space provided. If you believe the statement to be more false than true, write the letter "F."

1. _____   A team leader must be identified and agreed to before you arrive at the scene.

2. _____   An emergency operations plan is designed only for the local area.

3. _____   A technical rescue team is made up of OEC technicians.

4. _____   Not all positions in an incident command structure must be filled for every incident.

Short Answer

Complete this section with short written answers using the space provided.

1. List the key components of a mass-casualty incident.

_____

_____

_____

_____

_____

2. Describe an extrication area.

_____

_____

_____

_____

3. What is the role of a rescuer in a disaster?

_____

_____

6

Across

3. Zone for loading and moving of patients to definitive care

5. Person responsible for overall incident management

6. Important component of emergency operations plan

7. Incident command shared by various agencies

8. Widespread event that disrupts community resources and functions

9. Person responsible for protection against unseen hazards

Down

1. ICS

2. Designated field command center

3. Person responsible for sorting of patients

4. Avalanche rescue, climbing rescue, white-water rescue, etc.

Word Fun

www.OECzone.com
vocab explorer

The following crossword puzzle is an activity provided to reinforce correct spelling and understanding of medical terminology associated with emergency care. Use the clues in the column to complete the puzzle.

Calls to the Scene

The following case scenario will give you an opportunity to explore the concerns associated with patient management. Read the scenario, then answer the question in detail.

1. An avalanche has been reported just adjacent to your ski area boundary; however, it has come down into the area's parking lot and covered a number of vehicles. Your area has a written emergency operations plan.

   Identify specific concerns that involve immediate action decisions.

   _____

   _____

   _____

   _____

   _____

   _____

   _____

   _____

   _____

   _____

6

Workbook Activities

The following activities have been designed to help you. Your instructor may require you to complete some or all of these activities as a regular part of your OEC training program. You are encouraged to complete any activity that your instructor does not assign as a way to enhance your learning in the classroom.

Chapter Review

The following exercises provide an opportunity to refresh your knowledge of this chapter.

■ NOTES ■

Matching

Match each of the terms in the left column to the appropriate definition in the right column.

_____ **1.** Toddler

_____ **2.** Preschool-age children

_____ **3.** Adolescents

_____ **4.** Infancy

_____ **5.** Neonate

_____ **6.** Pediatrics

_____ **7.** Croup

_____ **8.** Wheezing

_____ **9.** Epiglottitis

_____ **10.** Rales

_____ **11.** Tonic-clonic movements

_____ **12.** Stridor

_____ **13.** Shock

_____ **14.** Apnea

_____ **15.** Febrile seizure

_____ **16.** Tripod position

_____ **17.** Child abuse

A. ages 12 to 18 years

B. ages 3 to 6 years

C. specialized medical practice devoted to the care of children

D. first month after birth

E. the first year of life

F. after infancy, until about age 3 years

G. leaning forward on two arms stretched forward

H. seizure relating to fever

I. rhythmic back and forth movement of an extremity with body stiffness

J. absence of breathing

K. infection of the airway below the level of the vocal chords

L. whistling sound made from air moving through narrowed bronchioles

M. infection of soft tissue in the area above the vocal chords

N. crackling sound caused by flow of air through liquid

O. insufficient blood to body organs

P. high-pitched sound caused by swelling around the vocal chords

Q. weak spots in the bone often injured as a result of trauma

Pediatric Outdoor Emergency Care

_____ **18.** Hyperventilation   **R.** improper or excessive action that injures or harms a child or infant

_____ **19.** Growth plates   **S.** rapid ventilation

Multiple Choice

Read each item carefully, then select the best response.

_____ **1.** In addition to the tongue, the _____ help(s) to produce a smaller opening to move air easily.

    A. tonsils

    B. adenoids

    C. soft pallet

    D. all of the above

_____ **2.** Anything that puts pressure on the abdomen of a young child can block the movement of the _____ and cause respiratory compromise.

    A. thorax

    B. air

    C. diaphragm

    D. lungs

_____ **3.** The primary method for the body to compensate for decreased oxygenation is to increase:

    A. the respiratory rate.

    B. the heart rate.

    C. the blood pressure.

    D. diaphragm contractions.

_____ **4.** Infants respond mainly to _____ stimuli.

    A. social

    B. mental

    C. physical

    D. all of the above

_____ **5.** As the work-of-breathing increases, you may see:

  A. faster breathing.

  B. retractions along the chest wall.

  C. the child sitting in a position to allow for more chest expansion.

  D. all of the above

_____ **6.** Anatomic differences between adults and children include all of the following except that the child's:

  A. heart is higher in the chest.

  B. lungs are smaller.

  C. opening to the trachea is lower in the neck.

  D. neck is shorter.

_____ **7.** Movement of the _____ dictates the amount of air a child can inspire.

  A. diaphragm

  B. ribs

  C. abdomen

  D. lungs

_____ **8.** Positioning the airway in a neutral sniffing position keeps the:

  A. trachea from kinking when the neck is hyperextended.

  B. trachea from kinking when the neck is flexed.

  C. neck in proper alignment if you have to immobilize the spine.

  D. all of the above

_____ **9.** Signs of complete airway obstruction include:

  A. inability to speak or cry.

  B. increasing respiratory difficulty, with stridor.

  C. cyanosis.

  D. all of the above

_____ **10.** Early signs of respiratory distress include all of the following except:

  A. combativeness.

  B. anxiety.

  C. cyanosis.

  D. restlessness.

_____ **11.** _____ is a continuous seizure, or multiple seizures without a return to consciousness, for 30 minutes or more.

  A. Status epilepticus

  B. Grand mal seizure

  C. Absence seizure

  D. Focal motor seizure

_____ **12.** Most pediatric seizures are due to _____, which is why they are called febrile seizures.

  A. infection

  B. fever

  C. ingestion

  D. trauma

_____ 13. Care of the actively seizing child includes all of the following except:

   A. assessing and managing the ABCs.

   B. noting the type of movement and position of the eyes.

   C. cooling the patient if there is fever.

   D. making sure the patient is protected from hitting anything.

_____ 14. _____ is an increase in body temperature caused by an inability of the body to cool itself.

   A. Fever

   B. Hyperthermia

   C. Hypothermia

   D. Thermoregulation

_____ 15. Common causes of shock in children include all of the following except:

   A. heart attack.

   B. head trauma.

   C. dehydration.

   D. pneumothorax.

_____ 16. Pediatric patients respond initially to fluid loss by:

   A. decreasing the heart rate.

   B. increasing respirations.

   C. showing signs of pink or red skin.

   D. decreasing blood pressure.

_____ 17. Life-threatening dehydration can overcome an infant in a matter of:

   A. minutes.

   B. hours.

   C. days.

   D. weeks.

_____ 18. Children differ from adults in that they have:

   A. less circulating blood volume.

   B. a larger body surface area in relation to body mass.

   C. more flexible and elastic bones.

   D. all of the above

_____ 19. When caring for children with sports-related injuries, you should remember to:

   A. elevate the extremities.

   B. assist ventilations.

   C. immobilize the cervical spine.

   D. remove all helmets.

_____ 20. Your single most important step in caring for a child with a head injury is to:

   A. immobilize the cervical spine.

   B. bandage all wounds.

   C. ensure an open airway.

   D. obtain a SAMPLE history.

_____ 21. Childrens' bones bend more easily than adults' bones and, as a result, incomplete or _____ fractures can occur.

   A. spiral

   B. comminuted

   C. greenstick

   D. compound

7

_____**22.** The principal injury from submersion is:

   A. lack of oxygen.

   B. neck and spinal cord injuries.

   C. drowning.

   D. hypothermia.

_____**23.** For children who have had traumatic injuries, use a child-sized BVM device at a rate of one breath every _____ seconds.

   A. 2

   B. 3

   C. 4

   D. 5

_____**24.** After difficult incidents involving children, _____ is helpful in working through the stress and trauma.

   A. having a drink

   B. talking with the family

   C. debriefing

   D. putting the incident out of your mind

Vocabulary

Define the following terms using the space provided.

1. Work-of-breathing (WOB):

_____

_____

_____

2. Altered level of consciousness:

_____

_____

_____

3. Epiglottitis:

_____

_____

_____

4. Shaken baby syndrome:

_____

_____

_____

Fill-in

Read each item carefully, then complete the statement by filling in the missing word.

1. _____ is an early sign that the child may be compensating for decreased perfusion.

2. Most _____ are able to think abstractly and can participate in decision-making.

3. The term _____ is used to describe a continuous seizure, or multiple seizures without a return to consciousness, for 30 minutes or more.

4. _____ indicates the amount of oxygen getting to the organs of the body.

5. A _____ is the result of disorganized electrical activity in the brain.

6. A child's _____ are softer and more flexible than an adult's and may compress the heart and lungs, causing serious injury with no obvious external damage.

7. Because a child's _____ is proportionately larger than an adult's, it exerts greater stress on the neck structures during a deceleration injury.

8. You should suspect a serious _____ _____ in any child who experiences nausea and vomiting after a traumatic event.

9. Children can lose a greater proportion of their blood volume than adults can before signs and symptoms of _____ develop.

10. _____ _____ are potential weak spots in the bone and are often injured as a result of trauma.

True/False

If you believe the statement to be more true than false, write the letter "T" in the space provided. If you believe the statement to be more false than true, write the letter "F."

1. _____ The skeletal system contains growth plates at the ends of long bones, which enable these bones to grow during childhood.

2. _____ Preschool-age children have a rich fantasy life, which can make them particularly fearful of pain and change involving their bodies.

3. _____ Normal respirations are a common sign of illness or injury in children.

4. _____ The parent or caregiver of a special needs child will be an important part of your assessment.

5. _____ Infants and small children are not very susceptible to temperature changes.

6. _____ When transporting children, do not allow the parent to hold the child during the actual transport.

7. _____ You must always assist ventilations in all pediatric patients who have respiratory rates greater than 60 breaths/min.

8. _____ Febrile seizures are self-limiting and do not need transport unless they recur.

9. _____ Alcohol applied to skin is a recommended method of cooling a patient.

10. _____ Children are simply little adults.

11. _____ Children may experience significant internal injuries with little or no obvious outside signs.

12. _____ Head injuries are uncommon in children.

13. _____ Children can lose a greater proportion of blood than adults before showing signs or symptoms of shock.

14. _____ Children have soft and flexible ribs.

Short Answer

Complete this section with short written answers using the space provided.

1. Discuss developmental considerations for the school-age child and approach for caregivers.

_____

_____

_____

_____

2. List the severity and body area involved for the three categories of burns in children.

_____

_____

_____

3. List ten common causes of altered level of consciousness in pediatric patients.

_____   _____

_____   _____

_____   _____

_____   _____

_____   _____

4. List four signs of increased work-of-breathing in children.

_____

_____

_____

_____

Word Fun

The following crossword puzzle is an activity provided to reinforce correct spelling and understanding of medical terminology associated with emergency care. Use the clues in the column to complete the puzzle.

CLUES

Across

1. Rapid rate of breathing
9. Able to think abstractly and participate in decisions
10. Absence of breathing
11. 25% blood volume loss significantly increased risk of this
12. Lack of this is the principal injury for submersion
13. Disorganized electrical activity in the brain

Down

1. Reduced rate of breathing
2. Leaning forward onto two arms stretched forward
3. Most important step in caring for a child with a head injury
4. Lower tip of sternum
5. "Terrible twos" stage
6. Specialized medical practice devoted to care of children
7. Growth of long bones occurs here
8. First year of life

Calls to the Scene

The following case scenarios provide an opportunity to explore the concerns associated with patient management. Read each scenario, then answer each question in detail.

1. You are dispatched to the children's center for an 8-year-old girl with a possible tibia fracture. Her teacher tells you that she tripped when she jumped out of a swing and twisted her leg when she landed. The child is lying on the ground and is fairly calm. You see obvious deformity to the lower left leg.

   How would you best manage this patient?

   _____

   _____

   _____

   _____

   _____

   _____

   _____

   _____

2. You are called to a child care center for a 3-year-old boy with difficulty breathing. The patient is still alert, but gasping for breath when you arrive. His respirations are 52 breaths/min and shallow.

   How would you best manage this patient?

   _____

   _____

   _____

   _____

   _____

   _____

   _____

   _____

   _____

   _____

3. You are dispatched to a residence for a possible drowning of a 7-year-old boy. When you arrive, the child is lying at the side of the pool where his father pulled him out. He is breathing shallowly at 8 breaths/min and has faint radial pulses. How would you best manage this patient?

_____

_____

_____

_____

_____

_____

_____

_____

Workbook Activities

The following activities have been designed to help you. Your instructor may require you to complete some or all of these activities as a regular part of your OEC training program. You are encouraged to complete any activity that your instructor does not assign as a way to enhance your learning in the classroom.

Chapter Review

The following exercises provide an opportunity to refresh your knowledge of this chapter.

NOTES

Matching
Match each of the priority terms in the right column to the appropriate triage injury in the left column.

_____ **1.** Mono skier

_____ **2.** ADD and dyslexia

_____ **3.** Disability

_____ **4.** Allergic to latex

_____ **5.** Disarticulation

_____ **6.** Cerebral palsy

_____ **7.** Outriggers

_____ **8.** Ataxia

_____ **9.** Three tracker

_____ **10.** Adaptive athlete

A. physically or mentally challenged and participates in a sport

B. amputation at a joint

C. sits in a bucket or seat that has only one ski or snowboard under the bucket

D. inability to walk

E. forearm crutches with short skis attached at the bottom

F. skis on one ski and uses outriggers on both arms

G. types of learning disorders

H. caused by anoxia or insufficient oxygen to brain cells

I. restriction or lack of ability to perform an activity in a manner considered normal

J. patients with spina bifida

Multiple Choice
Read each item carefully, then select the best response.

_____ **1.** What is the term adopted by the NSP to describe an individual who is physically or mentally challenged and participates in a sport?

A. impaired

B. disabled

C. handicapped

D. adaptive

Outdoor Adaptive Athletes

_____ **2.** Individuals with disabilities began participating in sports:

  A. following the 1960 Olympics.

  B. during the 1950s.

  C. after World War II.

  D. in 1990 after the Americans with Disabilities Act.

_____ **3.** To understand the special needs of adaptive athletes, it is important to know about their:

  A. mental conditions.

  B. physical conditions.

  C. age.

  D. both A and B

_____ **4.** Mentally challenged individuals may have several different conditions including:

  A. learning disabilities.

  B. mental retardation.

  C. cognitive and psychological disorders.

  D. all of the above

_____ **5.** The easygoing personalities of many individuals with Down syndrome makes:

  A. them good adaptive athletes.

  B. it possible that the rescuer will think they are not injured or ill.

  C. it difficult to assess patient condition.

  D. both B and C

_____ **6.** Individuals with psychosis can function reasonably well:

  A. because of available medications.

  B. for short periods of time.

  C. without ongoing treatment.

  D. when not dealing with others.

_____ **7.** A mentally challenged patient will usually have a supervising adult with him or her who can:

    A. ski with the patient.

    B. read the patient and assist the rescuer.

    C. provide information and interpretation of what is wrong with the patient for the rescuer.

    D. both B and C

_____ **8.** Physically challenged patients can make assessment:

    A. easy for the rescuer.

    B. a task that focuses on the patient's impairment.

    C. difficult for the rescuer.

    D. a task that requires little communication.

_____ **9.** Loss or absence of a limb can be the result of a:

    A. traumatic accident.

    B. surgical procedure.

    C. genetic anomaly.

    D. all of the above

_____ **10.** A broken femur on the same side as a below-knee amputation, when the patient is wearing a prosthesis, poses an interesting dilemma for the rescuer because:

    A. the patient has no feeling in the leg and doesn't know he or she is injured.

    B. traction will break the prosthesis.

    C. the prosthesis has no sensitivity.

    D. applying traction to the ankle of the prosthesis will pull off the artificial leg.

_____ **11.** Cerebral palsy is a disability:

    A. in which the body and its voluntary muscular coordination are impaired.

    B. that usually hampers normal mental activity.

    C. that results from a brain injury during early adolescence.

    D. that makes it easy to apply splints and cravats.

_____ **12.** Cerebral palsy is a condition that:

    A. results from insufficient oxygen to brain cells before, during, or shortly after birth.

    B. is categorized as spastic, athetoid, or dystonic.

    C. impacts individuals differently.

    D. all of the above

_____ **13.** Multiple sclerosis is a neurologic condition that:

    A. causes weakness, paralysis of the extremities, loss of stamina, and balance difficulties.

    B. affects the spinal nerves.

    C. can allow a patient to function almost normally during remission.

    D. both A and C

_____ **14.** A large population of mono- and bi- (sitting) skiers falls into two categories. These include adaptive athletes with:

    A. spinal cord injury and athletes with spina bifida.

    B. cerebral palsy and athletes with postpolio syndrome.

    C. multiple sclerosis and athletes with muscular dystrophy.

    D. learning disorders and athletes with cognitive disorders.

_____ **15.** In adaptive athletes with spina bifida, the area where the open spine was repaired is:

    A. not an area of concern for the rescuer.

    B. susceptible to injury.

    C. covered with a thinner layer of skin.

    D. both B and C

_____ **16.** Which of the following statements is true about full or partial loss of function in patients with spinal cord injury?

    A. Function can usually be returned with traction following treatment.

    B. Function is returned by correct anatomic alignment of the spine.

    C. Function occurs below the level of the injury to the cord.

    D. Function occurs above the level of injury to the cord.

_____ **17.** Which of the following statements is true about patients with spinal cord injury?

    A. Patients know when they are experiencing frostbite below the level of their spinal cord injury.

    B. Patients cannot sense hot or cold below the level of their spinal cord injury.

    C. Patients do not present concerns about hypothermia or hyperthermia for rescuers.

    D. Patients have lost mobility below the level of their injury site but can sense hot and cold.

_____ **18.** The number of visually impaired adaptive athletes is:

    A. increasing.

    B. decreasing.

    C. remaining constant.

    D. not being monitored.

_____ **19.** Rescuers treating adaptive athletes should be familiar with:

    A. braces used by athletes.

    B. appliances used by athletes.

    C. equipment used by adaptive athletes.

    D. all of the above

_____ **20.** Rescuers attempting to lift, evacuate, or transport adaptive athletes should:

    A. understand the handicap or disability of the athlete.

    B. be aware that blind skiers who must evacuate from a chair are usually very frightened.

    C. know how to attach evacuation lines/ropes to a sit-skier's bucket.

    D. all of the above

Vocabulary

Define the following terms using the space provided.

  1. Impairment:

_____

_____

_____

2. Disability:

_____

_____

_____

3. Mental retardation:

_____

_____

_____

4. Cognitive disability:

_____

_____

_____

5. Amputation:

_____

_____

_____

6. Spina bifida:

_____

_____

_____

Fill-in

Read each item carefully, then complete the statement by filling in the missing word.

1. Winter Paralympic events include both _____ and _____ skiers with various types of disability conditions.

2. To understand the special needs of adaptive athletes, it is important to know about their various _____ and _____ medical conditions.

3. The _____ of a mentally challenged patient is a good source of _____.

4. _____ is a common genetic condition resulting in mental and physical anomalies.

5. Physically challenged patients can make _____ difficult for the rescuer.

6. Progressive and irreversible muscle wasting is the hallmark of _____.

7. A large portion of mono- and bi- (sitting) skiers falls into two categories—those

   with _____ and _____.

8. Trauma to the _____ can damage the spinal cord.

9. Athletes with _____ and _____ can have emotional or psychological problems as well.

10. Adaptive athletes use _____, _____, and other equipment.

True/False
If you believe the statement to be more true than false, write the letter "T" in the space provided. If you believe the statement to be more false than true, write the letter "F."

1. _____ The Americans with Disabilities Act opened new frontiers for disabled persons.
2. _____ All people with learning disorders are mentally retarded.
3. _____ Individuals with psychosis are unable to function.
4. _____ Injured physically challenged patients are easy to assess.
5. _____ Upper extremity injuries occur to adaptive athletes who use outriggers.
6. _____ The number of visually impaired outdoor athletes is increasing.
7. _____ A stroke occurs when part of the brain receives an increase in blood supply.
8. _____ A stoma is an injury to the abdominal wall.
9. _____ Lift evacuation problems can arise with adaptive snow sports athletes.

Short Answer
Complete the section with short written answers using the space provided.

1. List the categories that a mentally challenged individual may fall into.

   _____

   _____

   _____

2. List types of lost function resulting from spinal cord injury.

   _____

   _____

   _____

7

3. Explain the purpose of a stoma.

_____

_____

_____

Word Fun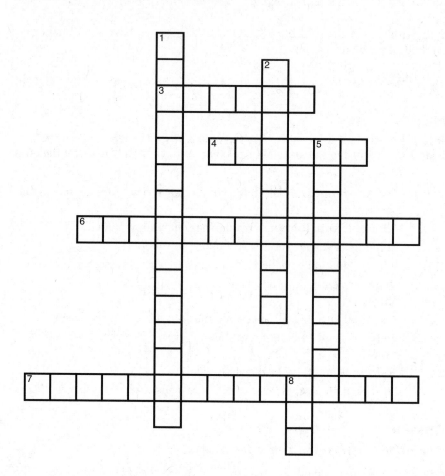

www.OECzone.com
vocab explorer

The following crossword puzzle is an activity provided to reinforce correct spelling and understanding of medical terminology associated with emergency care. Use the clues in the column to complete the puzzle.

■■■ CLUES ■■■

Across

3. Absence of oxygen

4. The inability to walk

6. A disability caused by insufficient oxygen to brain cells before, during, or shortly after birth

7. Amputation at a joint

Down

1. An individual who is physically or mentally challenged and participates in a sport

2. Restriction in or lack of ability to perform an activity

5. Loss or abnormality of psychological, physiologic, or anatomic structure or function

8. Attention-deficit disorder

Calls to the Scene

The following case scenarios provide an opportunity to explore the concerns associated with patient management. Read each scenario, then answer each question in detail.

1. You receive a call on your radio and are told that a skier has been reported down on your area's intermediate run. When you arrive on scene, you find a mono-skier who has collided with a tree and is lying on her right side. You find the skier conscious and alert. As you question the skier, you find she is a paraplegic adaptive athlete and is complaining of pain in her right arm. She also states that she thinks her legs hit the tree "pretty hard."

   How would you assess and best manage this patient?

   _____

   _____

   _____

   _____

   _____

   _____

   _____

   _____

2. You are working your shift in the patrol's clinic when a young man, whom you recognize from the area's cafeteria crew, walks in holding a cloth on his hand. Blood has begun to soak through the cloth. When you ask what has happened, the patient appears not to understand what you are asking. When he talks, his speech is difficult to understand. As you examine the patient for other injuries, you notice a hearing aid in the patient's ear. You realize that your patient is hearing impaired.

   In addition to dealing with your patient's injury, how would you communicate effectively with the patient?

   _____

   _____

   _____

   _____

   _____

   _____

   _____

7

Notes

Answer Key

Chapter 1: Introduction to Outdoor Emergency Care

Matching

1. F (page 5)
2. P (page 5)
3. G (page 5)
4. A (page 5)
5. C (page 20)
6. D (page 10)
7. I (page 7)
8. B (page 14)
9. E (page 7)
10. H (page 17)
11. J (page 14)
12. K (page 17)
13. N (page 17)
14. L (page 15)
15. M (pages 15–16)
16. O (page 7)

Multiple Choice

1. C – Quality control ensures that all staff members involved in caring for patients meet appropriate standards on each call. "Periodic" audits or reviews may be employed—these may be yearly, quarterly, or more frequently (A). EMT training in skills is a component of regulation and certification (B). Billing information (D) is an important aspect of documentation, but not a matter for the medical director in quality control. (page 10)

2. A – Ensuring your safety and that of your fellow OEC rescuers is a primary responsibility. (B), (C), and (D) are among the concerns upon arrival at the scene during scene size-up. (page 12)

3. B – The emergency care of patients occurs in three phases: the first phase consists of assessment, packaging and transport, the second phase continues care in the emergency department (C), and in the third phase the patient receives the necessary definitive care. Public recognition (A) and accurate dispatching (D) are components of access to the EMS System. (page 12)

4. B (page 6)

5. C (page 6)

6. B – The material and skills of the EMT-B training program was developed in the U.S. Department of Transportation 1994 EMT-Basic National Standard Curriculum. (A) The AAOS assists the development of EMS through research, quality standards, and publications. (C) The AHA conducts research, provides training standards, and certification in CPR. (D) The NSP represents the

snowsports and outdoor recreation community by providing quality education programs for rescuers working in the nonurban environment on the national, regional, and local levels. OEC training adheres to the U.S. DOT national standard curriculum for EMT-Bs for like topics. (page 5)

7. D – Negligence is proven when all four elements—duty, breach, cause, and damages—are met, whether consent was expressed (A) or implied, care was terminated or not (B), or how the patient was transported (C). (pages 14–18)

8. C – If you leave patients alone, you risk being accused of negligence or abandonment. (page 17)

9. B – Good Samaritan laws protect individuals who provide care within their scope of practice and in good faith. Proper performance of CPR (A), improvising BLS materials (C), and supportive care given to a patient with an advance directive or DNR (D) are each appropriate to the scope of practice of the OEC technician. (page 16)

10. D – Confidential information includes history, assessment, treatment, diagnosis, and mental or physical conditions (A, B, and C) and cannot be disclosed without authorization of the patient. The location of an emergency call is generally not considered to be confidential. (page 12)

11. D – Most experts agree that a complete and accurate record of an emergency incident is an important safeguard against legal complications. (page 18)

Vocabulary

1. Outdoor Emergency Care: An education program meeting U.S. DOT training standards for the EMT-B with modifications appropriate to the outdoor environment. (page 4)

2. First responder: The first trained individual, such as police officer, firefighter, or other rescuer, to arrive at the scene to provide initial medical assistance. (page 5)

3. OEC technician: An outdoor rescuer who is trained to provide emergency medical care in the field. (page 4)

4. Expressed consent: A type of consent in which a patient gives express authorization for provision of care or transport. (page 17)

5. Good Samaritan laws: Statutory provisions enacted by many states to protect citizens from liability for errors and omissions in giving good faith emergency medical care, unless there is wanton, gross, or willful negligence. (page 16)

6. Implied consent: Type of consent in which a patient who is unable to give consent is given treatment under the legal assumption that he or she would want treatment. (page 17)

7. Negligence: Failure to provide the same care that a person with similar training would provide. (page 15)

Fill-in

1. the U.S. DOT 1994 EMT-B national standard curriculum (page 5)

2. AED, medications (page 5)

3. local protocol (pages 10–11)

4. negligence (page 14)

5. stopping (page 14)

6. expressed, implied (page 17)

7. refuse treatment (page 16)

True/False

1. T (page 5)

2. T (page 11)

3. T (page 15)

4. F (page 18)

5. T (page 17)

Short Answer

1. The OEC technician provides basic life support skills and may also provide some ALS skills, such as advanced airways and defibrillation in the nonurban environment, and transports these patients to a location where EMT-Bs and ambulance services can provide safe transport to definitive care. (page 5)

2. -Ensuring your own safety and the safety of your fellow rescuers, the patient, and others at the scene

-Locating and safely securing the scene

-Sizing up the scene and situation

-Rapidly assessing the patient's gross neurologic, respiratory, and circulatory status

-Providing any essential immediate intervention

-Performing a thorough, accurate patient assessment

-Obtaining an expanded SAMPLE history

-Providing prompt, efficient, prioritized patient care based on your assessment

-Communicating effectively with and advising the patient of any procedures you will perform

-Properly interacting and communicating with EMS, fire, rescue, and law enforcement responders

-Identifying patients who require rapid packaging and initiating transport without delay

-Identifying patients who do not need emergency care and will benefit from further detailed assessment and care before they are moved and transported

-Properly packaging the patient

-Safely lifting and moving the patient

-Arranging safe appropriate transport to the hospital emergency department or other ordered facility

-Providing any additional assessment or treatment if time permits

-Monitoring the patient and checking vital signs

-Documenting all findings and care on the incident report

-Unloading the patient safely and, after giving a proper verbal report, transferring the patient's care to the EMS staff

-Safeguarding the patient's rights (page 12)

3. You must continue to care for the patient until the patient is transferred to another medical professional of equal or higher skill level, or another medical facility. (page 14)

Word Fun

Calls to the Scene

1. Decision making is very important. Prioritize heart attack over laceration; use oxygen; notify EMS in a timely manner; maintain communication with both patients. Have second patient help himself (direct pressure over wound with sterile dressings) and watch his friend while you make necessary calls. Make sure all names are documented in the report.

2. The child should be treated based on implied consent. A "loss of function" constitutes an emergency, and the child can be treated and transported without consent from the parent since not treating him could result in a loss of the extremity. The hospital will try to reach the child's mother once you arrive. You might also tell the other children to try and contact her and tell her to come to the hospital.

3. Assess the patient's mental status. If he is intoxicated or has an altered mental status, he should be treated under implied consent. If he is alert and oriented, you may attempt to talk him into being treated by explaining what you feel is necessary and what may happen if he does not receive care. If he has an altered mental status, wait for the ambulance and EMS, help law enforcement restrain the patient if necessary, and transport him to the hospital.

Chapter 2: The Well-Being of the Rescuer

Matching

1. D   (page 27)
2. A   (pages 42–43)
3. C   (page 55)
4. F   (page 51)
5. B   (page 55)
6. E   (page 55)
7. N   (page 55)
8. H   (page 43)

9. M   (page 29)
10. J   (page 55)
11. K   (page 55)
12. O   (page 55)
13. I   (page 28)
14. G   (page 28)
15. L   (pages 55–56)

Multiple Choice

1. C (page 33)
2. C (page 28)
3. D (page 44)
4. A – This is a presumptive sign. (page 44)
5. D (page 29)
6. C (page 30)
7. A (page 30)
8. D (page 29)
9. B (page 28)
10. A (page 46)
11. D (page 45)
12. B (pages 38–39)
13. B (pages 46–47)
14. D (pages 35–37)
15. D (page 47)
16. D (page 49)
17. A – Other factors that influence how a patient reacts to the stress of an incident involving injury include alcohol or substance abuse, history of chronic disease, mental disorders, reaction to medications, nutritional status, and feelings of guilt. (pages 49–50)
18. C – This is a sign, not a symptom. (page 51)
19. D (page 51)
20. A (page 39)
21. B (page 40)
22. C (page 54)
23. D (page 54)
24. C (page 54)
25. C (page 55)
26. B (page 54)
27. D – Modes of transmission also include oral contamination due to lack of, or improper, handwashing. (page 56)
28. B (page 60)
29. C (page 57)
30. C (pages 59–60)
31. B (page 58)

Vocabulary

1. Critical incident stress management (CISM): A process that confronts the responses to critical incidents and diffuses them, directing the emergency services personnel toward physical and emotional equilibrium. (page 51)
2. Posttraumatic stress disorder (PTSD): A delayed stress reaction to a prior incident. This delayed reaction is the result of one or more unresolved issues concerning the incident that might have been alleviated with the use of critical incident stress management. (page 51)
3. Critical incident stress debriefing (CISD): A confidential group discussion of a severely stressful incident that usually occurs within 24 to 72 hours of the incident. (page 54)
4. Conduction: The direct transfer of heat from a warm body to a cooler object. (page 29)
5. Convection: The transfer of heat when air that is cooler than body temperature moves across the body surface. (page 29)
6. Evaporation: The loss of heat when water or another volatile liquid on the body's surface is converted into vapor. (page 29)

7. Radiation: Heat loss from the body through infrared waves. (page 29)

8. Windchill: The relationship between actual temperature, wind velocity, and "effective" temperature at the skin surface. (page 31)

9. Layering principle: To prevent overheating or chilling by adding/subtracting layers of clothing. (page 34)

Fill-in

1. well-being (page 24)

2. emotional stress (page 20)

3. physician (page 45)

4. warm (page 44)

5. depression (page 47)

6. upper, lower extremities (page 43)

7. blood, semen, vaginal fluid (pages 55–56)

8. wash (page 59)

9. hydrogen peroxide (page 60)

True/False

1. T (page 43)

2. F (page 44)

3. F (page 44)

4. T (page 25)

5. T (page 45)

6. F (page 55)

7. F (pages 26–28)

8. T (page 53)

9. T (page 31)

10. T (page 63)

Short Answer

1. An infection control practice that assumes all body fluids are potentially infectious. (page 55)

2. -Oxygen

-Maintenance of body temperature

-Water

-Food

-Physical integrity

-Confidence, the will to survive (page 24)

3. -Rate and depth of breathing increases.

-Blood absorbs oxygen more efficiently.

-Blood carries oxygen more efficiently.

-Heart and skeletal muscle action become more efficient. (page 27)

4. -Muscular activity

-Eating—heat from hot food and drink

-Food—energy

-Stove, fire, sun (pages 32–33)

5. -Shivering

-Foot stamping and other semiresponsive activity (pages 28–29)

6. -Add clothing.

-Seek shelter. (page 30)

7. -Decrease sweating.

-Shunt blood away from the shell.

-Decrease body surface area. (page 30)

8. -Attain and maintain a high state of physical fitness. Allow time for acclimatization.

-Maximize body heat loss by exposing as much skin to the air as possible, wearing loose, light colored, cotton clothing; maintain hydration to promote sweating; and acclimatize.

-Minimize heat gain from the environment by wearing protective clothing, seek shade during the heat of the day, avoid touching hot objects, and do not lie directly on the ground.

-Minimize body heat production by decreasing muscular activity. (page 39)

9. To reduce heat loss from radiation and convection, wear a hat. Up to 70% of the heat produced by the body can be lost from an uncovered head. (page 31)

10. -Light in weight

-High in energy

-Not require cooking or complicated preparation

-Resistant to spoilage (page 40)

11. -Carbohydrates

-Proteins

-Fat

-Minerals

-Vitamins

-Water (page 39)

12. -A warm-up period

-Selected calisthenics

-A period of rhythmical, nonstop training

-A cooling-down period (page 43)

13. -Rubber or latex gloves

-Goggles

-Pocket mask

-Face shield (page 56)

14. 1. Use soap and water.

2. Rub hands together for at least 10 to 15 seconds to work up a lather.

3. Rinse hands and dry with a paper towel.

4. Use paper towel to turn off faucet. (page 56)

15. -Thin inner layer

-Thermal middle layer

-Outer layer (pages 36–37)

Word Fun

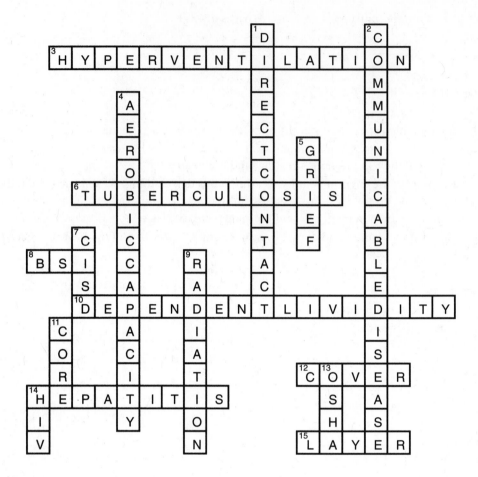

Calls to the Scene

1. -Since winds will be high and it may rain/snow/sleet, prepare to layer clothing. By layering you can stay the warmest and driest.

   -Start with polypropylene long underwear. Outerwear should include wind or rain pants.

   -Definitely have a hat, gloves, and waterproof boots with good traction in case trails get slick.

   -Equipment should include shelter such as a tent and ground cloth for extra insulation.

2. -BSI precautions

   -Prevent further heat loss

   -Transport immediately

   -Monitor vital signs

3.

Insufficient oxygen in the outside air	-High altitude
	-Burial in a snow or dirt avalanche
	-Poorly ventilated snow cave or other confined space
	-Malfunction of underwater breathing apparatus
	-Near drowning
	-Smoke or other substance in the air replaces oxygen

Obstruction of the upper airway	-Relaxation of the tongue or pharyngeal tissue in an unresponsive person -Aspirated food, vomitus, dentures, or other foreign material -Injury to the face or neck
Obstruction of the lower airway	-Inhaled foreign body -Inability to cough up blood, pus, or mucus

Interference with lung function
    Acute
 	
    Chronic
	Acute
	-Filling of the alveoli with pus, blood, or fluid, as in pneumonia, lung hemorrhage, or pulmonary edema
	-Partial or total collapse of the lung because of blood, fluid, or air pressing on the outside of the lung
	-Spasm and thickening of bronchial walls and plugging of small bronchi with mucus, as in an asthma attack
	Chronic
	-Thickening of the alveoli walls, as in pulmonary fibrosis
	-Loss of some alveoli, enlargement of others, and narrowing of the bronchi, as in emphysema
	-Replacement of lung tissue by tumor (benign or malignant)

Interference with chest integrity or function	-Paralysis of the nerve supply to the diaphragm and/or chest muscles, as in spinal cord injury -Crushing injury to the chest, as in flail chest caused by multiple rib fractures -Open chest wounds
Interference with the brain's control of breathing	-Head injury -Meningitis -Stroke -Poisoning overdose of depressants

Abnormal function of the circulatory system
    Illness
 	
    Injury
	Illness
	-Heart attack
	-Chronic heart failure
	-Fluid in the sac around the heart
	-Blood clot in the lung blocking blood flow through its vessels (pulmonary embolus)
	Injury
	-Shock
	-Direct injury to the heart or blood vessels

Interference with the blood's oxygen-carrying capacity	-Anemia -Carbon monoxide poisoning

Skill Drills

1. Skill Drill 2-1: Proper Glove Removal Technique (page 58)

   1. Partially remove the first glove by pinching at the wrist. Be careful to touch only the outside of the glove.
   2. Remove the second glove by pinching the exterior with the partially gloved hand.
   3. Pull the second glove inside out toward the fingertips.
   4. Grasp both gloves with your free hand, touching only the clean, interior surfaces.

Chapter 3: Interfacing with EMS and Other Medical Personnel

Matching

1. B   (page 70)
2. F   (page 72)
3. A   (page 72)
4. E   (page 75–76)

5. G   (page 75)
6. D   (page 76)
7. H   (pages 77–78)
8. C   (page 78)

Multiple Choice

1. B   (page 78)
2. A   (page 81)
3. D   (page 73)
4. C   (page 73)
5. A   (page 75)

Vocabulary

1. Advanced life support (ALS): Advanced lifesaving procedures, such as cardiac monitoring, administration of IV fluids and medications, and use of advanced airway adjuncts. (page 73)
2. Basic life support (BLS): Noninvasive emergency lifesaving care that is used to treat airway obstruction, respiratory arrest, or cardiac arrest. (page 73)
3. Standard of training: The knowledge and skills required to facilitate training rescuers to operate in a variety of situations, using an assortment of equipment and techniques. (page 74)
4. Standard of care: What a specific area or rescue group has chosen to use as its methods (protocols) for providing care to ill and injured patients. (page 74)
5. First responder: The first medically trained individual, such as a patroller, search and rescue personnel, police officer, or other rescuer, to arrive at the scene of an emergency to provide initial medical assistance. (page 74)

Fill-in

1. Documentation (page 78)
2. EMS providers (page 71)
3. dispatch (page 76)
4. transport (page 77)
5. rescuer (or patrol) (page 77)

True/False

1. T (pages 73–74)
2. F (page 80)
3. T (page 74)
4. F (pages 79–80)
5. T (page 73)

Short Answer

1. -Training

   -Establish guidelines/protocols for various treatment options on the hill and in the aid room.

   -Provide advice on medical issues. (page 80)

2. -The OEC technician/rescuer uses a set of training standards that follows the EMT-B's urban training but focuses on care in a unique outdoor environment, generally some distance from a higher level of care, using different transportation methods. General protocols/guidelines are established through local medical advisors. Concentration is on prehospital emergency care in nonurban settings, stabilization, and getting the patient to and into the EMS system.

   -EMS incorporates a direct contact with a medical control physician or facility, following direct orders or preauthorized protocols for encountered situations to provide on-scene medical stabilization and transport to definitive care. (pages 73–74)

3. -Responses will vary depending on local situations and protocols. Students should discuss specifics with their instructors and the rescue groups they will be working with and gain a solid understanding regarding the contacts and parameters for working with these systems. (pages 75–79)

Word Fun

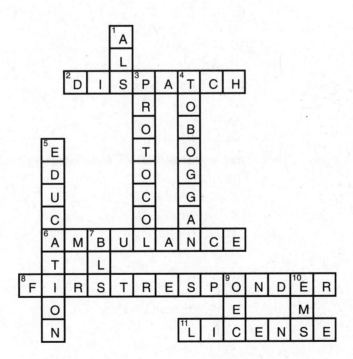

Calls to the Scene

1. -Ask the physician's specialty.

-Assure the physician that you are well trained to handle this emergency, but invite the doctor to assist you with patient care.

-If the physician is willing to assist, provide careful instructions on what you want him to do.

-If the physician insists on taking over, explain that he would assume *all* responsibility for the care and transport of this patient off the mountain and be required to sign documentation to that effect.

2. -Plan a training agenda that includes, but is not limited to:

- discussions of the interface between the rescue group and EMS.
- an exchange of training on various equipment and protocols, eg, splints, stretchers, AEDs, ALS procedures.
- demonstrations of rescuer techniques not used by the EMS services, eg, lift evacuation, cliff rescue, helicopter evacuation, search and rescue.
- demonstrations of EMS techniques not common for the outdoor rescuer, eg, loading and unloading patients from ambulances.
- a review of mass-casualty plans involving multiple services.h
- a review of ways to resolve problems that might crop up in the future.

-Arrange for medical directors from both sides to meet and review protocols.

-Coordinate a social activity, such as a lunch, after-training cocktails, or a barbecue.

Chapter 4: Human Anatomy and Physiology

Matching

1. F	(page 87)	
2. K	(page 114)	
3. D	(page 86)	
4. G	(page 87)	
5. E	(page 87)	
6. L	(page 114)	
7. A	(page 87)	
8. C	(page 87)	
9. M	(page 114)	
10. J	(page 87)	
11. O	(page 114)	
12. B	(page 87)	
13. H	(pages 86–87)	
14. N	(page 114)	
15. I	(pages 86–87)	
16. B	(page 98)	
17. B	(page 98)	
18. A	(pages 99–100)	
19. B	(page 98)	

20. B	(page 98)	
21. A	(page 99)	
22. A	(page 99)	
23. A	(page 102)	
24. B	(page 103)	
25. B	(page 103)	
26. A	(page 102)	
27. A	(page 102)	
28. C	(page 103)	
29. B	(page 102)	
30. C	(page 103)	
31. A	(page 102)	
32. C	(page 103)	
33. A	(page 92)	
34. C	(page 116)	
35. E	(page 118)	
36. B	(pages 118–119)	
37. F	(page 116)	
38. D	(page 118)	

Multiple Choice

1. B – The parts that lie closer to the midline are called medial (inner) structures. (page 87)

2. C – Distal describes structures that are farther from the trunk or nearer to the free end of the extremity. (page 87)

3. B – Cricoid cartilage, a firm ridge of cartilage inferior to the thyroid cartilage, may be difficult to palpate. (page 91)

4. C – Smooth muscle carries out much of the automatic work of the body; therefore, it is also called involuntary muscle. (page 103)

5. D – The spinal column is the central supporting structure of the body and is composed of 33 bones, each called a vertebra. (page 92)

6. C – Much like the skull, each pelvic bone is formed by the fusion of three separate bones. These three bones are called the ilium, the ischium, and the pubis. (page 97)

7. B – Protecting the opening of the trachea is a thin, leaf-shaped valve called the epiglottis. (page 104)

8. B – The endocrine system is a complex message and control system that integrates many body functions. It releases substances called hormones, either by target organs or directly. (page 121)

9. D – The pulmonary artery begins at the right side of the heart and carries oxygen-poor blood to the lungs. (page 112)

10. C – The three major types of nerves are sensory nerves, motor nerves, and connecting nerves. Sensory nerves carry information from the body to the central nervous system. Motor nerves carry information from the central nervous system to the muscles of the body. Connecting nerves do just what their name implies: they connect the sensory and motor nerves. (page 118)

Labeling

1. Directional Terms (page 87)

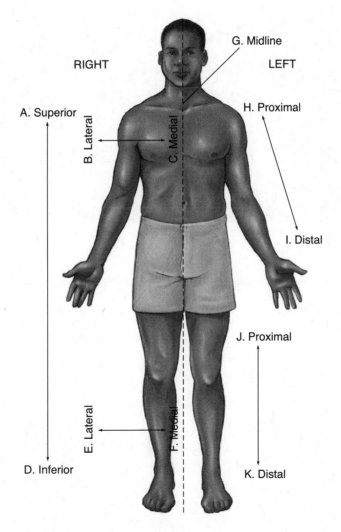

2. Anatomic Positions (page 89)

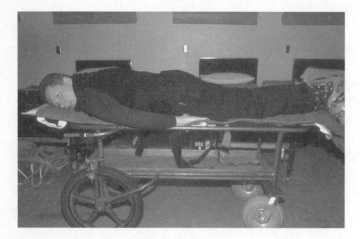

Prone

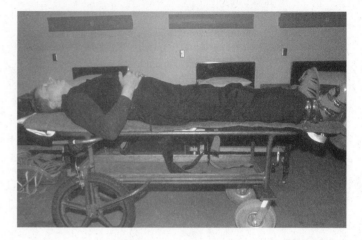

Supine

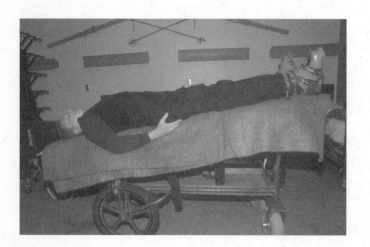

Shock position (modified Trendelenburg's position)

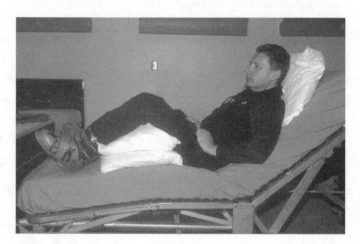

Fowler's position

3. The Skeletal System (page 90)

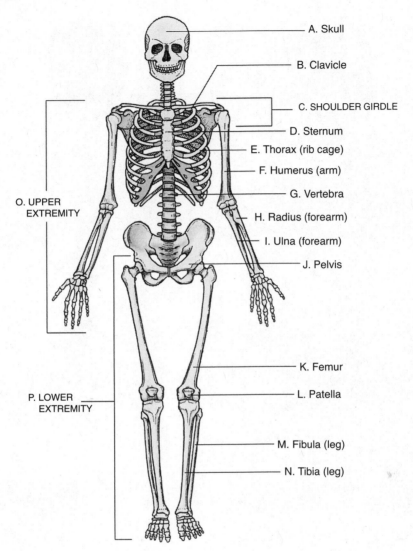

A. Skull
B. Clavicle
C. SHOULDER GIRDLE
D. Sternum
E. Thorax (rib cage)
F. Humerus (arm)
G. Vertebra
H. Radius (forearm)
I. Ulna (forearm)
J. Pelvis
K. Femur
L. Patella
M. Fibula (leg)
N. Tibia (leg)
O. UPPER EXTREMITY
P. LOWER EXTREMITY

4. The Skull (page 90)

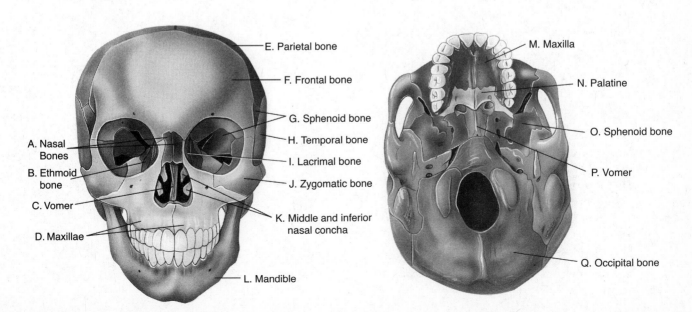

E. Parietal bone
F. Frontal bone
G. Sphenoid bone
H. Temporal bone
I. Lacrimal bone
J. Zygomatic bone
K. Middle and inferior nasal concha
A. Nasal Bones
B. Ethmoid bone
C. Vomer
D. Maxillae
L. Mandible
M. Maxilla
N. Palatine
O. Sphenoid bone
P. Vomer
Q. Occipital bone

5. The Spinal Column (page 92)

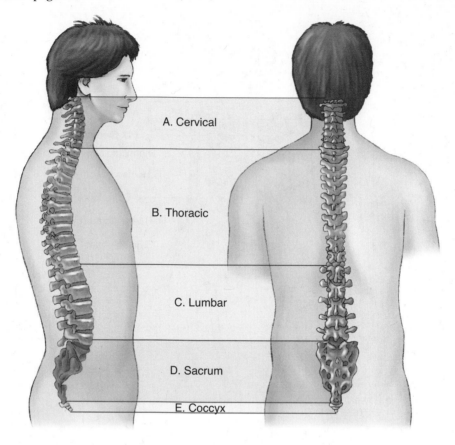

A. Cervical

B. Thoracic

C. Lumbar

D. Sacrum

E. Coccyx

6. The Thorax (page 93)

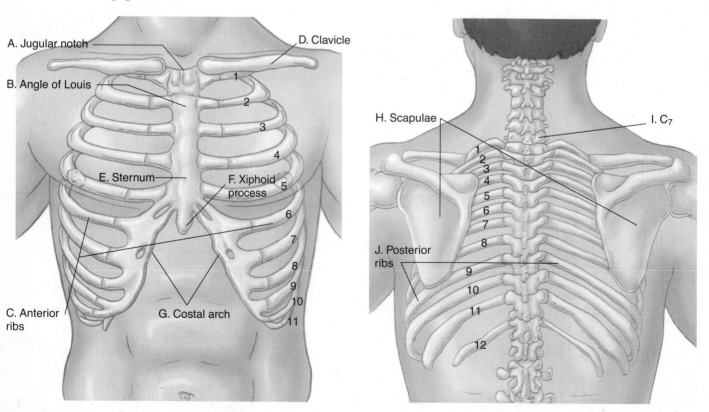

A. Jugular notch

B. Angle of Louis

E. Sternum

F. Xiphoid process

C. Anterior ribs

G. Costal arch

D. Clavicle

H. Scapulae

I. C_7

J. Posterior ribs

7. The Pelvis (page 97)

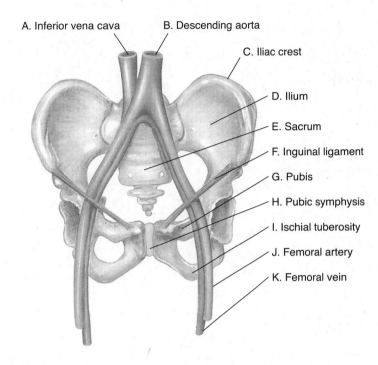

A. Inferior vena cava
B. Descending aorta
C. Iliac crest
D. Ilium
E. Sacrum
F. Inguinal ligament
G. Pubis
H. Pubic symphysis
I. Ischial tuberosity
J. Femoral artery
K. Femoral vein

8. The Lower Extremity (page 98)

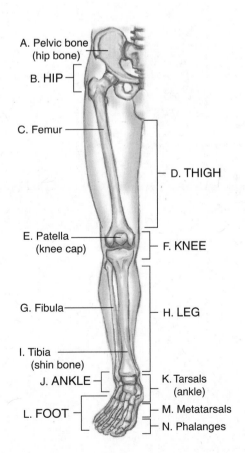

A. Pelvic bone (hip bone)
B. HIP
C. Femur
D. THIGH
E. Patella (knee cap)
F. KNEE
G. Fibula
H. LEG
I. Tibia (shin bone)
J. ANKLE
K. Tarsals (ankle)
L. FOOT
M. Metatarsals
N. Phalanges

9. The Shoulder Girdle (page 99)

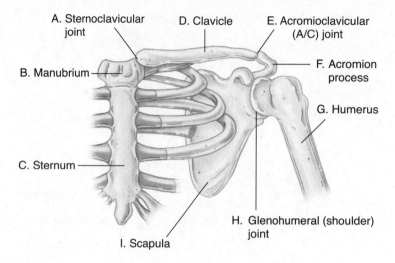

A. Sternoclavicular joint
D. Clavicle
E. Acromioclavicular (A/C) joint
B. Manubrium
F. Acromion process
G. Humerus
C. Sternum
H. Glenohumeral (shoulder) joint
I. Scapula

10. The Upper Extremity (page 100)

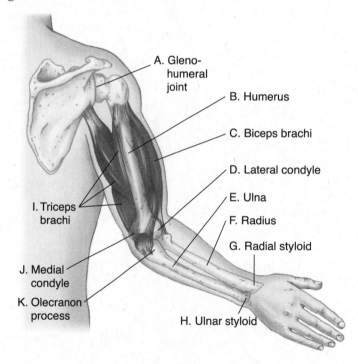

A. Glenohumeral joint
B. Humerus
C. Biceps brachi
D. Lateral condyle
E. Ulna
F. Radius
G. Radial styloid
I. Triceps brachi
J. Medial condyle
K. Olecranon process
H. Ulnar styloid

11. Wrist and Hand (page 100)

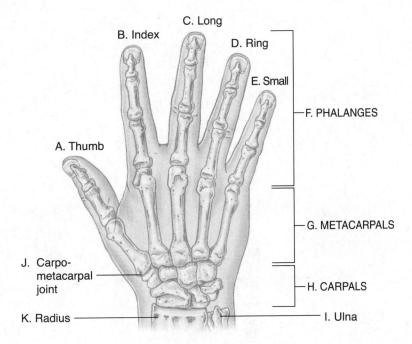

C. Long

B. Index

D. Ring

E. Small

F. PHALANGES

A. Thumb

G. METACARPALS

J. Carpo-
metacarpal
joint

H. CARPALS

K. Radius

I. Ulna

12. The Respiratory System (page 104)

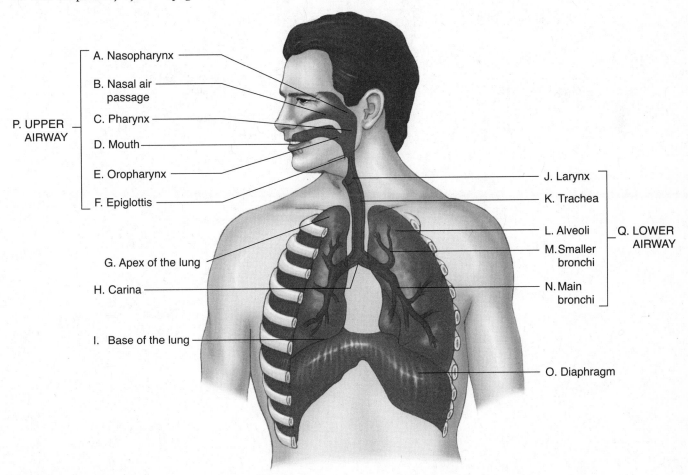

P. UPPER
AIRWAY

A. Nasopharynx

B. Nasal air
passage

C. Pharynx

D. Mouth

E. Oropharynx

F. Epiglottis

J. Larynx

K. Trachea

L. Alveoli

M. Smaller
bronchi

Q. LOWER
AIRWAY

N. Main
bronchi

G. Apex of the lung

H. Carina

I. Base of the lung

O. Diaphragm

13. The Circulatory System (page 110)

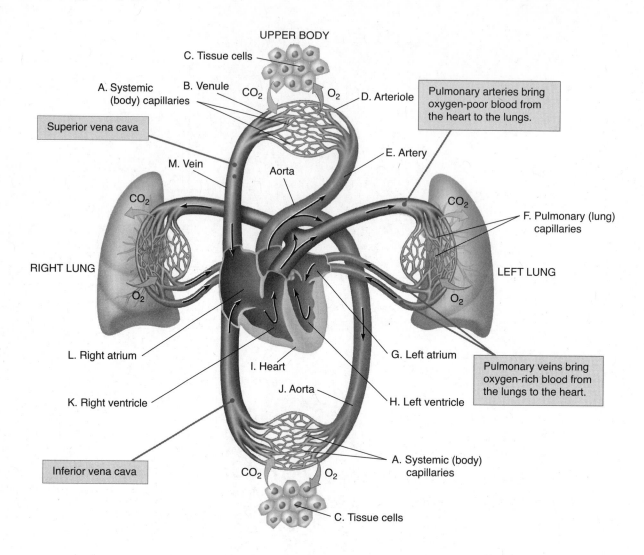

UPPER BODY

C. Tissue cells

A. Systemic (body) capillaries

B. Venule

CO_2

O_2

D. Arteriole

Pulmonary arteries bring oxygen-poor blood from the heart to the lungs.

Superior vena cava

E. Artery

M. Vein

Aorta

CO_2

CO_2

F. Pulmonary (lung) capillaries

RIGHT LUNG

LEFT LUNG

O_2

O_2

L. Right atrium

G. Left atrium

I. Heart

Pulmonary veins bring oxygen-rich blood from the lungs to the heart.

J. Aorta

K. Right ventricle

H. Left ventricle

Inferior vena cava

A. Systemic (body) capillaries

CO_2

O_2

C. Tissue cells

14. Electrical Conduction (page 112)

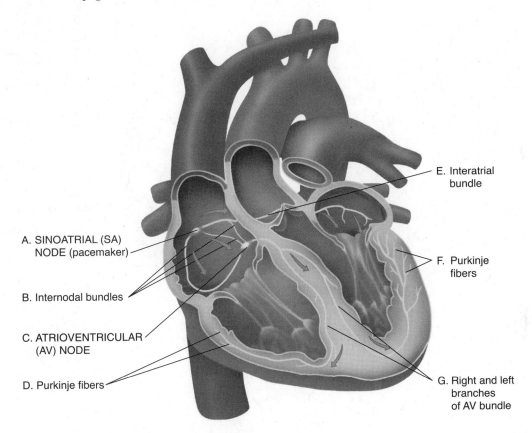

A. SINOATRIAL (SA) NODE (pacemaker)

B. Internodal bundles

C. ATRIOVENTRICULAR (AV) NODE

D. Purkinje fibers

E. Interatrial bundle

F. Purkinje fibers

G. Right and left branches of AV bundle

15. Central and Peripheral Pulses (page 115)

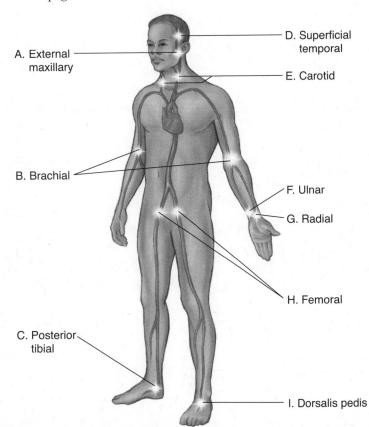

A. External maxillary

B. Brachial

C. Posterior tibial

D. Superficial temporal

E. Carotid

F. Ulnar

G. Radial

H. Femoral

I. Dorsalis pedis

16. The Brain (page 117)

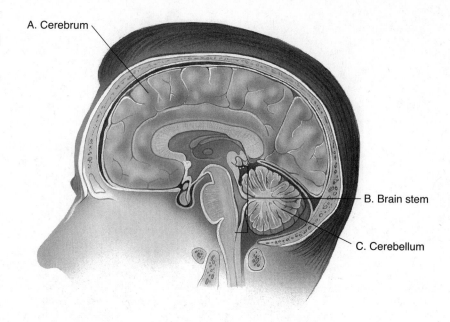

A. Cerebrum
B. Brain stem
C. Cerebellum

17. Anatomy of the Skin (page 120)

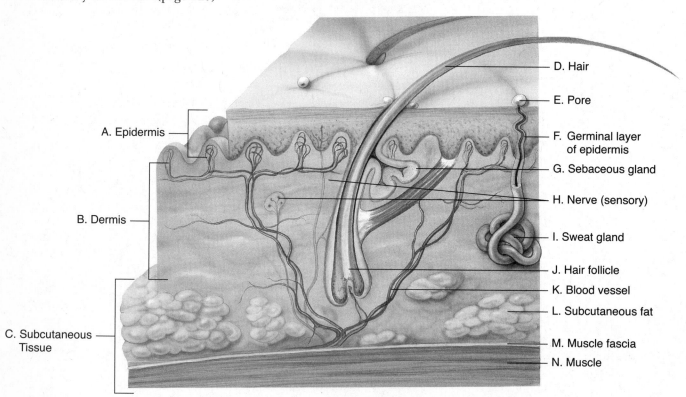

A. Epidermis
B. Dermis
C. Subcutaneous Tissue
D. Hair
E. Pore
F. Germinal layer of epidermis
G. Sebaceous gland
H. Nerve (sensory)
I. Sweat gland
J. Hair follicle
K. Blood vessel
L. Subcutaneous fat
M. Muscle fascia
N. Muscle

18. The Male Reproductive System (page 126)

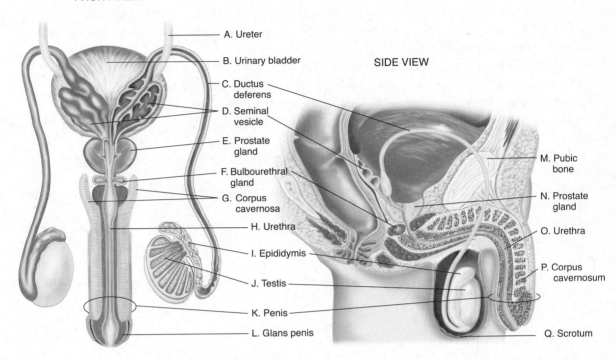

FRONT VIEW

A. Ureter

B. Urinary bladder

SIDE VIEW

C. Ductus deferens

D. Seminal vesicle

E. Prostate gland

M. Pubic bone

F. Bulbourethral gland

N. Prostate gland

G. Corpus cavernosa

H. Urethra

O. Urethra

I. Epididymis

J. Testis

P. Corpus cavernosum

K. Penis

L. Glans penis

Q. Scrotum

19. The Female Reproductive System (page 127)

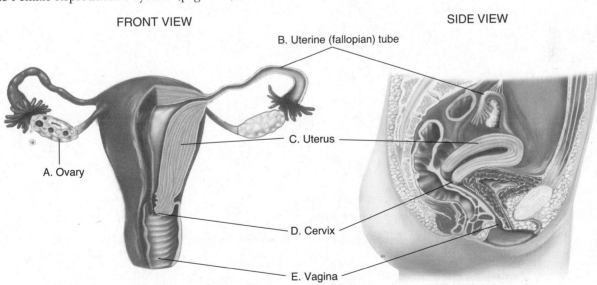

FRONT VIEW

SIDE VIEW

B. Uterine (fallopian) tube

C. Uterus

A. Ovary

D. Cervix

E. Vagina

Vocabulary

1. Perfusion: The circulation of blood within an organ or tissue in adequate amounts to meet the cells' current needs. (page 116)
2. Agonal respirations: Irregular, gasping respirations, sometimes heard in dying patients. (page 110)
3. Autonomic nervous system: The part of the nervous system that regulates many body functions that are not under voluntary control. (page 116)
4. Pleural space: Potential space between the parietal and visceral pleura. (page 106)
5. Trendelenburg's position: The body is supine with the head lower than the feet. (page 88)
6. Fowler's position: Patient is sitting up or semi-sitting with the knees bent. (page 88)
7. Somatic nervous system: The part of the nervous system that regulates activities over which there is involuntary control. (page 116)
8. Endocrine system: A complex message and control system that integrates many body functions, including the release of hormones. (page 121)
9. Peripheral nervous system: The part of the nervous system that consists of 31 pairs of spinal nerves and 12 pairs of cranial nerves. These may be sensory or motor nerves. (page 118)
10. Epiglottis: The leaf-shaped valve that allows air to pass into the trachea, but prevents food or liquid from entering the airway. (page 104)
11. Metabolism: Chemical reactions that occur in the body. (page 119)
12. Brain stem: The area of the brain that lies deep within the cranium and is the best-protected part of the central nervous system. It controls vital body functions. (page 117)

Fill-in

1. 7 (page 92)
2. mandible (page 91)
3. 5 (page 105)
4. 12 (page 94)
5. 33 (page 92)
6. larynx (page 105)
7. talus (page 98)
8. floating ribs (page 94)

True/False

1. F   (page 114)
2. T   (page 98)
3. T   (pages 99–100)
4. F   (page 111)
5. F   (page 94)

Short Answer

1. Plasma – a sticky, yellow fluid that carries the blood cells and nutrients

   Red blood cells – give blood its red color and carry oxygen

   White blood cells – play a role in the body's immune defense mechanism against infection

   Platelets – essential in the formation of blood clots (pages 114–115)
2. Cervical spine – 7

   Thoracic spine – 12

   Lumbar spine – 5

   Sacrum – 5

   Coccyx – 4 (page 92)
3. RUQ – liver, gallbladder, portion of the colon

   LUQ – stomach, spleen, portion of the colon

   RLQ – large intestine, small intestine, appendix, ascending colon

   LLQ – large intestine, small intestine, descending and the sigmoid portions of the colon (page 88)

4. 1. superior and inferior
    vena cava
  2. right atrium
  3. right ventricle
  4. pulmonary artery
  5. lungs

  6. pulmonary vein
  7. left atrium
  8. left ventricle
  9. aorta (pages 111-112)

Word Fun

Calls to the Scene

1. Lacerated liver, gall bladder, small intestine, large intestine, pancreas, diaphragm, right lung if the pathway is up, right kidney depending on the severity of the pole jab, as well as involvement of the other four quadrants based on the direction of travel of the blade.

   The description would be a puncture wound or severe bruise.

2. Angulation and deformity, possibly with crepitus, to the left forearm, proximal to his left wrist or distal to his left elbow.

3. Deformity to left tibia/fibula with swelling. Possible fracture.

Chapter 5: Baseline Vital Signs and SAMPLE History

Matching

1. N (page 139)
2. E (page 143)
3. D (page 145)
4. L (page 140)
5. A (page 142)
6. H (page 149)
7. K (page 143)
8. F (page 141)

9. M (page 140)
10. O (page 141)
11. B (page 141)
12. G (page 145)
13. I (page 145)
14. C (page 141)
15. J (page 140)

Multiple Choice

1. D – When assessing the patient, look (A), listen (B), and feel (C), and think. (page 134)
2. C (page 135)
3. A – Dizziness (A) is a symptom. (page 135)
4. D (page 136)
5. B (page 136)
6. D – In addition, you should evaluate skin temperature and condition in adults. (page 136)
7. A – Inspiration is active (B). Oxygen is drawn in (C). (page 136)
8. D (pages 136–137)
9. D – The normal rate is 12 to 20 breaths/min. 15 to 30 breaths/min (B) is the rate for children. 25 to 50 breaths/min (C) is the rate for infants. (page 137)
10. D (page 138)
11. B (page 138)
12. C (page 138)
13. B – Dyspnea (B) is a symptom. (page 138)
14. C (page 139)
15. C (page 139)
16. A (page 139)
17. D (page 140)
18. B (page 140)
19. D (page 140)
20. D (page 140)
21. D (page 140)
22. D (page 141)
23. B (page 141)
24. D (page 141)
25. D (page 141)
26. B (page 142)
27. A (page 142)
28. D (page 142)
29. B (page 142)
30. A (page 143)
31. C (page 144)
32. A (page 145)
33. B (page 146)
34. C (page 147)
35. D (page 147)
36. D (page 148)
37. C (page 149)

Vocabulary

1. Glasgow Coma Scale: A method of assessing a patient's level of consciousness by scoring the patient's response to eye opening, motor response, and verbal response. (page 147)
2. AVPU scale: A method of assessing a patient's level of responsiveness by determining whether the patient is awake or alert, responsive to verbal stimulus or pain, or is unresponsive. (page 146)
3. Chief complaint: The reason a patient called for help. Also, the patient's response to questions such as, "What's wrong?" or "What happened?" (page 135)

4. Stridor: Harsh, high-pitched, crowing inspiratory sound, such as the sound often heard in acute laryngeal (upper airway) obstruction. (page 138)

Fill-in

1. Tidal volume (page 139)
2. conjunctiva (page 140)
3. deductive (page 134)
4. symptom (page 135)
5. spontaneous respirations (page 136)
6. Vital signs (page 136)
7. quality (page 137)
8. labored breathing (page 138)
9. fluid (page 138)
10. perfusion (page 140)

True/False

1. T   (page 139)
2. T   (page 145)
3. F   (page 145)
4. T   (page 138)
5. T   (page 137)
6. F   (page 139)
7. F   (page 140)
8. T   (page 140)
9. T   (page 141)
10. F   (page 141)
11. F   (page 147)
12. F   (page 137)

Short Answer

1. 1. Pulse
   2. Respirations
   3. Pupils
   4. Blood pressure
   5. Skin
   6. Level of responsiveness
   7. Capillary refill (page 136)
2. 1. Flushed (red)
   2. Pale (white, ashen, or graying)
   3. Jaundice (yellow)
   4. Cyanotic (blue-gray) (page 141)
3. 1. Rate
   2. Rhythm
   3. Quality
   4. Depth (tidal volume)
   5. Effort (pages 136–139)
4. Pressure exerted against the walls of the artery when the left ventricle contracts (page 143)
5. Pressure remaining against the walls of the artery when the left ventricle is at rest (page 143)
6. 1. Rate
   2. Strength
   3. Regularity (page 140)
7. 1. Color
   2. Temperature
   3. Moisture (pages 140–141)
8. Gently compress the fingertip until it blanches. Release the fingertip, and count until it returns to its normal pink color. (pages 141–142)

9. Pupils Equal And Round, Regular in size, react to Light (page 148)

10. A sign is a condition that can be seen, heard, felt, smelled, or measured. A symptom is something that the patient reports to you as a problem or feeling. (page 135)

Word Fun

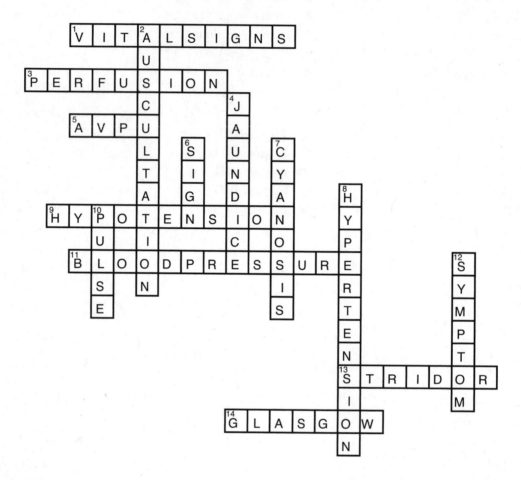

Calls to the Scene

1. -BSI precautions.

-Place patient in the position of comfort.

-Obtain a SAMPLE history.

-Apply high-flow oxygen via nonrebreathing mask, call 9-1-1 if available, or closely observe breathing.

-Obtain baseline vital signs.

-Monitor patient and repeat vital signs every 15 minutes.

-Arrange for normal transport.

2. -BSI precautions.

-Place patient in position of comfort.

-Call 9-1-1 (if available) or closely observe breathing.

-Apply high-flow oxygen via nonrebreathing mask.

-Obtain baseline vital signs.

-Obtain SAMPLE history.

-Monitor patient and repeat vital signs every 15 minutes.

-Arrange for normal transport.

3. -BSI precautions.

-Open and assess the airway.

-If not breathing, ventilate twice either by mouth-to-mouth or BVM device.

-Apply high-flow oxygen via nonrebreathing mask or BVM (if available).

-Coordinate transport to definitive care.

-Assess carotid pulse.

-If no pulse, initiate chest compressions.

-If patient has a pulse, treat for shock and rapid transport.

-Place patient in shock position and cover to keep warm.

-Continue assessment and obtain SAMPLE history.

-Monitor vital signs and take a complete set every 5 minutes.

Skill Drills

1. **Skill Drill 5-1: Obtaining a Blood Pressure by Auscultation or Palpation (page 144)**

1. Apply the cuff snugly.
2. Palpate the brachial artery.
3. Place the stethoscope and grasp the ball-pump and turn-valve.
4. Close the valve and pump to 20 mm Hg above the point at which you stop hearing pulse sounds. Note the systolic and diastolic pressures as you let air escape slowly.
5. Open the valve and quickly release the remaining air.
6. When using the palpation method, you should place your fingertips on the radial artery so that you feel the radial pulse.

Section 2 Airway

Chapter 6: Airway

Matching

1. C	(page 158)	**7.** A	(page 158)
2. I	(page 159)	**8.** F	(page 158)
3. H	(page 160)	**9.** L	(page 156)
4. G	(page 158)	**10.** D	(page 156)
5. K	(page 161)	**11.** J	(page 161)
6. E	(page 158)	**12.** B	(page 163)

Multiple Choice

1. D – Normally the air we breathe contains 21% oxygen and 78% nitrogen (A). (B) is the amount of oxygen left after a rescue breath has been delivered. (C) is the amount of oxygen delivered by the rescuer during rescue breathing. (page 159)

2. B – Opening the airway to relieve obstruction can often be done using the head tilt–chin lift maneuver for patients who have not sustained trauma. Therefore, this procedure is not "always" used. (A), (C), and (D) are each true. (pages 164–165)

3. B – An adult who is breathing normally will have respirations of 12 to 20 breaths per minute. (page 162)

4. D – (A), (B), and (C) are among the conditions associated with hypoxia. (pages 161–162)

5. A – When the level of carbon dioxide becomes too high, the brain stem sends nerve impulses down the spinal cord that cause the diaphragm and intercostal muscles to contract, increasing respirations. (B), (C), and (D) do not affect respirations. (page 161)

6. A – (B), (C), and (D) are among the signs of inadequate breathing in an adult. Warm, dry skin (A) indicates adequate circulation and perfusion. (pages 162–163)

7. C – To select the proper size for an oropharyngeal airway, measure from the patient's earlobe to the corner of the mouth on the side of the face. (A), (B), and (D) are incorrect. (page 167)

8. D – It may be very difficult to maintain a proper seal between the mask and the face. It is not practical for the rescuer to accurately measure tidal volumes (A). Positioning the patient's head (B) is easily accomplished with the head tilt–chin lift or modified jaw-thrust maneuver. All BVM devices should have the ability to perform under extreme environmental conditions (C). (page 181)

9. C – As you are assisting ventilations with a BVM device, you should evaluate how well the patient is breathing. You will know that artificial ventilation is not adequate if the patient's chest does not rise and fall with each ventilation. Inflation of the cheeks (A) may indicate obstruction of the air passage, requiring closer attention. Signs of spontaneous breathing (B) indicate how well the patient is breathing, but not how well the rescuer is assisting ventilations. Gurgling (D) indicates the need for immediate suctioning of the oral airway. (pages 182–183)

10. D – Do not suction an adult for more than 15 seconds. (A), (B), and (C) are incorrect. (page 170)

Labeling

1. Upper and Lower Airways (page 157)

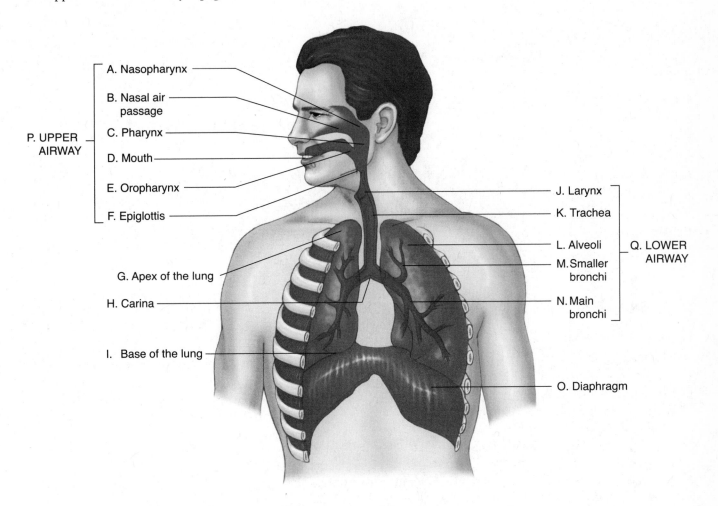

P. UPPER AIRWAY

A. Nasopharynx

B. Nasal air passage

C. Pharynx

D. Mouth

E. Oropharynx

F. Epiglottis

G. Apex of the lung

H. Carina

I. Base of the lung

J. Larynx

K. Trachea

L. Alveoli

M. Smaller bronchi

N. Main bronchi

O. Diaphragm

Q. LOWER AIRWAY

2. Thoracic Cage (page 157)

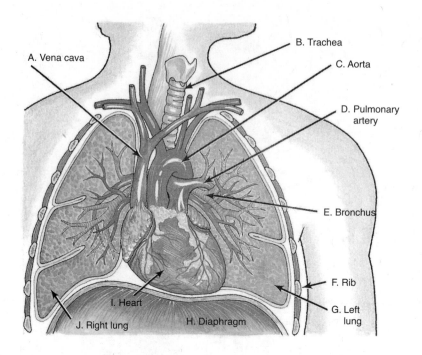

3. Cellular Exchange (page 160)

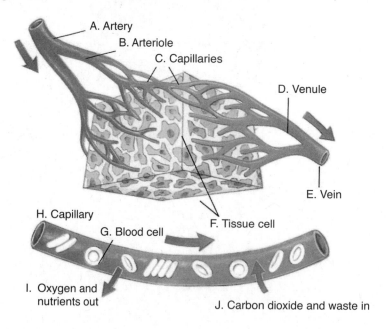

4. Pulmonary Exchange (page 160)

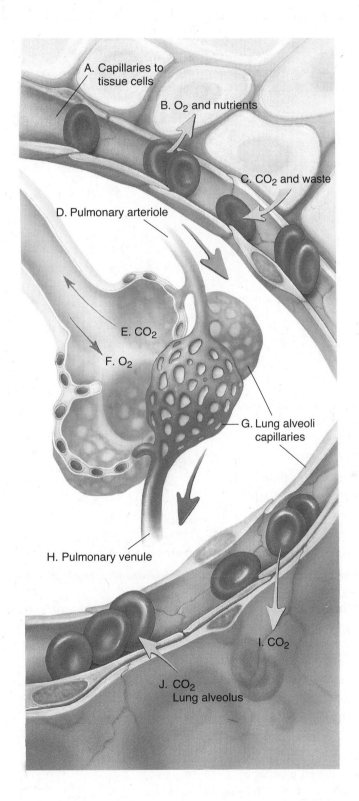

A. Capillaries to tissue cells

B. O_2 and nutrients

C. CO_2 and waste

D. Pulmonary arteriole

E. CO_2

F. O_2

G. Lung alveoli capillaries

H. Pulmonary venule

I. CO_2

J. CO_2 Lung alveolus

Vocabulary

1. Gag reflex: Normal reflex mechanism that causes retching when the soft palate or the back of the throat is touched. (page 166)

2. Gastric distention: Air filling the stomach during artificial ventilation due to high volume and pressure. (page 183)

3. Bag-valve-mask device: A device with a face mask attached to a ventilation bag containing a reservoir and connected to oxygen; delivers more than 90% supplemental oxygen. (page 180)

Fill-in

1. trachea (page 156)
2. higher (page 159)
3. 21, 78 (page 159)
4. carbon dioxide (page 161)
5. diaphragm, intercostal muscles (page 158)
6. low oxygen, high carbon dioxide (page 161)
7. hypoxia (page 161)

True/False

1. F   (page 166)
2. T   (page 177)
3. F   (page 167)
4. F   (pages 173, 176)
5. F   (page 174)

Short Answer

1. Nervousness, tachycardia, irritability, fear, apprehension. (Other signs: Mental status changes, use of accessory muscles for breathing, breathing difficulty, possible chest pain.) (page 161)

2. Adults: 12 to 20 breaths/min

   Children: 15 to 30 breaths/min

   Infants: 25 to 50 breaths/min (page 162)

3. Give slow, gentle breaths. (page 184)

4. 1. Kneel above the patient's head.

   2. Extend the patient's neck unless you suspect a cervical spine injury.

   3. Open the mouth and suction as needed. Insert an airway adjunct as needed.

   4. Select a proper-sized mask.

   5. Position the mask on the patient's face.

   6. Use the C-clamp technique to hold the mask, then squeeze the bag every 5 seconds for adults, every 3 seconds for children and infants. (pages 181–182)

5. 1. Respiratory rate of less than 8 breaths/min or greater than 24 breaths/min

   2. Accessory muscle use

   3. Skin pulling in around the ribs during inspiration

   4. Pale, cyanotic, or cool (clammy) skin

   5. Irregular pattern of inhalation and exhalation

   6. Lung sounds that are decreased, unequal, or "wet"

   7. Labored breathing

   8. Shallow and/or uneven chest movement

   9. Two- or three-word sentences spoken (pages 162–163)

6. They are the secondary muscles of respiration. They are not used in normal breathing. They include:

   1. Sternocleidomastoid (neck)

   2. Pectoralis major (chest)

   3. Abdominal muscles (page 162)

7. When the patient has severe trauma to the head or face. (page 168)

8. 1. Select the proper-size airway and apply a water-soluble lubricant.

2. Place the airway in the larger nostril with the curvature following the curve of the floor of the nose.

3. Advance the airway gently.

4. Continue until the flange rests against the skin. (pages 168–169)

9. Tonsil tips are best because they have a large diameter and do not collapse. In addition, they are curved, which allows easy, rapid placement. (page 170)

10. 15 seconds. (page 171)

Word Fun

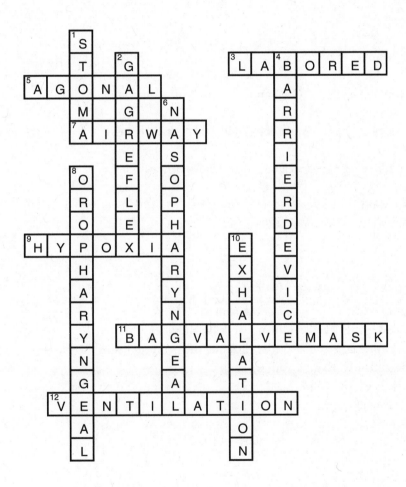

Calls to the Scene

1. -BSI precautions

-Maintain cervical spine stabilization.

-Immediately open the airway with a modified jaw thrust.

-Suction to remove obstruction.

-Assess the airway for breathing (rate, rhythm, quality) and provide oxygen via nonrebreathing mask or BVM.

-Continue initial assessment, rapid extrication, and arrange for rapid transport.

2. -BSI precautions

-Assess breathing for rate, quality, and degree of distress.

-Give 100% oxygen via nonrebreathing mask or BVM as appropriate.

-Transport in position of comfort.

-Arrange for rapid transport.

3. -BSI precautions

-Open the airway and attempt to ventilate.

-If air does not go in, reposition the airway and attempt to ventilate.

-If air still does not go in, treat child for a foreign body airway obstruction.

-Deliver 5 back blows and 5 chest thrusts.

-Look in the mouth to see if there is a visible obstruction that can be removed.

-If not, attempt to ventilate.

-If air does not go in, continue sequence as above while transporting.

-Arrange for rapid transport.

-If obstruction is cleared, ventilate and assess circulation.

-Continue to treat according to AHA guidelines.

Skill Drills

1. Skill Drill 6-1: Positioning an Unconscious Patient (page 164)

1. Support the head while your partner straightens the patient's legs.
2. Have your partner place his or her hand on the patient's far shoulder and hip.
3. Roll the patient as a unit with the person at the head calling the count to begin the move.
4. Open and assess the patient's airway and breathing status.

Section 3 Patient Assessment

Chapter 7: Patient Assessment

Matching

1. O   (page 202)
2. B   (page 240)
3. K   (page 238)
4. L   (page 209)
5. A   (page 237)
6. E   (page 239)
7. J   (page 209)
8. M   (page 216)

9. I   (page 224)
10. N   (page 224)
11. G   (page 200)
12. D   (page 227)
13. C   (page 224)
14. F   (page 218)
15. H   (page 204)

Multiple Choice

1. C – Level of responsiveness is determined during the "initial assessment." (pages 204, 206)
2. D – Possible dangers you may observe in scene size-up also include leaking gasoline or diesel fuel, hostile bystanders/potential for violence, fire or smoke, possible hazardous or toxic materials, other dangers at crash or rescue scenes and crime scenes. (page 202)
3. B (page 201)
4. C (pages 222–224)
5. D (page 200)
6. A (page 211)
7. C (page 200)
8. D (page 237)
9. D (page 215)
10. C (page 202)
11. B – The pupils are assessed during the detailed exam. (page 237)
12. D – An altered mental status may also be caused by stroke, cardiac problems, or drug use. (page 212)
13. A – Tightness in the chest is a symptom. (page 208)
14. B – The tongue becomes an obstruction due to the relaxation of the muscles. (page 207)
15. D (pages 207–208)
16. D (page 209)
17. B (page 218)
18. A (pages 239–240)
19. C (page 239)
20. D (page 237)
21. D (page 237)
22. B – Only apply an AED if the patient is unresponsive, apneic, and pulseless. (page 209)
23. C – (A,B,D) are all treatments. (page 201)
24. D (page 218)
25. B (page 200)
26. C (page 209)
27. B – AVPU (A) evaluates level of responsiveness in the initial assessment, OPQRST (C) evaluates pain, and SAMPLE (D) provides the necessary history. (page 211)

28. C – Once the c-collar is in place it should not be removed and does not allow for palpation of the neck and cervical spine. (page 232)

29. A – (B,C) evaluate sensation, not motor function. (pages 239–240)

30. C (page 215)

31. B – If the impact is minor and their ABCs are intact with no other complaint, they do not require a rapid trauma assessment and rapid transport. (page 210)

32. C (page 224)

33. B (page 224)

34. D – When assessing a chief complaint of chest pain, also evaluate blood pressure and look for trauma to the chest. (page 225)

35. D (page 215)

36. B (page 211)

37. D – When performing the detailed physical exam, depending on what you learn, you should also be prepared to perform spinal immobilization, and provide transport to an appropriate facility, or call for ALS backup. (page 230)

38. D (page 238)

39. B – A diagnosis cannot be made in the field. (page 198)

40. D – When reevaluating interventions, also take a moment to ensure that the airway is still open. (page 242)

Vocabulary

1. Intervention: An urgent measure that interrupts assessment in order to care for a condition that threatens life or limb and requires immediate care. (page 200)

2. Recovery position: The preferred body position for an unresponsive patient with no suspected spine injury. (page 200)

3. Mechanism of injury: The way in which traumatic injuries occur; the forces that act on the body to cause damage. (page 200)

4. Golden Hour: The time from injury to definitive care, during which treatment of shock or traumatic injuries should occur because survival potential is the best. (page 201)

Fill-in

1. body substance isolation (page 202)

2. Rate, rhythm, strength (page 242)

3. general impression (page 204)

4. life-threatening (page 204)

5. airway (pages 206–207)

6. reevaluate (page 207)

7. initial assessment (page 210)

True/False

1. F (page 204)

2. T (page 198)

3. F (page 242)

4. T (page 198)

5. T (page 209)

6. T (page 230)

7. T (page 201)

Short Answer

1. 1. Detect life-threatening conditions rapidly and care for them immediately.

2. Determine whether you need to attend to any other problems.

3. Evaluate and facilitate the rapid transport of the patient to enter the EMS system or to get to definitive medical care.

4. Do nothing that would make the patient worse. (page 198)

2. To identify and initiate treatment of immediate or potential life threats. (page 204)

3. Immediate assessment of the environment, the patient's presenting signs and symptoms, and the patient's chief complaint. (page 204)

4. A-Airway

B-Breathing

C-Circulation (page 205)

5. 1. Identify the patient's chief complaint.

2. Understand the circumstances surrounding the chief complaint.

3. Direct further physical examination. (page 218)

6. Deformities, Contusions, Abrasions, Punctures/penetrations, Burns, Tenderness, Lacerations, Swelling (page 211)

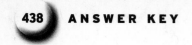

Word Fun

```
              ¹R A L E ²S     ³G
              A           A    U
              D           M    A
          ⁴B S I       ⁵O P Q R S T
            A T           L    D
            T         ⁶C ⁷R E P I T U S
          ⁸M O I         H    N
            O N          O    G     ⁹F
            N            N          O
                         C          C
          ¹⁰H Y P O T H E R M I A    L
                         I          L
```

Calls to the Scene

1. -BSI precautions

-Maintain cervical spine control

-Immediately manage the airway by suction and oxygen

-Control bleeding

-Rapid survey and transport

This patient is a load-and-go based on:

 Mechanism of injury

 Level of responsiveness

 Airway compromise

2. -BSI precautions.

-Scene size-up. Move patient if necessary.

-Form general impression. Stabilize ABCs if necessary.

-Perform focused history and physical exam: determine chief complaint, obtain vitals and SAMPLE history.

-Transport to aid room.

-Perform detailed physical exam.

-Monitor patient until ambulance arrives.

3. -BSI precautions.

-Stabilize ABCs if needed.

-Perform focused history and physical exam for responsive medical patients.

-Determine chief complaint, baseline vitals, and SAMPLE history.

-Transport to aid room for detailed physical exam.

Skill Drills

1. Skill Drill 7-1: Performing a Rapid Body Survey (page 214)

1. Assess the head.

2. Assess the neck.

3. Assess the chest.

4. Assess the abdomen.

5. Assess the pelvis.
6. Assess the lower extremities.
7. Assess the upper extremities.
8. Assess the back.

2. **Skill Drill 7-2: Performing a Focused History and Physical Exam: Responsive Trauma Patient (pages 220–221)**

1. Ensure scene safety and patient responsiveness. Recheck ABCs.
2. Institute BSI precautions and obtain the patient's consent for treatment.
3. Determine the patient's chief complaint.
4. Assess the patient's head, neck, and back if a loss of responsiveness or spine or head injury is suspected.
5. Assess the patient's pulse, skin temperature, and breathing rate. Obtain SAMPLE history.
6. Perform a focused assessment of the injured site (chief complaint).
7. Expose only what is necessary to determine the essential emergency care.
8. Splint and/or provide appropriate care of injuries.

3. **Skill Drill 7-4: Performing the Detailed Physical Exam (pages 234–236)**

1. Observe the patient's face.
2. Inspect the eyelids and the area around the eyes.
3. Examine the eyes for redness, contact lenses. Check pupil function.
4. Look behind the ear for Battle's sign.
5. Check the ears for drainage or blood.
6. Observe and palpate the head.
7. Palpate the zygomas and maxillae.
8. Palpate the mandible
9. Assess the mouth.
10. Inspect the neck.
11. Palpate the neck, front and back.
12. Observe for jugular vein distention.
13. Inspect the chest and observe breathing motion.
14. Gently palpate the ribs.
15. Listen to anterior breath sounds (midaxillary, midclavicular).
16. Listen to posterior breath sounds (bases, apices).
17. Observe the abdomen and pelvis.
18. Gently palpate the abdomen.
19. Gently compress the pelvis from the sides.
20. Gently press the iliac crests.
21. Assess the lower extremities.
22. Assess distal circulation, motor, and sensory functions in the lower extremities.
23. Assess the upper extremities.
24. Assess distal circulation, motor, and sensory functions in the upper extremities.
25. Log roll the patient. Inspect and palpate the back.

Chapter 8: Bleeding

Matching

1. J   (page 250)
2. E   (page 250)
3. K   (page 250)
4. F   (page 251)
5. C   (page 250)
6. H   (page 250)
7. B   (page 254)

8. I   (page 261)
9. M   (page 258)
10. A   (page 261)
11. D   (page 255)
12. L   (page 253)
13. G   (page 254)

Multiple Choice

1. D (page 250)
2. D (page 250)
3. C (page 250)
4. C (page 250)
5. B – Blood returns to the heart from the lungs via the pulmonary veins. (page 250)
6. A – Arteries carry blood away from the heart. The pulmonary arteries carry blood away from the heart to the lungs to be oxygenated. (page 250)
7. D – The left ventricle is the thickest chamber of the heart because it must pump blood throughout the body. (page 251)
8. B (page 251)
9. D – The muscles at the arterial ends of the capillaries also dilate and constrict in response to heat and cold. (page 252)
10. C (page 252)
11. B (page 252)
12. C – The lungs (A) and kidneys (B) require a constant blood supply. (page 253)
13. C (page 253)
14. A – Shock is also called hypoperfusion. (page 253)
15. D (page 253)
16. B (page 254)
17. D – They may also present with an altered mental status, cool/clammy skin, and cyanosis. (page 254)
18. A (page 254)
19. B (page 254)
20. C (page 254)
21. C (page 254)
22. D (pages 254–255)
23. B (page 255)
24. C (page 255)
25. A (page 256)
26. A (page 256)
27. C (page 257)
28. C (page 257)
29. D – Never cover a tourniquet (B). Wide padding may actually help protect the tissues and help with arterial compression (C). (page 258)
30. D – Also, facial injuries, hypertension, and digital trauma. (page 260)
31. B (page 260)

32. B (pages 260–261)

33. D – Nontraumatic internal bleeding in the abdomen can also result from irritable bowel syndrome. (page 260)

34. D – (A), (B), and (C) are signs, not symptoms. (pages 260–261)

35. D – Also includes hematuria, hematemesis, nonmenstrual vaginal bleeding, and pain, tenderness, bruising, guarding, or swelling. (pages 260–261)

36. C – Blood pressure changes (D) are a late sign. (page 261)

Labeling

1. The Left and Right Sides of the Heart (page 251)

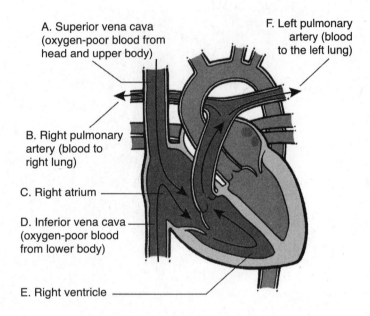

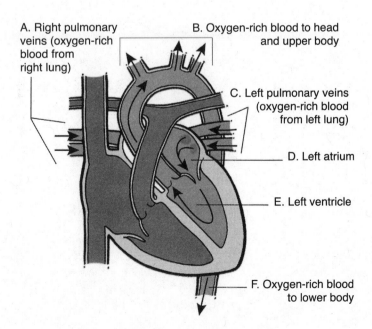

2. Perfusion (page 253)

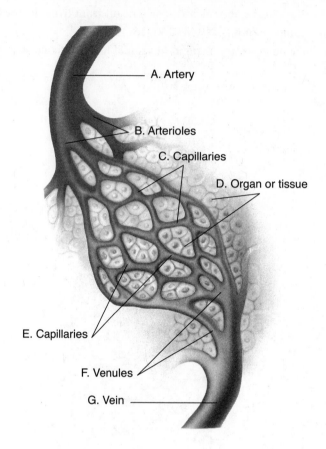

3. Arterial pressure points (page 257)

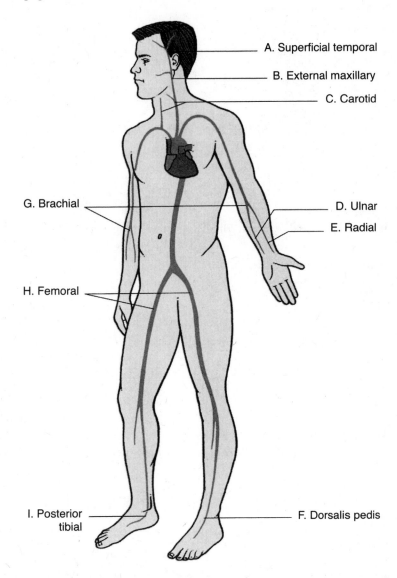

A. Superficial temporal
B. External maxillary
C. Carotid
G. Brachial
D. Ulnar
E. Radial
H. Femoral
I. Posterior tibial
F. Dorsalis pedis

Vocabulary

1. Perfusion: Circulation of blood within an organ or tissue in adequate amounts to meet the cells' current needs for oxygen, nutrients, and waste removal. (page 252)

2. Shock: A condition in which the circulatory system fails to provide sufficient circulation for every body part to perform its function. Low blood volume results in inadequate perfusion, also known as hypovolemic shock. (page 253)

3. Melena: Black, foul smelling, tarry stool that contains digested blood. (page 261)

4. Hematemesis: Vomited blood (page 261)

5. Hemoptysis: Bright red blood coughed up by a patient. (page 261)

Fill-in

1. perfusion (page 252)

2. involuntary (page 250)

3. lungs (page 251)

4. hypoperfusion (page 253)

5. inferior (page 250)

6. white cells, red cells, platelets, and plasma (page 252)

7. oxygenated, deoxygenated (page 250)

8. heart, brain, lungs, and kidneys (page 253)

9. 4 to 6 (page 253)

True/False

1. F   (pages 254–255)   **4.** F   (page 258)

2. F   (page 254)   **5.** T   (page 258)

3. T   (page 255)   **6.** F   (page 256)

Short Answer

1. It redirects blood away from nonessential organs to the heart, brain, lungs, and kidneys. (page 253)

2. Artery: Bright red, spurting

Vein: Dark color with steady flow

Capillary: Darker color, oozes (pages 254–255)

3. 1. Direct pressure and elevation

2. Pressure dressings

3. Pressure points (for upper and lower extremities)

4. Splints

5. Air splints

6. PASG

7. Tourniquets (page 255)

4. 1. Change in mental status (restlessness, anxiety, combativeness)

2. Weakness, fainting, or dizziness on standing (early sign) or at rest (later sign)

3. Tachycardia

4. Thirst

5. Nausea and vomiting

6. Cold, moist (clammy) skin

7. Shallow, rapid breathing

8. Dull eyes

9. Slightly dilated pupils, slow to respond to light

10. Capillary refill in infants and children of more than 2 seconds

11. Weak, rapid (thready) pulse

12. Decreasing blood pressure

13. Altered level of consciousness (page 254)

5. 1. BSI precautions

2. Maintain the airway.

3. Administer high-flow oxygen.

4. Control all obvious external bleeding.

5. Apply splints to extremity, if a limb is involved.

6. Monitor and record the patient's vital signs.

7. Give the patient nothing by mouth.

8. Elevate the legs 6" to 12" in nontrauma patients.

9. Keep the patient warm.

10. Provide immediate transport. (page 261)

Word Fun

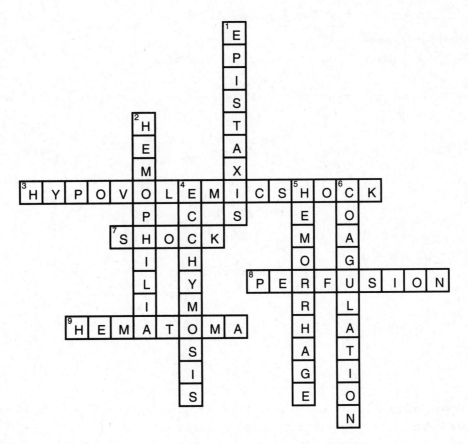

Calls to the Scene

1. -BSI precautions.
   -Control bleeding with direct pressure, elevation, pressure point, and a tourniquet as a LAST resort.
   -Apply high-flow oxygen.
   -Place patient in the position of comfort.
   -Monitor vital signs.
   -Arrange for rapid transport.

2. -BSI precautions.
   -High-flow oxygen.
   -Maintain c-spine immobilization and place patient in the Trendelenburg's position.
   -Cover to keep warm.
   -Consider the mechanism of injury.
   -Monitor vital signs.
   -Arrange for rapid transport.

3. -BSI precautions.
   -Control bleeding with direct pressure, elevation, pressure point, or tourniquet as a LAST resort.
   -Apply high-flow oxygen and treat for shock as signs and symptoms present.
   -Monitor vital signs.
   -Arrange for normal transport unless patient shows signs and symptoms of shock.

Skill Drills

1. **Skill Drill 8-1: Controlling External Bleeding (page 256)**

1. Apply **direct pressure** over the wound.
   Elevate the injury above the **level** of the **heart** if no **fracture** is suspected.
2. Apply a **pressure dressing**.
3. Apply pressure at the appropriate **pressure point** while continuing to hold **direct pressure** and **elevation**.

Chapter 9: Shock

Matching

1. B (page 266)	**6.** A (page 270)	
2. G (page 266)	**7.** F (page 269)	
3. H (page 266)	**8.** I (page 270)	
4. C (page 266)	**9.** D (page 271)	
5. E (page 266)		

Multiple Choice

1. D (page 266)
2. B (page 266)
3. D (page 266)
4. C – It is accomplished by vessel constriction or dilation, together with sphincter constriction or dilation. (page 266)
5. D – Adequate waste removal is primarily through the lungs. (page 266)
6. D – C is peripheral vasoconstriction. (page 267)
7. D (pages 267–268)
8. C – Sepsis (A) and metabolic (B) shock may result in fluid loss or poor pump function. Hypovolemia (D) is due to fluid loss. (page 269)
9. A (page 268)
10. B (page 268)
11. C (page 269)
12. A (page 269)
13. C (page 269)
14. D (page 269)
15. A (page 269)
16. B (pages 268–269)
17. A (page 270)
18. A (page 270)
19. D (page 270)
20. B (page 271)
21. D – Anaphylactic shock is caused by an allergic reaction to a substance, can develop in minutes, and can be fatal. (page 270)
22. B (page 273)
23. C – Because the first 60 minutes after the injury are critical, rapid evaluation, stabilization, and transport are important. (page 273)
24. B (page 273)
25. D – With too little circulating blood, additional oxygen may be lifesaving. (page 275)
26. B (page 277)

Vocabulary

1. Edema: The presence of abnormally large amounts of fluid between cells in body tissues, causing swelling of affected areas. (page 268)
2. Hypothermia: A condition in which the internal body temperature falls below 95°F/35°C, usually as a result of prolonged exposure to cool or freezing temperatures. (page 269)
3. Shock: A condition in which the circulatory system fails to provide sufficient circulation to enable every body part to perform its function. (page 266)
4. Autonomic nervous system: The part of the nervous system that regulates involuntary functions, such as digestion and sweating. (page 266)
5. Cyanosis: Bluish color of the skin resulting from poor oxygenation of the circulating blood. (page 270)
6. Dehydration: Loss of water from the tissues of the body. (page 268)
7. Sensitization: Developing a sensitivity to a substance that initially caused no allergic reaction. (page 270)

Fill-in

1. Hypoperfusion (page 266)
2. contraction (page 266)
3. nonessential, essential (page 266)
4. perfusion (page 266)
5. heart, vessels, blood (page 266)
6. shock (hypoperfusion) (page 266)
7. Sphincters, constrict, dilate (page 266)
8. Diastolic, systolic (page 266)
9. Blood (page 266)
10. involuntary (page 266)

True/False

1. T   (page 270)
2. T   (page 268)
3. T   (page 266)
4. F   (page 266)
5. F   (page 271)
6. T   (page 276)
7. T   (page 269)

Short Answer

1. Causes: allergic reaction (most severe form)

   Signs/Symptoms: Can develop within seconds; mild itching/rash; burning skin; vascular dilation; generalized edema; profound coma; rapid death

   Treatment: Manage airway. Assist ventilations. Administer high-flow oxygen. Determine cause. Assist with administration of epinephrine. Transport promptly. (pages 270, 274–275)

2. Causes: Inadequate heart function; disease of muscle tissue; impaired electrical system; disease or injury

   Signs/Symptoms: Chest pains; irregular pulse; weak pulse; low blood pressure; cyanosis (lips, under nails); anxiety

   Treatment: Position comfortably. Administer high-flow oxygen. Assist ventilations. Transport promptly.
   (pages 268, 274–275)

3. Causes: Loss of blood or fluid

   Signs/Symptoms: Rapid, weak pulse; low blood pressure; change in mental status; cyanosis (lips, under nails); cool, clammy skin; increased respiratory rate

   Treatment: Secure airway. Assist ventilations. Administer high-flow oxygen. Control external bleeding. Elevate legs. Keep warm. Transport promptly. (pages 268–269, 274–275)

4. Causes: Severe chest injury, airway obstruction

   Signs/Symptoms: Rapid, weak pulse; low blood pressure; change in mental status; cyanosis (lips, under nails); cool, clammy skin; increased respiratory rate

   Treatment: Secure airway. Clear air passages. Assist ventilations. Administer high-flow oxygen. Transport promptly. (pages 270, 274–275)

5. Causes: Damaged cervical spine, which causes widespread blood vessel dilation

   Signs/Symptoms: Bradycardia (slow pulse); low blood pressure; signs of neck injury

   Treatment: Secure airway. Spinal immobilization. Assist ventilations. Administer high-flow oxygen. Transport promptly. (pages 270, 274–275)

6. Causes: Temporary, generalized vascular dilation; anxiety; bad news; sight of injury/blood; prospect of medical treatment; severe pain; illness; tiredness

   Signs/Symptoms: Rapid pulse; normal or low blood pressure

   Treatment: Determine duration of unconsciousness. Record initial vital signs and mental status. Suspect head injury if patient is confused or slow to regain consciousness. Transport promptly. (pages 270, 274–275)

7. Causes: Severe bacterial infection

   Signs/Symptoms: Warm skin; tachycardia; low blood pressure

   Treatment: Transport promptly. Administer high-flow oxygen. Provide full ventilatory support. Elevate legs. Keep patient warm. (pages 270, 274–275)

8. 1. Poor pump function

   2. Blood or fluid loss from blood vessels

   3. Poor vessel function (blood vessels dilate) (page 267)

Word Fun

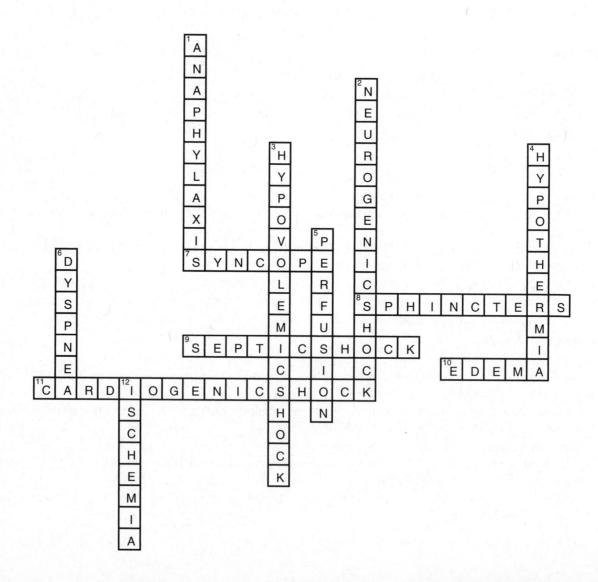

Calls to the Scene

1. -BSI precautions.
   -Treat for shock (neurogenic).
   -High-flow oxygen.
   -Place patient in Trendelenburg's position.
   -Keep patient warm.
   -Arrange for rapid transport.
   -Monitor vital signs continually en route.

2. -BSI precautions.
   -Treat for shock (hypovolemic).
   -High-flow oxygen via BVM.
   -Place patient in Trendelenburg's position.
   -Keep patient warm with consideration for burned areas.
   -Arrange for rapid transport.
   -Monitor vital signs continually en route.

3. -BSI precautions.
   -Treat for anaphylactic shock.
   -Apply high-flow oxygen while inquiring if the patient has an EpiPen.
   -Obtain orders and assist the mother with administering the EpiPen.
   -Monitor vital signs.
   -Arrange for rapid transport.

Skill Drills

1. **Skill Drill 9-1: Treating Shock (page 272)**

   1. Keep the patient supine, open the airway, and check breathing and pulse.
   2. Control obvious external bleeding.
   3. Splint any broken bones or joint injuries.
   4. Give high-flow oxygen if you have not already done so, and place blankets under and over the patient.
   5. If no fractures are suspected, elevate the legs 6" to 12".

Section 4 Medical Emergencies

Chapter 10: Respiratory Emergencies

Matching

1. B   (page 292)
2. D   (page 287)
3. H   (pages 288–289)
4. J   (pages 290–291)
5. L   (page 293)
6. C   (page 291)
7. G   (page 287)

8. E   (page 288)
9. M   (page 300)
10. A   (page 290)
11. K   (page 294)
12. F   (page 292)
13. I   (page 294)

Multiple Choice

1. D (page 287)
2. C (page 284)
3. D (page 286)
4. C – This will replace the carbon dioxide content in the arterial blood. (page 286)
5. B – Rapid and deep breathing helps to blow off excess carbon dioxide (page 286)
6. A – Pale or cyanotic skin (B), pursed lips and nasal flaring (C), and cool, damp skin (D) are signs of inadequate breathing. (page 286)
7. D (page 287)
8. B (page 287)
9. A (page 287)
10. B – Epiglottitis (A) and colds (C) create obstruction of the flow of air in the major passages. (page 287)
11. A (page 287)
12. D (page 289)
13. D (page 289)
14. C (page 290)
15. A (page 290)
16. D (page 290)
17. B – Blood pressure (A) of COPD patients is normal. The pulse (C) of COPD patients is rapid and occasionally irregular. (page 291)
18. C (page 291)
19. C (page 292)
20. B (page 292)
21. D (page 293)
22. C (page 293)
23. A (page 293)
24. D (page 294)
25. B (page 294)
26. B (page 295)
27. C (page 295)
28. D (page 296)
29. D (page 296)

30. D (page 297)
31. D (page 298)
32. C (page 301)

Labeling

The Upper Airway (page 285)

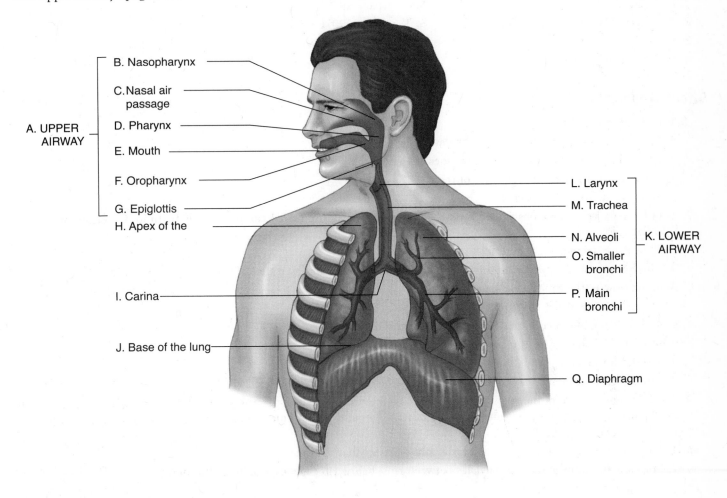

A. UPPER AIRWAY
- B. Nasopharynx
- C. Nasal air passage
- D. Pharynx
- E. Mouth
- F. Oropharynx
- G. Epiglottis
- H. Apex of the
- I. Carina
- J. Base of the lung

K. LOWER AIRWAY
- L. Larynx
- M. Trachea
- N. Alveoli
- O. Smaller bronchi
- P. Main bronchi
- Q. Diaphragm

Vocabulary

1. Stridor: High-pitched, rough barking inspiratory sound often heard with upper airway obstruction. (page 289)
2. Croup: Inflammation and swelling of the lining of the larynx. (page 289)
3. Rales: Crackling, rattling breath sounds. (page 291)
4. Rhonchi: Coarse, gravelly breath sounds. (page 291)
5. Diphtheria: An infectious disease in which a membrane lining the pharynx is formed that can severely obstruct passage of air into the larynx. (page 288)
6. Chronic obstructive pulmonary disease (COPD): A slow process of dilation and disruption of the airways and alveoli, caused by chronic bronchial obstruction. (page 290)

Fill-in

1. carbon dioxide (page 286)
2. oxygen (page 287)
3. Oxygen, oxygen (page 284)

4. alveoli (page 284)

5. trachea (page 284)

6. 8, 24 (page 286)

7. carbon dioxide (page 284)

True/False

1. F   (page 290)

2. T   (page 291)

3. F   (page 292)

4. F   (page 292)

5. T   (page 294)

6. T   (page 290)

7. F   (pages 291–292)

Short Answer

1. 1. Normal rate and depth

2. Regular pattern of inhalation and exhalation

3. Good audible breath sounds on both sides of the chest

4. Regular rise and fall on both sides of the chest

5. Pink, warm, dry skin (page 286)

2. 1. Pulmonary vessels are obstructed from absorbing oxygen and releasing carbon dioxide by fluid, infection, or collapsed air spaces.

2. Alveoli are damaged.

3. Air passages obstructed by muscle spasm, mucus, weakened airway walls

4. Blood flow to the lungs obstructed

5. Pleural space is filled with air or excess fluid (page 286)

3. 1. Patient is unable to coordinate administration and inhalation

2. Inhaler is not prescribed for patient.

3. You did not obtain permission from medical control or local protocol.

4. Patient has already met maximum prescribed dose before your arrival. (page 297)

4. An ongoing irritation of the respiratory tract; excess mucus production obstructs small airways and alveoli. Protective mechanisms are impaired. Repeated episodes of irritation and pneumonia can cause scarring and alveolar damage, leading to COPD. (page 290)

5. 1. Respiratory rate of slower than 8 breaths/min or faster than 24 breaths/min

2. Muscle retractions above the clavicles between ribs, below rib cage, especially in children

3. Pale or cyanotic skin

4. Cool, damp (clammy) skin

5. Shallow or irregular respirations

6. Pursed lips

7. Nasal flaring (pages 286–287)

6. A condition characterized by a chronically high blood level of carbon dioxide in which the respiratory center no longer responds to high blood levels of carbon dioxide. In these patients, low blood oxygen causes the respiratory center to respond and stimulate respiration. If the arterial level of oxygen is then raised, as happens when the patient is given additional oxygen, there is no longer any stimulus to breathe; both the high carbon dioxide and low oxygen drives are lost. (page 287)

Word Fun

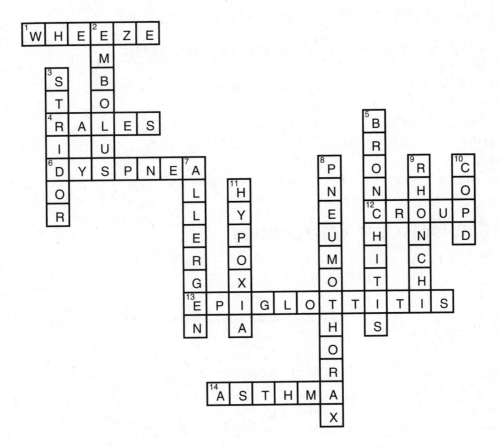

Calls to the Scene

1. -BSI precautions
   -Ask if patient has an inhaler
   -Obtain SAMPLE history
   -Transport in position of comfort
   -Maintain a clear airway
   -High-flow oxygen as needed

2. -BSI precautions
   -Place patient in position of comfort.
   -Administer high-flow oxygen.
   -Try to calm the patient and talk her into slowing her respirations.
   -Monitor vital signs
   -Arrange for normal transport.

3. -BSI precautions
   -Place patient in position of comfort.
   -Reassure patient in a calm manner
   -Supply supplemental oxygen
   -Monitor vital signs, watch for signs of fainting
   -Stabilize knee as conditions allow.
   -Transport to aid room.

Skill Drills

Skill Drill 10-1: Assisting a Patient with a Metered-Dose Inhaler (page 299)

1. Check that you have the right **medication**, the right **patient**, and the right **route**.
2. Remove oxygen mask.
   Hand inhaler to the patient. Instruct the patient about breathing and **lip seal**.
   Use a **spacer** if the patient has one.
3. Instruct the patient to press the inhaler and inhale.
   Instruct the patient about **breath holding**.
4. Reapply **oxygen**.
   After a few **breaths**, have the patient repeat the **dose** if order/protocol allows.

Chapter 11: Cardiovascular Emergencies

Matching

1.	K	(page 306)	**8.**	L	(page 306)
2.	D	(page 307)	**9.**	C	(page 310)
3.	N	(page 307)	**10.**	E	(page 309)
4.	F	(page 307)	**11.**	B	(page 314)
5.	M	(page 307)	**12.**	H	(page 311)
6.	J	(page 308)	**13.**	I	(page 313)
7.	G	(page 306)	**14.**	A	(page 313)

Multiple Choice

1. D – The number of deaths can also be reduced with increased numbers of lay people trained in CPR. (page 306)
2. D (page 306)
3. A (page 308)
4. B – Pulmonary veins transport blood from the lungs, where it has picked up oxygen. (page 306)
5. A (page 307)
6. B (page 307)
7. C (page 308)
8. C (page 308)
9. A – White blood cells (B) help fight infection. Platelets (C) help blood to clot. Veins (D) carry deoxygenated blood back to the heart. (page 308)
10. C (page 308)
11. C – Diastolic blood pressure is the resting phase of the ventricles. (pages 308–309)
12. A (page 310)
13. B (page 311)
14. B (page 311)
15. D (page 311)
16. B (page 311)
17. D – It is usually felt in the midchest, under the sternum, but may radiate. (page 311)
18. D (page 311)
19. C (page 312)
20. C (page 312)

21. C – (A) and (B) refer to angina. (page 312)

22. D (pages 312–313)

23. D (page 312)

24. A – Asystole (B) is absence of electrical activity. Ventricular stand still (C) is the same thing as asystole. Ventricular tachycardia (D) is a rapid heart rate greater than 100 beats/min. (page 313)

25. B (page 313)

26. A (page 314)

27. D (page 314)

28. B (page 314)

29. A (page 314)

30. C (page 313)

31. B – AVPU (A) is used to assess level of consciousness. SAMPLE (B) is used to assess history. CHART (D) is used for documentation. (page 312)

32. D (page 314)

33. B (page 318)

34. D (page 318)

35. C (page 319)

36. C (page 320)

37. B (page 320)

38. C (page 320)

39. D (pages 319–320)

Labeling

1. The Right and Left Sides of Heart (page 307)

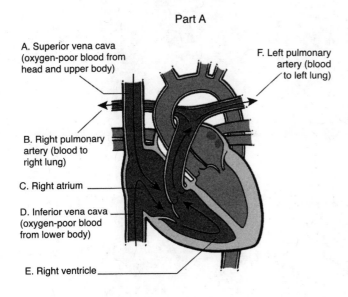

Part A

A. Superior vena cava (oxygen-poor blood from head and upper body)

F. Left pulmonary artery (blood to left lung)

B. Right pulmonary artery (blood to right lung)

C. Right atrium

D. Inferior vena cava (oxygen-poor blood from lower body)

E. Right ventricle

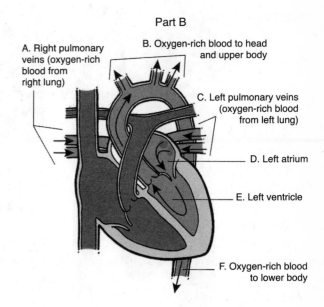

Part B

A. Right pulmonary veins (oxygen-rich blood from right lung)

B. Oxygen-rich blood to head and upper body

C. Left pulmonary veins (oxygen-rich blood from left lung)

D. Left atrium

E. Left ventricle

F. Oxygen-rich blood to lower body

2. Electrical Conduction (page 308)

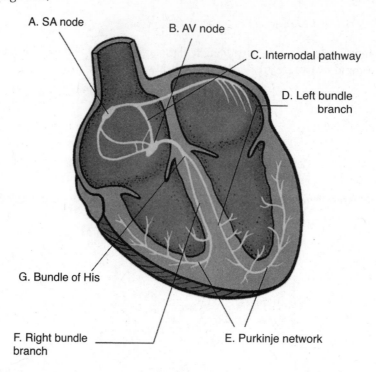

A. SA node

B. AV node

C. Internodal pathway

D. Left bundle branch

G. Bundle of His

F. Right bundle branch

E. Purkinje network

3. Pulse Points (page 310)

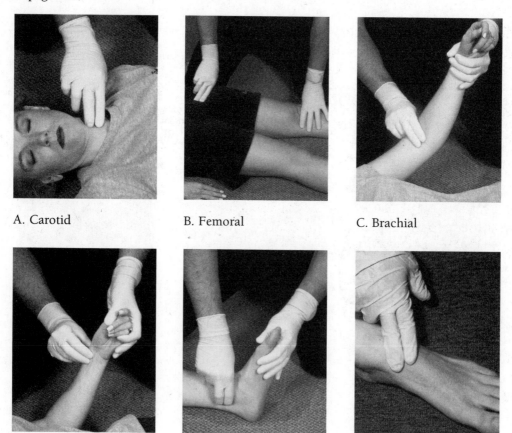

A. Carotid

B. Femoral

C. Brachial

D. Radial

E. Posterior tibial

F. Dorsalis pedis

Vocabulary

1. Angina pectoris: Transient chest discomfort caused by partial or temporary blockage of blood flow to heart muscle. (page 311)
2. Ventricular fibrillation: Disorganized, ineffective twitching of the ventricles, resulting in no blood flow to the heart. (page 313)
3. Cardiogenic shock: Body tissues do not get enough oxygen because the heart lacks enough power to force the proper volume of blood through the circulatory system. (page 313)
4. Acute myocardial infarction (AMI): Heart attack; death of myocardium following obstruction of blood flow to the heart muscle. (page 311)
5. Cardiac arrest: A state in which the heart fails to generate an effective and detectable blood flow. (page 311)
6. Congestive heart failure (CHF): A disorder in which the heart loses part of its ability to effectively pump blood, usually as a result of damage to the heart muscle and usually resulting in a backup of fluid into the lungs. (page 314)

Fill-in

1. septum (page 306)
2. aorta (page 306)
3. right (page 306)
4. AV (page 307)
5. dilation (page 307)
6. Red blood (page 308)
7. Diastolic (page 309)
8. four (page 306)
9. left (page 306)

True/False

1. F (page 306)
2. F (page 307)
3. T (page 310)
4. F (page 311)
5. T (page 311)
6. F (page 312)
7. T (page 316)
8. F (page 319)
9. T (page 311)
10. F (page 308)

Short Answer

1. Angina pectoris: A characteristic type of pain that occurs when the heart muscle is temporarily starved for oxygen. It usually appears during physical exertion or emotional stress, when the heart requires more oxygenated blood than the narrowed coronary arteries can deliver. (page 311)
2. Cardiac arrest, cardiogenic shock, pulmonary edema (page 313)
3. 1. Pain described as squeezing or crushing, or a sensation of pressure
   2. Pain beneath the sternum, typically radiating to the throat, jaw, left shoulder, and left arm. The pain occasionally radiates to both shoulders, both arms and the epigastrium.
   3. Anxiety and fear of death
   4. Respiratory distress
   5. Pale, cold clammy skin
   6. The pulse can be normal or subnormal.
   7. Blood pressure can be normal or abnormal.
   8. The patient usually prefers to sit up.
   9. Complications: cardiac arrest, cardiogenic shock, and pulmonary edema (page 312)

4. 1. Place pads correctly.

2. Make sure no one is touching the patient.

3. Do not defibrillate a patient who is in pooled water.

4. Dry the chest before defibrillating a wet patient.

5. Do not defibrillate a patient who is touching metal that others are touching.

6. Remove nitroglycerin patches and wipe the area with a dry towel before defibrillation. (page 325)

5. 1. It may or may not be caused by exertion, but can occur at any time.

2. It does not resolve in a few minutes.

3. It may or may not be relieved by rest or nitroglycerin. (page 312)

6. 1. Cardiac arrest

2. Cardiogenic shock

3. Pulmonary edema (page 313)

7. 1. Sudden onset of weakness, nausea, or sweating without an obvious cause

2. Chest pain/discomfort that does not change with each breath

3. Pain in lower jaw, arms, or neck

4. Sudden arrhythmia with syncope

5. Pulmonary edema

6. Sudden death

7. Increased and/or irregular pulse

8. Normal, increased, or decreased blood pressure

9. Normal or labored respirations

10. Pale or gray skin

11. Feelings of apprehension (pages 312–313)

Word Fun

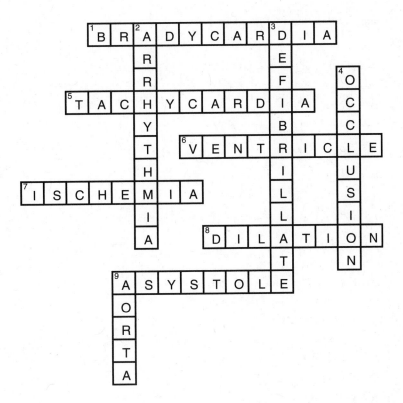

Calls to the Scene

1. -BSI precautions
   -Place patient in the position of comfort.
   -High-flow oxygen via nonrebreathing mask
   -Monitor vital signs.
   -Arrange for normal transport
2. -BSI precautions
   -Explain the need for seeking medical attention.
   -Place patient in position of comfort.
   -High-flow oxygen via nonrebreathing mask
   -Monitor vital signs.
   -Check a SAMPLE history and assist patient with nitroglycerin after contacting medical control if he currently has a prescription.
   -Arrange for rapid transport
3. -Stroke.
   -BSI precautions.
   -Call for transport (9-1-1).
   -Perform initial assessment.
   -Perform ABCs and insert an oral airway if needed.
   -Obtain a SAMPLE history. Make sure there are no other injuries.
   -Administer high-flow oxygen.
   -Transport to aid room, keeping head slightly elevated.
   -Perform detailed physical exam and obtain vitals.
   -Monitor patient's ABCs closely until ambulance arrives.

Skill Drills

1. Skill Drill 11-1: Integrating the AED and CPR (page 322)

1. Stop CPR if in progress.

   Assess responsiveness.

   Check breathing and pulse.

   If unresponsive and not breathing adequately, give two slow ventilations.

2. If pulseless, begin CPR.

   Prepare the AED pads.

   Turn on the AED; begin narrative if needed.

3. Apply AED pads.

   Stop CPR.

4. Verbally and visually clear the patient.

   Push the analyze button if there is one.

   Wait for the AED to analyze rhythm.

   If no shock advised, perform CPR for 1 minute.

   If shock advised, recheck that all are clear and push the shock button.

   Push the analyze button, if needed, to analyze rhythm again.

   Press the shock button if advised (second shock).

   Push the analyze button, if needed, to analyze rhythm again.

   Press the shock button if advised (third shock).

5. Check pulse.

   If pulse is present, check breathing.

6. If breathing adequately, give oxygen and transport. If not, open airway, ventilate, and transport.

   If no pulse, perform CPR for 1 minute.

   Clear the patient and analyze again.

   If necessary, repeat one cycle of up to three shocks.

   Transport and call medical control.

   Continue to support breathing or perform CPR, as needed.

Chapter 12: Neurologic Emergencies

Matching

1. D (page 334)
2. G (page 335)
3. E (page 335)
4. B (page 334)
5. I (page 335)
6. F (page 334)
7. J (page 336)
8. C (page 336)
9. M (page 337)
10. H (page 339)
11. L (page 340)
12. K (page 336)
13. A (page 340)

Multiple Choice

1. D (pages 337–338)
2. A – The cerebellum (B) controls muscle and body coordination. The cerebrum (C) controls emotion, thought, touch, movement, and sight. (page 334)
3. A (page 334)

4. C – (page 335)

5. C – A hemorrhagic stroke (A) is bleeding in the brain. Atherosclerosis (B) is usually the cause of the blockage. A cerebral embolism (D) may be the cause of the blockage. (page 336)

6. A – (B and C) may also result in a hemorrhagic stroke, but (D) leads to ischemic stroke. (page 336)

7. B (page 336)

8. B (page 336)

9. D (page 337)

10. A (page 337)

11. D – Epilepsy (A) is congenital in origin. A brain tumor (B) is a structural cause. A seizure due to a fever (C) is a febrile seizure. (page 337)

12. D (page 338)

13. D (page 338)

14. C – Unequal pupils may be seen in conjunction with a head injury, but they are not the cause of the altered mental status. (page 339)

15. B – A patient who has had a stroke may be alert and attempting to communicate normally, whereas a patient with hypoglycemia almost always has an altered or decreased level of consciousness. (pages 339–340)

16. C (page 339)

17. D (page 340)

18. B – Aphasia (A) is an inability to produce or understand speech. With expressive aphasia (C), the patient will be able to understand the question but cannot produce the right sounds in order to answer. With dysarthria (D), they will understand language and be able to speak, but their words may be slurred and hard to understand. (page 340)

19. A (page 341)

20. B – The airway is assessed first with any patient. (page 341)

21. D (page 342)

22. A – Key physical tests for patients suspected of having a stroke include tests of speech, facial movement, and arm movement. (page 342)

23. C – A score of 11-13 indicates moderate to severe dysfunction. A score of 14-15 indicates mild dysfunction (B). A score of 10 or less indicates severe dysfunction (D). (page 343)

24. C (pages 343–344)

25. B – The body is attempting to rid itself of excessive buildup of acid. (page 344)

26. C (page 345)

27. D (page 346)

Labeling

1. Brain (page 335)

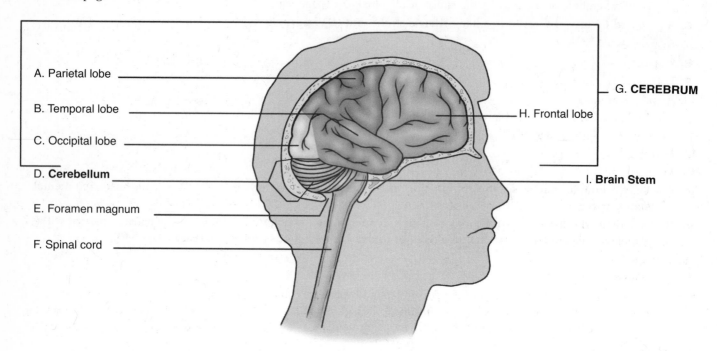

A. Parietal lobe

B. Temporal lobe

C. Occipital lobe

D. **Cerebellum**

E. Foramen magnum

F. Spinal cord

G. **CEREBRUM**

H. Frontal lobe

I. **Brain Stem**

2. Spinal Cord (page 335)

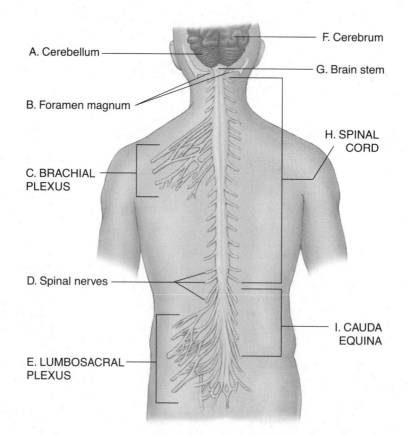

A. Cerebellum

B. Foramen magnum

C. BRACHIAL PLEXUS

D. Spinal nerves

E. LUMBOSACRAL PLEXUS

F. Cerebrum

G. Brain stem

H. SPINAL CORD

I. CAUDA EQUINA

Vocabulary

1. Cerebrovascular accident (CVA): An interruption of blood flow to the brain that results in the loss of brain function. (page 335)
2. Ischemic stroke: Occurs when blood flow to a particular part of the brain is cut off by blockage inside a blood vessel. (page 336)
3. Transient ischemic attack (TIA): Stroke symptoms that resolve spontaneously within 24 hours. (page 337)
4. Hemorrhagic stroke: Occurs as a result of bleeding inside the brain. (page 336)
5. Generalized seizure: Neurologic emergency characterized by unconsciousness and a generalized twitching of all the body's muscles that lasts several minutes or longer. (page 337)
6. Absence seizure: Seizure characterized by a brief lapse of attention during which the patient simply stares or does not respond to anyone. (page 337)
7. Atherosclerosis: A disorder in which cholesterol and calcium build up inside the walls of blood vessels, forming plaque, which eventually leads to partial or complete blockage of blood flow. (page 336)
8. Cerebral embolism: Obstruction of a cerebral artery caused by a clot that was formed elsewhere in the body and traveled to the brain. (page 336)
9. Febrile seizure: Convulsion that results from a sudden high fever, particularly in children. (page 338)
10. Thrombosis: Clotting of the cerebral arteries that may result in the interruption of cerebral blood flow and subsequent stroke. (page 336)

Fill-in

1. twelve (page 335)
2. cerebellum (page 334)
3. emotion and thought (page 334)
4. head (page 335)
5. three (page 334)
6. nerves (page 335)
7. opposite (page 334)
8. cerebrum (page 334)
9. Incontinence (page 338)
10. brain (page 334)
11. epidural (page 341)
12. hemiparesis (page 339)
13. altered mental status (page 340)

True/False

1. F   (page 338)
2. F   (pages 337–338)
3. T   (page 338)
4. F   (page 339)
5. T   (page 341)
6. F   (page 342)
7. F   (page 342)

Short Answer

1. 1. Facial droop—Ask patient to show teeth or smile.
   2. Arm drift—Ask patient to close eyes and hold arms out with palms up.
   3. Speech—Ask patient to say, "The sky is blue in Cincinnati." (pages 342–343)

2. Newer clot-busting therapies may be helpful in reversing damage in certain kinds of strokes, but treatment must be started within 3 hours after onset of the event. (page 346)

3. 1. Remove clothing.

   2. Spray/wipe with tepid water, particularly about the head/neck.

   3. Fan moistened areas. (page 346)

4. A period of time after a seizure, generally lasting from 5 to 30 minutes, that is characterized by some degree of altered mental status and labored respirations. (pages 338–339)

5. Infarcted cells are dead. Ischemic cells are still alive, although they are not functioning properly because of hypoxia. (page 335)

6. 1. Hypoglycemia

   2. Postictal state

   3. Subdural or epidural bleeding (page 341)

Word Fun

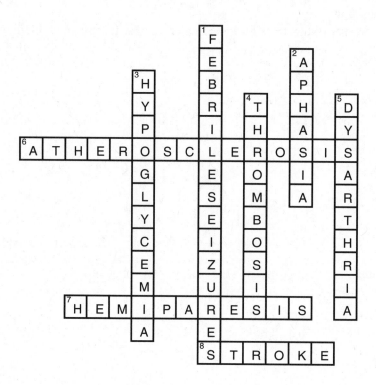

Calls to the Scene

1. -BSI precautions

   -Stabilize ABCs

   -Rapid body survey and SAMPLE history

   -Rapid transport to aid room keeping head slightly elevated

   -High-flow oxygen.

   -Monitor vital signs.

   -Transport to definitive care.

2. -BSI precautions

   -Maintain the airway—high-flow oxygen.

   -Suction if necessary or position lateral recumbent to clear secretions.

   -Check glucose level.

   -Arrange for rapid transport.

3. -BSI precautions

-Initial assessment procedures

-Focused history, SAMPLE, care for laceration

-Depending on location, walk or transport patient to aid room.

-Detailed physical exam.

-Advise patient regarding concussion and suggest no exercise for day.

-Monitor vitals.

-Reassess.

Chapter 13: Common Medical Emergencies

Matching

1. C	(page 358)	**10.** G	(page 360)
2. A	(page 352)	**11.** M	(page 365)
3. B	(page 353)	**12.** N	(page 366)
4. D	(page 353)	**13.** L	(page 367)
5. F	(page 360)	**14.** K	(page 374)
6. H	(page 359)	**15.** Q	(page 379)
7. J	(page 361)	**16.** R	(page 379)
8. E	(page 361)	**17.** O	(page 384)
9. I	(page 360)	**18.** P	(page 389)

Multiple Choice

1. A – To gauge the degree of distention, simply look at the patient's abdomen. (page 354)

2. B – The kidneys, genitourinary structures, and large vessels (inferior vena cava, abdominal aorta) are found in the retroperitoneal space. The stomach, gall bladder, liver, pancreas, and uterus (answers A, C, D) are all found within the peritoneum. The adrenal glands (D) sit atop the kidneys in the retroperitoneal space. (page 354)

3. C – The patient with peritonitis usually has abdominal pain, even when lying quietly. The patient may have difficulty breathing and may take rapid, shallow breaths because of the pain. (page 353)

4. C – Rebound tenderness and fever are signs and symptoms associated with inflammation of the peritoneum. The patient usually has abdominal pain, even when resting (A), and will present with hypotension and tachycardia (B) if associated with shock/fluid loss. (pages 353–354)

5. C – The acute abdomen is associated with possible fluid loss and bleeding. You should anticipate the possible development of hypovolemic shock and be prepared to provide prompt treatment. (page 353)

6. C – The central problem in diabetes is the lack or ineffective action of insulin. (page 359)

7. D – Insulin is a hormone that is normally produced by the pancreas that enables glucose to enter the cells. (page 359)

8. D – Diabetic coma occurs in the patient who is not under medical treatment, who takes insufficient insulin, who markedly overeats, or who is undergoing some sort of stress, such as infection, illness, overexertion, fatigue, or drinking alcohol. (page 361)

9. B – A sweet or fruity (acetone) odor on the breath is caused by the unusual waste products in the blood (ketones). (page 361)

10. B – Insulin shock develops much more quickly than diabetic coma. In some instances, it can occur in a matter of minutes. (page 361)

11. D – Glucose is the major source of energy for the body, and all cells need it to function properly. A constant supply to the brain is as important as oxygen. (page 360)

12. A – Diabetic coma occurs in the patient who takes insufficient insulin. Too much insulin (B) results in insulin shock. (page 361)

13. B – If unable to perform a blood glucose test, you must always suspect hypoglycemia in any patient with altered mental status. (page 363)

14. C – The first step in caring for any patient is to perform an initial assessment to verify that the airway is open. All the others (A, B, D) are secondary to airway. (page 363)

15. D – You must use your knowledge of the signs and symptoms to decide whether the problem is diabetic coma or insulin shock when dealing with an unresponsive diabetic patient. However, this assessment should not prevent you from providing prompt treatment and transport (A, B, C). (page 363)

16. A – The only contraindications to glucose are an inability to swallow or unconsciousness, since aspiration can occur. (page 363)

17. D – Maintain the airway and provide prompt transport to the hospital. (page 363)

18. D – All of the others (A, B, C) are signs of diabetic ketoacidosis. (pages 361–362)

19. C – Dehydration can be indicated by sunken eyes. Good skin turgor (A), would indicate sufficient hydration and elevated blood pressure (B), could indicate overhydration. (page 361)

20. A – Diabetes may mask signs and symptoms of other problems. Any diabetic complaining of "not feeling well," with no mechanism of injury, should have their glucose level evaluated to rule out hypo- or hyperglycemia, followed by the appropriate medical assessment (B). As long as the mental status is intact, oral glucose (D) is not immediately indicated, nor is rapid transport to the closest facility (C). Transport, whether slow or rapid, should always be to the closest most appropriate facility. (pages 362–363)

21. C – If the patient has an altered mental status, a glucose test should be performed to rule out possible diabetic complications. (page 363)

22. D (page 363)

23. A – Medical protocols usually recommend sugar cubes, granulated sugar, honey, candy, oral glucose gel, etc. Do not give sugar-free drinks that are sweetened with saccharin or other synthetic sweetening compounds (B, C, D), as they will have little or no effect. (page 365)

24. A – (B) The tip is placed against the lateral thigh. (C) Needles are never to be recapped. (pages 369–370)

25. A – Rocky Mountain spotted fever and Lyme disease are both spread through the tick's saliva, which is injected into the skin when the tick attaches itself. (page 375)

26. D – Additional signs, which may or may not occur, include weakness, sweating, fainting, and shock. (page 374)

27. C – (A) Suffocating it with gasoline or (B) trying to burn it with a lighted match will only succeed in burning the patient. (C) Pulling it straight out will usually remove the whole tick. (page 376)

28. B – The wasp's stinger is unbarbed, meaning that it can inflict multiple stings. (page 366)

29. D – Anaphylaxis typically involves multiple organ systems. Wheezing and urticaria are common signs. (page 366)

30. D – The patient may also experience sudden pain, redness, and itching. (page 366)

31. D – It is also important to determine what the effects of the exposure have been and how they have progressed, what interventions have been completed, and if the patient has prescribed medication for allergic reactions. (page 368)

32. D (page 374)

33. D – Epinephrine constricts the blood vessels, which raises blood pressure. Epinephrine also raises the pulse rate, inhibits allergic reactions, and dilates the bronchioles. (page 369)

34. B – Epinephrine (C) should only be administered in extreme reaction cases, and the patient with no signs or symptoms should be placed in the position of comfort (A). (page 369)

35. D – Assess ABCs (A) in all patients. Take the plant with you (B) for identification of the poison, and always provide prompt transport (C) for suspected or known poisonings. (page 380)

36. B – Alcohol dulls the sense of awareness (A) and decreases reaction time (C). (page 383)

37. B – (A) and (C) are symptoms of poisoning by botulism. (page 389)

38. A (page 385)

39. D – These would be unusual responses to the drug and require assessment in an emergency department. (page 386)

40. D – Carbon monoxide is odorless and can produce severe hypoxia without damaging the lungs. (pages 381–382)

41. B – (A) is not a sign or symptom, but part of the interview process. (C) Dyspnea is a systemic rather than localized problem. (page 382)

42. C (page 381)

43. A – Move the patient into fresh air (A) immediately. Rescuers should wear SCBAs (B) if indicated by the situation. (pages 380–381)

44. D (page 380)

45. C – Most poisons do not have a specific antidote (A). Syrup of ipecac (D) is only used for specific instances. Oxygen (B) is never contraindicated, but it will not solve the problem this patient is experiencing. (page 380)

Labeling

1. Solid Organs (page 355)

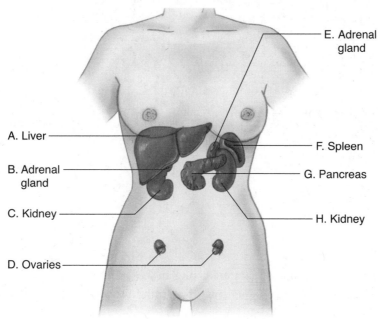

A. Liver
B. Adrenal gland
C. Kidney
D. Ovaries
E. Adrenal gland
F. Spleen
G. Pancreas
H. Kidney

2. Hollow Organs (page 355)

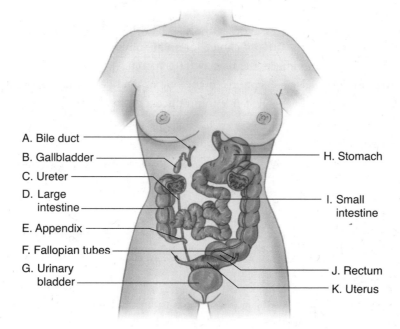

A. Bile duct
B. Gallbladder
C. Ureter
D. Large intestine
E. Appendix
F. Fallopian tubes
G. Urinary bladder
H. Stomach
I. Small intestine
J. Rectum
K. Uterus

3. Retroperitoneal Organs (page 355)

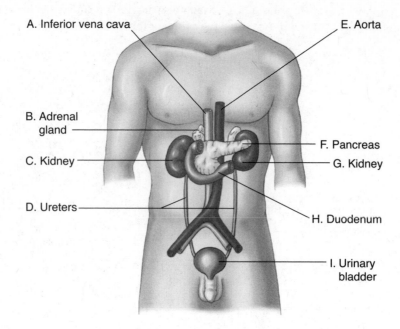

A. Inferior vena cava

E. Aorta

B. Adrenal gland

C. Kidney

D. Ureters

F. Pancreas

G. Kidney

H. Duodenum

I. Urinary bladder

Vocabulary

1. Acute abdomen: Sudden onset of abdominal pain indicating an irritation of the peritoneum. (page 352)

2. *Giardia lamblia*: Common cause of diarrhea in persons who drink untreated surface water in the back country. (page 356)

3. Anaphylaxis: An extreme, possibly life-threatening systemic allergic reaction that may include shock and respiratory failure. (page 366)

4. Histamine: A substance released by the immune system in allergic reactions that is responsible for many of the symptoms of anaphylaxis. (page 365)

5. Epinephrine: A substance produced by the body (adrenaline), and a drug produced by pharmaceutical companies that increases pulse rate and blood pressure; the drug of choice for an anaphylactic reaction. (page 369)

6. Envenomation: When an insect bites and injects the bite with its venom. (page 366)

7. Hallucinogen: An agent that produces false perceptions in any one of the five senses. (page 386)

8. Substance abuse: The knowing misuse of any substance to produce a desired effect. (page 378)

Fill-in

1. sugar, insulin (page 361)

2. bronchial passages (page 368)

3. barbed (page 367)

4. imminent death (page 368)

5. ABCs (page 380)

6. 5 to 10 minutes, 15 to 20 minutes (page 382)

7. respiratory depression (page 384)

8. ingestion (page 379)

9. ignite (page 382)

True/False

1. F (page 352)
2. F (page 354)
3. F (page 354)
4. T (page 361)
5. T (page 359)
6. T (page 359)
7. F (page 374)
8. F (page 377)

9. T (page 365)
10. F (page 368)
11. F (page 377)
12. F (pages 357–358)
13. F (page 380)
14. F (page 381)
15. T (page 384)

Short Answer

1. No. It is too complex and treatment is the same. (page 354)
2. Do not attempt to diagnose the cause.
   - Clear and maintain the airway.
   - Anticipate vomiting.
   - Administer oxygen.
   - Nothing by mouth.
   - Document pertinent information.
   - Anticipate shock.
   - Keep comfortable.
   - Monitor vital signs.
   (pages 358–359)
3. Insulin shock; it develops rapidly as opposed to diabetic coma, which takes longer to develop. (pages 361–363)
4. 1. Insect bites/stings
   2. Medications
   3. Plants
   4. Food
   5. Chemicals (page 366)
5. Respiratory: Sneezing or itchy, runny nose; chest or throat tightness; dry cough; hoarseness; rapid, noisy, or labored respirations; wheezing and/or stridor
   Circulatory: Decreased blood pressure; increased pulse (initially); pale skin and dizziness; loss of consciousness and coma (page 369)
6. 1. Calm the patient. Have the patient lie flat and stay quiet.
   2. Wash the bite area with soapy water.
   3. Splint the extremity.
   4. Mark the skin with a pen to monitor advancing swelling.
   5. Monitor vital signs.
   6. If there are signs of shock, place the patient in the shock position and give oxygen.
   7. Evacuate the patient promptly to the next level of care. (pages 373–374)
7. 1. Limit further discharge of nematocysts.
   2. Keep the patient calm.
   3. Reduce motion of the extremity.
   4. Apply alcohol (isopropyl or rubbing, or any kind available).
   5. Remove remaining tentacles by carefully scraping.
   6. If necessary, immerse injury in hot water for 30 minutes.
   7. Transport. (pages 377–378)

8. 1. Ingestion

2. Inhalation

3. Injection

4. Absorption (page 379)

9. 1. What substance did you take?

2. When did you take it or become exposed to it?

3. How much did you ingest?

4. What actions have been taken?

5. How much do you weigh? (page 378)

Word Fun

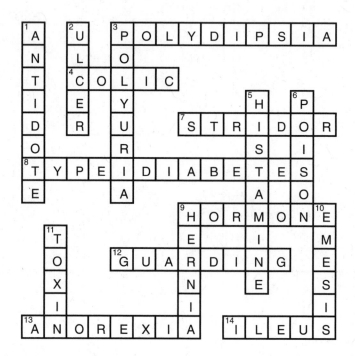

Calls to the Scene

1. -BSI precautions

-Possible appendicitis.

-Place patient in the position of comfort.

-Apply high-flow oxygen.

-Keep patient warm.

-Arrange for rapid transport.

-Obtain a SAMPLE history.

-Document OPQRST.

-Monitor patient closely.

2. -BSI precautions

-Consider cervical spine immobilization.

-Apply high-flow oxygen.

-Try to obtain a SAMPLE history, but do not delay treatment or transport.

-Attempt to obtain a blood glucose level.

-Give sugar or oral glucose following local protocols.

-Monitor the patient.

3. -BSI precautions

-Check the EpiPen for clarity, expiration date, etc.

-Assist the patient to administer the EpiPen following local protocols.

-Promptly dispose of the auto-injector.

-Apply high-flow oxygen.

-Arrange for rapid transport.

-Monitor the patient and assess vital signs frequently

4. -BSI precautions

-Assess the ABCs.

-Keep the patient as calm as possible.

-Take the plant, or at least part of it, with you for identification.

-Monitor the vital signs and provide support en route.

-Arrange for rapid transport.

Skill Drills

1. **Skill Drill 13-1: Administering Glucose (page 364)**

1. Make sure that the tube of glucose is intact and has not **expired**.
2. Squeeze the entire tube of oral glucose onto the **bottom third** of a **bite stick** or tongue depressor.
3. Open the patient's **mouth**. Place the tongue depressor on the **mucous membranes** between the cheek and the gum with the **gel side** next to the cheek.

2. **Skill Drill 13-2: Using an Auto-Injector (page 370)**

1. Remove the auto-injector's **safety cap**.
2. Place the tip of the auto-injector against the **lateral** thigh.
3. Help the patient push the **auto-injector** firmly against the **thigh** and hold it in place until all the medication is injected.

Comparison Table (page 362)

	Diabetic Coma	Insulin Shock
History		
Food intake	Excessive	Insufficient
Insulin dosage	Insufficient	Excessive
Onset	Gradual	Rapid, within minutes
Skin	Warm and dry	Pale and moist
Infection	Common	Uncommon
Gastrointestinal Tract		
Thirst	Intense	Absent
Hunger	Absent	Intense
Vomiting	Common	Uncommon
Respiratory System		
Breathing	Rapid, deep (Kussmaul respirations)	Normal or rapid
Odor of breath	Sweet, fruity	Normal
Cardiovascular System		
Blood pressure	Normal to low	Low
Pulse	Normal or rapid and full	Rapid, weak
Nervous System		
Consciousness	Restless merging to coma	Irritability, confusion, seizure, or coma
Urine		
Sugar	Present	Absent
Acetone	Present	Absent
Treatment		
Response	Gradual, within 6 to 12 hours following medication and fluid	Immediately after administration of glucose

Chapter 14: Snowsports and Mountain Biking Emergencies

Matching

1. B   (page 404)
2. D   (page 402)
3. A   (page 402)
4. C   (page 400)
5. F   (page 402)
6. E   (page 403)

Multiple Choice

1. B (page 398)
2. C (page 400)
3. D (pages 405–407)
4. A (page 408)
5. D (page 409)

Vocabulary

1. Acromioclavicular separations: The joint between the clavicle and the acromion of the scapula at the point of the shoulder. (pages 401, 403)
2. Anterior cruciate ligament (ACL): A bank of thick, strong, fibrous tissue that originates in the groove between the femoral condyles, cross each other in an X, and fit into the tibial plateau. (page 400)
3. Medial collateral ligament (MCL): Condensation or thickening of the medial joint capsule of the knee that provides medial stability to the knee joint; attached at its midportion to the medial meniscus; most frequently injured knee ligament in snowsports. (page 401)
4. Phantom foot syndrome: A mechanism responsible for anterior cruciate ligament injury when the tail of the ski acts as a lever pointing in a direction opposite to that of the foot. Occurs when the thigh rotates internally when the knee is hyperflexed, as when novices try to stop by sitting down. (page 400)

Fill-in

1. skier's thumb (page 401)
2. falls, collisions (page 399)
3. documentation (page 409)
4. Ability, experience (page 400)
5. knee (page 400)
6. head, chest (page 402)

True/False

1. F (page 399)
2. F (page 398)
3. T (page 401)
4. T (page 406)
5. F (page 408)
6. T (page 409)

Short Answer

1. -soft-tissue injuries
   -lower extremity fractures, sprains
   -head, spine
   -chest, abdominal trauma injuries
   -shoulder injuries
   -skier's thumb
   -knee: MCL, ACL (pages 399–401)

2. -abrasions

-contusions

-lacerations

-fractures

-concussions (page 409)

3. -extremities (especially lower)

-spinal injuries (compression trauma)

-head and neck trauma

-avalanche burial and drowning

-overuse injuries (page 408)

4. A disease of the hands and feet, characterized by intermittent spasm of the small arteries of the fingers and toes caused by exposure to cold. (page 408)

5. A sprain or fracture of the structures at the base of the thumb. Occurs when a skier tries to break a fall with an outstretched hand while holding a ski pole. The thumb is abducted on impact. (page 401)

6. Characterized by pain in the big toe caused by repeated dorsiflexion. (page 405)

7. Fracture of the talus (the support structure for both the tibia and fibula). (page 402)

8. -Stay in good physical condition all year long.

-Get good equipment and take care of it.

-Know your bindings and test them regularly.

-Use devices to prevent runaway and buried skis and snowboards.

-Avoid slopes and snow conditions that you cannot handle.

-Be aware of your surroundings.

-Avoid alcohol and drugs.

-Stay well nourished.

-Rest, warm up, and eat when tired and cold.

-Dress for a variety of conditions.

-Be familiar with the outdoor recreation area.

-Avoid skiing or snowboarding alone, if possible.

-Follow your responsibility code, and urge others to do the same.

-Carry emergency survival equipment when out of bounds.

-Use high-quality eyewear.

-Whenever wearing a helmet, make sure it fits, is comfortable, and provides adequate protection. (pages 405–407)

Word Fun

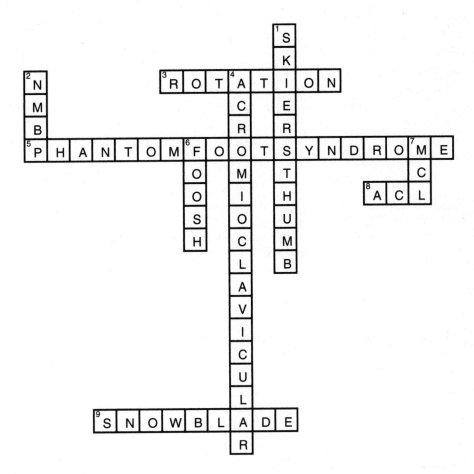

Calls to the Scene

1. **(Probable injuries)**
-Probable multiple rib fractures, left lateral chest
-Probable ruptured spleen with progressive hypovolemic shock
-Probable distal radius fracture, left wrist
-Possible compression fracture, midthoracic spine

(Emergency care procedures)
-Scene safety; call for and question witnesses.
-Perform a rapid trauma assessment; rapid body survey.
-Obtain an initial set of vital signs, and repeat frequently.
-Call for extra hands and equipment.
-Apply a splint to the left forearm, wrist, and hand while awaiting help, checking CMS before and after immobilization.
-Administer oxygen by nonrebreathing facemask as soon as available at 12–15 L/min.
-When extra help arrives apply a cervical collar, and while maintaining spinal integrity perform "jams and pretzels" to bring the rider into the #2 position.
-While continuing to stabilize the cervical spine, logroll the rider onto a backboard; place rolled blankets under both knees to maintain knee flexion.
-Obtain a set of vital signs, and distal upper- and lower-extremity CMS after transfer to the backboard.
-Secure the rider to the backboard and apply a cervical immobilization device.
-Load rider into the toboggan, with the head facing downhill, and transport promptly.

2. (Probable injuries)

-Probable displaced distal right humerus fracture "near the elbow joint," with neurovascular compromise (brachial artery and nerve compression)

-Mild hypothermia

(**EMS interface/communications**)

-9-year-old female with:

a. an apparent fracture deformity just above the right elbow, diminished sensation in the right palm, and loss of radial pulse at the right wrist

b. mild hypothermia, with an estimated core body temperature above 90° F

c. no evidence of loss of responsiveness

d. no other significant injuries noted

-Estimated body weight—70 lb

-Accompanied by parent/guardian

-Emergency care rendered up to the time of transfer: application of long arm splint with sling and swathe to left upper extremity; active and passive rewarming with blankets and hot water bottles

-To reduce the risk of aspiration, do not give the patient any food or drink.

-Vital signs at the time of transfer

Chapter 15: Environmental Emergencies

Matching

1. G (page 426)

2. H (page 431)

3. E (page 431)

4. A (page 441)

5. K (page 414)

6. C (page 423)

7. B (page 431)

8. F (page 415)

9. J (page 431)

10. I (page 431)

11. D (page 437)

Multiple Choice

1. C – Confusion is seen in moderate hypothermia. (pages 415–416)

2. D (pages 417–418)

3. A – It is necessary to assess the trunk of the body to get a true feel for the extent of the cold emergency. The cooler the core temperature, the more serious the emergency. (page 418)

4. C – The golden rule of hypothermia states, "They are not dead until they are warm and dead." Patients may survive even severe hypothermia if proper emergency measures are carried out. (page 415)

5. D (page 419)

6. B – The patient could be bradycardic and initiating chest compressions could cause cardiac arrhythmias. (page 419)

7. D (page 417)

8. B (page 422)

9. C – (A), (B), and (D) are all localized signs and symptoms. (page 418)

10. A – (B), (C), and (D) are conditions that result from hyperthermia. (page 431)

11. D (page 432)

12. D (page 431)

13. A (page 431)

14. D (page 432)

15. A – The patient should also be transported if the level of consciousness decreases; if the temperature remains elevated; or if the person is very young, elderly, or has any underlying medical condition, such as diabetes, cardiovascular disease, or another worrisome condition. (page 434)

16. A (page 434)

17. D (page 434)

18. B (page 437)

19. D (page 437)

20. A – Take care to stabilize and protect the patient's spine since associated cervical spine injuries are possible. (page 438)

21. C (page 438)

22. D (page 438)

23. D (page 438)

24. B – (A) Heat is transferred from the body to the water, resulting in hypothermia. (C) Hypothermia lowers the metabolic rate in an effort to preserve body heat. (page 418)

25. B (page 428)

26. A – The skin, joints, and vision are areas with signs and symptoms of air embolism. (page 443)

27. D (page 443)

28. A – The brain and spinal cord require a constant supply of oxygen. (page 443)

29. B (page 445)

Vocabulary

1. HACE: High-altitude cerebral edema. A serious complication of acute mountain sickness characterized by swelling of the brain, ataxia, and altered mental status.(page 426)

2. Decompression sickness: Condition seen in divers in which gas, usually nitrogen, forms bubbles that obstruct blood vessels. (page 444)

3. Heat exhaustion: The result of the body losing so much water and so many electrolytes through very heavy sweating that hypovolemia occurs. (page 432)

4. Frostbite: The most serious local cold injury. Because the tissues are actually frozen, the freezing permanently damages the cells. (page 422)

5. Near drowning: Survival, at least temporarily, after suffocation in water. (page 437)

6. HAPE: High-altitude pulmonary edema. A type of high-altitude illness characterized by the lungs filling with fluid. (page 426)

Fill-in

1. moderate to severe (page 416)

2. ascent (page 443)

3. rewarming (pages 424–425)

4. self-protection (page 425)

5. Shivering (page 414)

6. to open the airway (pages 421–422)

7. mild (page 416)

True/False

1. T   (page 419)

2. F   (pages 415–416)

3. T   (page 431)

4. T   (page 431)

5. T   (page 431)

6. F   (page 426)

7. T   (page 426)

8. T   (page 434)

Short Answer

1. 1. Move the patient out of the hot environment and into a cooler environment.

2. Set air conditioning to maximum cooling.

3. Remove patient's clothing.

4. Administer high-flow oxygen.

5. Apply cool packs to patient's neck, groin, and armpits.

6. Cover patient with wet towels, or spray with cool water and fan.

7. Keep fanning.

8. Transport immediately.

9. Notify the hospital. (page 434)

2. An air embolism is a bubble of air in the blood vessels caused by breath-holding during rapid ascent. The resulting high pressure in the lungs causes alveolar rupture. (page 443)

3. Do not stand in or near a body of water. Take shelter away from high points, exposed ridges, solitary trees, and trees taller than surrounding trees. (pages 436–437)

4. 1. Remove the patient from the cold.

2. Handle injured part gently and protect from further injury.

3. Remove wet or restricting clothing. (pages 424–425)

5. 1. Do not break blisters.

2. Do not rub or massage area.

3. Do not apply heat or rewarm unless instructed by medical control.

4. Do not allow patient to stand or walk on a frostbitten foot. (pages 424–425)

6. Blotching; froth at nose and mouth; severe pain in muscles, joints, abdomen; dyspnea and/or chest pain; dizziness; nausea; vomiting; dysphasia; difficulty with vision; paralysis and/or coma; and irregular pulse with possible cardiac arrest. (page 444)

Word Fun

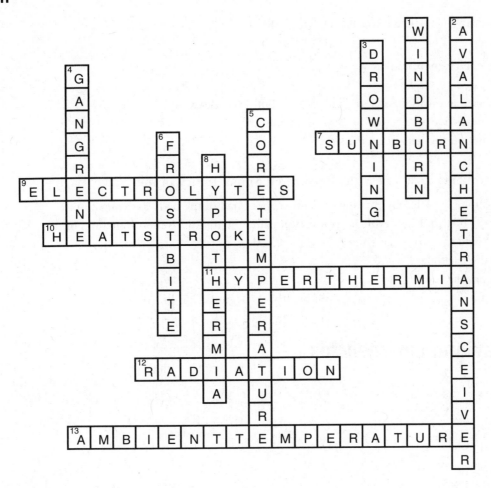

Calls to the Scene

1. -You suspect acute mountain sickness.
   -BSI precautions.
   -Administer oxygen at 1 to 2 liters/min.
   -Transport the patient to a lower altitude.
   -Recommend rest and a light diet before resumption of skiing.
   -HACE or HAPE may develop.
   -No hospital care is necessary if symptoms subside.
2. -BSI precautions.
   -Assess and maintain airway.
   -Immobilize and splint fractured humerus.
   -Eliminate or reduce heat loss and stabilize hypothermia.
   -Reposition the patient to minimize surface contact.
   -Prepare for rapid evacuation.
   -Do not try to warm externally.
3. -BSI precautions.
   -Remove the patient from the hot environment, preferably into an air-conditioned vehicle or facility.
   -Have the patient lie down with knees pulled up to relieve pressure on the abdomen.
   -Replace fluid loss with water, diluted Gatorade, etc.
   -Transport if patient still complains of cramps after this treatment.
   -Monitor vital signs.

Skill Drills

1. Skill Drill 15-1: Treating for Heat Exhaustion (page 433)

1. Remove **extra clothing**
2. Move the patient to a **cooler environment**.
   Give **oxygen**.
   Place the patient in a **supine** position, elevate the legs, and **fan** the patient.
3. If the patient is **fully alert**, give an electrolyte solution by mouth.
4. If nausea develops, **position** the patient on the side.

2. Skill Drill 15-2: Stabilizing a Patient with a Suspected Spinal Injury in the Water (page 439)

1. Turn the patient to a supine position by rotating the entire upper half of the body as a single unit.
2. As soon as the patient is turned, begin artificial ventilation using the mouth-to-mouth method or a pocket mask.
3. Float a buoyant backboard under the patient.
4. Secure the patient to the backboard.
5. Remove the patient from the water.
6. Cover the patient with a blanket and apply oxygen if breathing. Begin CPR if breathing and pulse are absent.

Chapter 16: Behavioral Emergencies

Matching

1. C (pages 452–453)
2. F (page 456)
3. B (page 453)
4. D (page 453)
5. E (page 453)
6. A (page 452)

Multiple Choice

1. D (page 452)
2. B – A and C are both indications that the patient may indeed have a behavioral problem. (page 452)
3. D (page 453)
4. B (page 452)
5. A (page 453)
6. B (page 453)
7. A (pages 452–453)
8. D (page 453)
9. C – A, B, and D would have no influence on the mental status because they are all normal measures. (page 453)
10. D – All are correct because anything that creates a temporary or permanent dysfunction of the brain may cause organic brain syndrome. (page 453)
11. A – (B) and (C) are both diseases or dysfunction of the brain. Schizophrenia (A) cannot be identified as a problem with the brain itself. (page 453)
12. B – (A) All findings should be documented objectively; (C) Quote the patient's own words using quotation marks. (page 453)

13. D – (A) Scene safety is top priority on any call; (B) It may take longer to assess, listen to, and prepare the patient for transport; (C) Help the patient to prepare by dressing and gathering appropriate belongings to take to the hospital. (page 454)

14. B – (A), (C), and (D) are all important aspects of the assessment, but scene safety (B) is first on any call. (page 455)

15. D (page 456)

Vocabulary

1. Mental disorder: An illness with psychological or behavioral symptoms that may result in an impairment in functioning, caused by a social, psychological, genetic, physical, chemical, or biological disturbance. (page 453)

2. Activities of daily living (ADL): The basic activities a person usually accomplishes during the normal day. (pages 452–453)

3. Altered mental status: A change in the way a person thinks or behaves. (page 454)

4. Implied consent: When a patient is not mentally competent to grant consent for emergency medical care, the law assumes that there is implied consent. Consent is implied because of the necessity for immediate emergency treatment. (page 456)

Fill-in

1. Behavior (page 452)

2. behavioral crisis (pages 452–453)

3. depression (page 453)

4. Organic brain syndrome (page 453)

5. coping mechanisms (page 455)

True/False

1. T   (page 453)

2. F   (page 453)

3. F   (page 453)

4. F   (page 457)

5. F   (page 454)

6. F   (page 456)

7. F   (page 452)

8. F   (page 453)

Short Answer

1. A behavioral crisis is a temporary change in behavior that interferes with ADL or that is unacceptable to the patient or others. A mental health problem is this kind of behavioral change recurring on a regular basis. (pages 452–453)

2. 1. Improper functioning of the central nervous system.

  2. Drugs or alcohol

  3. Psychogenic circumstances (page 453)

3. 1. Be prepared to spend extra time.

  2. Have a definite plan of action.

  3. Identify yourself calmly.

  4. Be direct.

  5. Assess the scene.

  6. Stay with the patient.

  7. Encourage purposeful movement.

  8. Express interest in the patient's story.

  9. Do not get too close to the patient.

  10. Avoid fighting with the patient.

  11. Be honest and reassuring.

  12. Do not judge. (page 454)

Word Fun

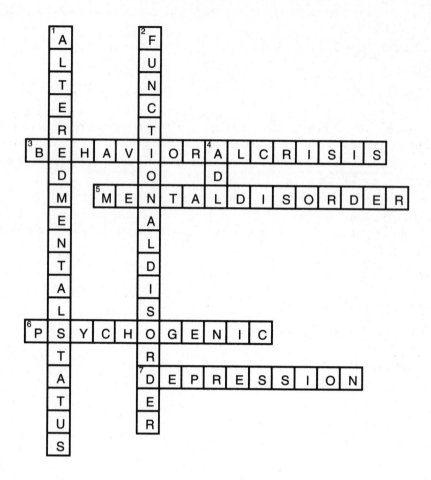

Calls to the Scene

1. -BSI precautions.
   -Call for police back up.
   -Calmly speak to the aggressive man without being judgmental.
   -Stay out of his "personal space"—leave yourself an out.
   -Try to obtain the person's consent for treatment and transport.
2. -BSI precautions.
   -Be understanding and listen.
   -Explain to the patient that she needs medical care.
   -Monitor vital signs and reassure patient.
   -Arrange for transportation to definitive care.

Chapter 17: Obstetrics and Gynecological Emergencies

Matching

1. D (page 462)

2. C (page 462)

3. L (page 462)

4. B (page 463)

5. N (page 462)

6. H (page 462)

7. M (page 462)

8. E (page 463)

9. F (page 462)

10. O (pages 474–475)

11. K (page 475)

12. I (page 463)

13. A (page 469)

14. G (page 474)

15. J (page 464)

Multiple Choice

1. D (pages 469–470)

2. B (page 469)

3. B – Aggressive suctioning of the baby's mouth and oropharynx before delivery of the baby may prevent meconium aspirations and respiratory distress. (page 469)

4. C – By suctioning the nose first (B), the baby may be stimulated to breathe and aspirate fluid into its lungs. (page 470)

5. D (page 470)

6. B (page 471)

7. A (page 472)

8. C (page 472)

9. D (page 473)

10. D – 90 compressions to 30 ventilations. (page 474)

11. A (page 475)

12. D (pages 475–476)

13. D (page 463)

14. B (page 463)

15. D (page 462)

16. A (page 463)

17. C (page 463)

18. C (page 463)

19. B – (A), (C), and (D) are signs of preeclampsia. (page 464)

20. B (page 464)

21. B (page 465)

22. D (page 466)

23. C – Never leave the mother once the decision has been made to deliver at the scene (A). The only acceptable reasons for inserting fingers into the vagina are a breech delivery (to provide an airway) and prolapsed cord (B). (page 467)

24. A (page 464)

25. D (page 464)

26. D (page 475)

27. C (page 464)

28. B (page 464)

29. A (page 464)

Tables

Apgar Scoring System

Area of Activity	Score		
	2	1	0
Appearance	Entire infant is pink.	Body is pink, but hands and feet remain blue.	Entire infant is blue and pale.
Pulse	More than 100 beats/min	Fewer than 100 beats/min	Absent pulse.
Grimace or Irritability	Infant cries and tries to move foot away from finger snapped against its sole.	Infant gives a weak cry in response to stimulus.	Infant does not cry or react to stimulus.
Activity or Muscle Tone	Infant resists attempts to straighten out hips and knees.	Infant makes weak attempts to resist straightening.	Infant is completely limp, with no muscle tone.
Respiration	Rapid respirations	Slow respirations	Absent respirations

(page 473)

Labeling

1. Anatomic Structures of the Pregnant Woman (page 462)

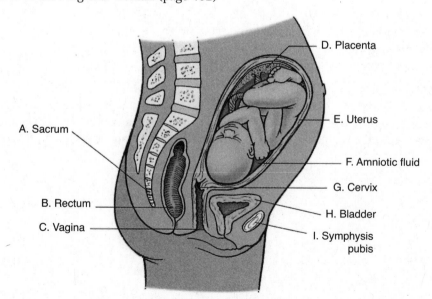

A. Sacrum
B. Rectum
C. Vagina
D. Placenta
E. Uterus
F. Amniotic fluid
G. Cervix
H. Bladder
I. Symphysis pubis

Vocabulary

1. Primigravida: A woman who is experiencing her first pregnancy. (page 463)
2. Multigravida: A woman who has had previous pregnancies. (page 463)
3. Ectopic pregnancy: A pregnancy that develops outside the uterus, typically in a fallopian tube. (page 464)
4. Crowning: The appearance of the top of the infant's head at the vaginal opening during labor. (page 463)
5. APGAR score: A scoring system for assessing the status of a newborn that assigns a number value to each of five areas of assessment. (page 472)
6. Bloody show: A plug of pink-tinged mucus that is discharged when the cervix begins to dilate. (page 462)

Fill-in

1. placenta (page 471)
2. arteries, vein (page 463)
3. 500 to 1,000 mL (page 463)
4. 36, 40 (page 463)
5. trimesters (page 463)
6. body fluids (page 463)
7. ectopic pregnancy (page 464)
8. resuscitate (page 465)
9. fontanels (page 469)

True/False

1. T (page 462)
2. F (page 463)
3. F (page 463)
4. F (page 463)
5. F (page 465)
6. T (page 474)
7. T (page 470)
8. F (page 471)
9. F (page 471)
10. T (page 475)
11. T (page 477)

Short Answer

1. Early: spontaneous abortion (miscarriage) or ectopic pregnancy
   Later: Placenta previa or placenta abruptio (page 464)
2. On the left side, to prevent supine hypotensive syndrome (low blood pressure occurring from the weight of the fetus compressing the inferior vena cava) (page 464)
3. 1. Uterine contractions
   2. Bloody show
   3. Rupture of amniotic sac (page 463)
4. 1. When delivery can be expected in a few minutes.
   2. When some natural disaster or catastrophe makes it impossible to reach the hospital.
   3. When no transportation is available. (pages 465–466)
5. Exert gentle pressure on the head as it emerges to prevent rapid expulsion with a strong contraction. (page 469)
6. The brain is covered by only skin and membrane at the fontanels. (page 469)
7. Exerting gentle pressure horizontally across the perineum with a sterile gauze pad may reduce the risk of perineal tearing. (page 469)
8. 1. During a breech delivery to protect the infant's airway
   2. When the umbilical cord is prolapsed (pages 475–476)

Word Fun

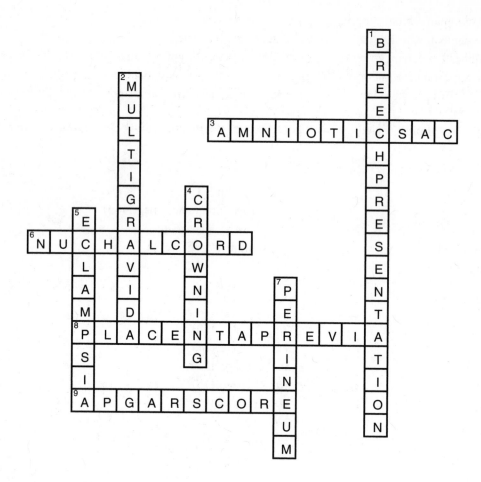

Calls to the Scene

1. -BSI precautions.
  -Place the mother on her left side.
  -Maintain the airway, suctioning as needed.
  -Provide high-flow oxygen.
  -Monitor vital signs.
  -Protect the mother from harm if seizing starts again.
  -Arrange for rapid transport.

2. -BSI precautions.
  -Place patient on her left side.
  -Give high-flow oxygen. The baby needs extra oxygen if the placenta is abruptio, or there are other serious conditions.
  -Place a sterile pad or sanitary napkin over the vagina.
  -Take any clots to the hospital.
  -Arrange for prompt transport.

3. -BSI precautions.
  -Position the mother for delivery and apply high-flow oxygen.
  -As crowning occurs, use a clamp to puncture the sac, away from the baby's face.
  -Push the ruptured sac away from the infant's face as the head is delivered.
  -Clear the baby's mouth and nose immediately.
  -Continue with the delivery as normal.

Skill Drills

1. Skill Drill 17-1: Delivering the Baby (page 468)

1. Support the **bony** parts of the head with your hands as it emerges.
   Suction fluid from the **mouth**, then **nostrils**.
2. As the **upper shoulder** appears, guide the head **down** slightly, if needed to deliver the **shoulder**.
3. Support the head and upper body as the **lower shoulder** delivers, guiding the head **up** if needed.
4. Handle the slippery delivered infant firmly but gently, keeping the neck in **neutral** position to **maintain** the airway.
5. Place clamps **2"** to **4"** apart and **cut** between them.
6. Allow the **placenta** to deliver itself. Do not pull on the **cord** to speed delivery.

Section 5 Trauma

Chapter 18: Mechanisms and Patterns of Injury

Matching

1. F   (page 488)
2. E   (page 487)
3. D   (page 486)

4. B   (page 487)
5. A   (page 488)
6. C   (page 488)

Multiple Choice

1. B – Thermal energy causes burns. (page 487)
2. C (page 487)
3. C – Energy can be neither created nor destroyed. (page 487)
4. B (page 487)
5. A (page 487)
6. C (page 487)
7. C (page 489)
8. C (page 491)
9. D (page 487)
10. A (pages 488–489)
11. C (page 494)
12. B (page 493)
13. D – Significant mechanisms of injury also include severe deformities of the frontal part of the vehicle, with or without intrusion to the passenger compartment. (page 495)
14. C (page 490)
15. D (page 491)
16. B – You should still suspect that other serious injuries to the extremities and to internal organs have occurred. (page 489)
17. A (page 493)
18. B (page 493)
19. D (page 493)
20. D (page 488)

Vocabulary

1. Newton's First Law of Motion: Objects at rest tend to stay at rest, and objects in motion tend to stay in motion unless acted upon by some force. (page 487)
2. Distraction trauma: Trauma caused by stretching. (page 490)
3. Velocity: Speed. The magnitude of velocity is the body's speed, and the direction of velocity is the body's direction of motion. (page 487)

Fill-in

1. kinetic (page 487)
2. compression (page 488)
3. Traumatic injury (page 487)
4. $KE = \frac{1}{2} MV^2$ (page 487)
5. crushing (page 490)
6. acceleration (page 488)
7. penetrating trauma (page 488)

True/False

1. F (page 487)
2. F (page 487)
3. T (page 486)
4. T (page 490)
5. T (page 493)
6. T (page 487)

Short Answer

1. Potential energy is the product of mass (weight), force of gravity, and height, and is mostly associated with the energy of falling objects. (page 487)
2. 1. Fallen from a height that is 2 to 3 times the body height
   2. Involved in a moderate- to high-speed accident
   3. Hit by a vehicle going 25 mph or more
   4. Colliding with another skier/snowrider at high speed
   5. Gunshot wound
   6. Person in shock or respiratory distress
   7. Unresponsive due to head injury
   8. Buried in an avalanche
   9. Struck by a fallen object (page 495)
3. 1. The height of the fall
   2. The surface struck
   3. The part of the body that hits first, followed by the path of energy displacement (page 493)
4. -Estimated speed of travel, distance of fall, speed of the striking object
   -Characteristics of the ground or any other surface impacted by the patient.
   -Forces inflicted on the patient's body
   -Types of trauma involved
   -Visible injuries
   -Type of internal injuries possible
   -Signs of developing shock
   -Likelihood of spinal injury (page 493)
5. 1. Rotational
   2. Bending
   3. Penetrating
   4. Compression
   5. Distraction (stretching) (pages 488–490)

Word Fun

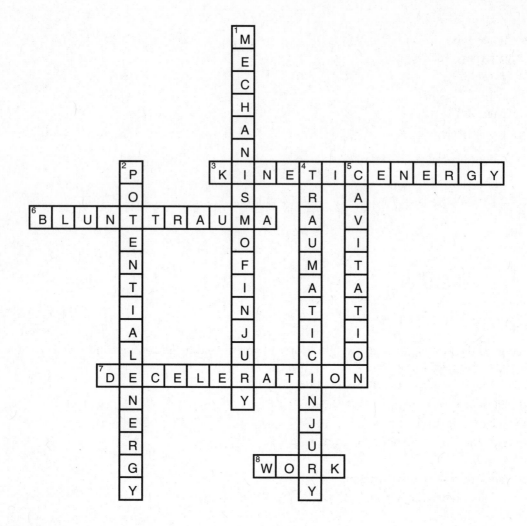

Calls to the Scene

1. **(Type of trauma and injury)**
   -Rotational trauma
   -Hyperflexion injury
   -Compression trauma
   -BSI precautions.
   (Emergency care)
   -Maintain cervical spine control.
   -Apply high-flow oxygen.
   -Keep a high index of suspicion for life-threatening injuries.
   -Monitor vital signs.
   -Arrange for rapid transport.
2. -BSI precautions.
   -Maintain cervical spine control.
   -Apply high-flow oxygen.
   -Fully immobilize the patient and splint the leg.
   -Stabilize on backboard.
   -Monitor vital signs.
   -Arrange for normal transport off mountain.

Chapter 19: Soft-Tissue Injuries

Matching

1. G (page 500)
2. B (page 500)
3. D (page 500)
4. F (page 500)
5. I (page 500)
6. L (page 503)
7. E (page 504)
8. J (page 507)
9. A (page 505)
10. C (page 504)
11. K (page 508)
12. H (page 507)

Multiple Choice

1. C (page 500)
2. B (page 500)
3. B (page 500)
4. A (page 500)
5. B (page 501)
6. C (page 502)
7. B (page 502)
8. B (page 502)
9. D (page 502)
10. C (page 502)
11. C (pages 502–503)
12. C (page 503)
13. B (page 503)
14. A (page 503)
15. D (page 504)
16. B (page 504)
17. A (page 509)
18. D (page 505)
19. A (page 506)
20. D (page 506)
21. D (page 506)
22. B (page 507)
23. C – Never touch exposed organs (A). Use moist sterile dressings (B). Never use adherent dressings (D). (page 508)
24. C – Hypovolemic shock (A) does not result from air being sucked in. Tracheal deviation (B) results from a tension pneumothorax. Subcutaneous emphysema (D) results from air outside the vessels. (page 510)
25. D (page 511)
26. D – Factors in helping to determine the severity of a burn also include whether or not there are any preexisting medical conditions or other injuries, and if the patient is younger than 5 years of age or older than 55 years of age. (page 511)
27. C (page 512)
28. B (page 512)
29. C (page 512)
30. D (page 512)
31. D – Significant airway burns may also be associated with soot around the nose and mouth. (page 513)
32. B – Personal safety always comes first. (page 517)
33. D – Apply high-flow oxygen (A). Be prepared to defibrillate (B). (page 517)
34. A – An occlusive dressing must be airtight; gauze pads (A) are not. (page 507)
35. D (page 519)

Labeling

1. The Skin (page 501)

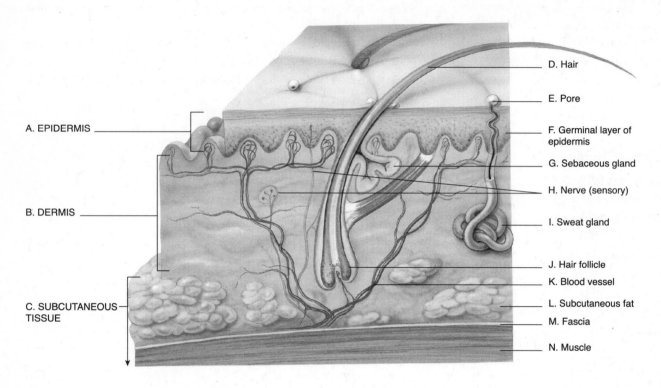

A. EPIDERMIS

B. DERMIS

C. SUBCUTANEOUS TISSUE

D. Hair

E. Pore

F. Germinal layer of epidermis

G. Sebaceous gland

H. Nerve (sensory)

I. Sweat gland

J. Hair follicle

K. Blood vessel

L. Subcutaneous fat

M. Fascia

N. Muscle

2. The Rule of Nines (page 514)

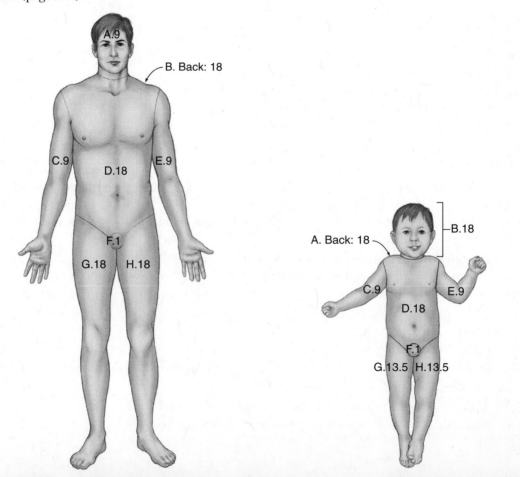

A.9

B. Back: 18

C.9

D.18

E.9

F.1

G.18

H.18

A. Back: 18

B.18

C.9

D.18

E.9

F.1

G.13.5

H.13.5

Vocabulary

1. Partial-thickness burn: A burn affecting the epidermis and some portion of the dermis; characterized by red, moist, mottled skin with blisters present. (page 512)
2. Closed injury: Injury in which damage occurs beneath the skin or mucous membrane, but the surface remains intact. (page 501)
3. Evisceration: An open wound in the abdominal cavity in which organs protrude through the wound. (page 508)
4. Compartment syndrome: Swelling in a confined space that produces dangerous pressure. (page 502)
5. Contamination: The presence of infective organisms or foreign bodies such as dirt, gravel, or metal. (page 503)

Fill-in

1. moist (page 500)
2. cool (page 500)
3. dermis (page 500)
4. subcutaneous (page 500)
5. constrict (page 501)
6. bacteria, water (page 501)
7. dermis (page 500)
8. temperature (page 501)
9. epidermis, dermis (page 500)
10. radiated (page 501)

True/False

1. T (page 512)
2. F (page 512)
3. T (page 512)
4. T (page 513)
5. T (page 511)
6. T (pages 513)
7. F (page 514)
8. T (page 517)
9. T (page 519)
10. T (page 507)
11. F (page 508)
12. F (page 519)
13. T (page 519)
14. F (page 502)
15. F (page 502)

Short Answer

1. 1. superficial
   2. partial-thickness
   3. full-thickness (page 512)
2. 1. closed
   2. open
   3. burns (page 501)
3. I=ice
   C=compression
   E=elevation
   S=splinting (page 503)
4. -Full- or partial-thickness burns covering more than 20% of total body surface area
   -Burns involving the hands, feet, face, airway, or genitalia (page 512)
5. Brush off dry chemicals and/or remove clothing, then flush the burned area with large amounts of water. (page 516)
6. First, there may be deep tissue injury not visible on the outside. Second, there is a danger of cardiac arrest from the electrical shock. (pages 517–518)
7. A wound caused by a penetrating object into the chest that causes air to enter the chest. The air enters the chest area through the wound, but remains in the pleural space and the lung does not expand. With exhalation, air passes back through the wound, making a "sucking" sound. (page 507)
8. 1. Control bleeding
   2. Protect from further damage
   3. Prevent further contamination and infection (page 519)

9. 1. Abrasions

2. Lacerations

3. Avulsions

4. Penetrating (page 502)

10. 1. Depth (superficial/partial/full)

2. Extent (% of body burned)

3. Involvement of critical areas (face, upper airway, hands, feet, genitalia)

4. Preexisting medical conditions or other injuries

5. Age younger than 5 years or older than 55 years (page 511)

Word Fun

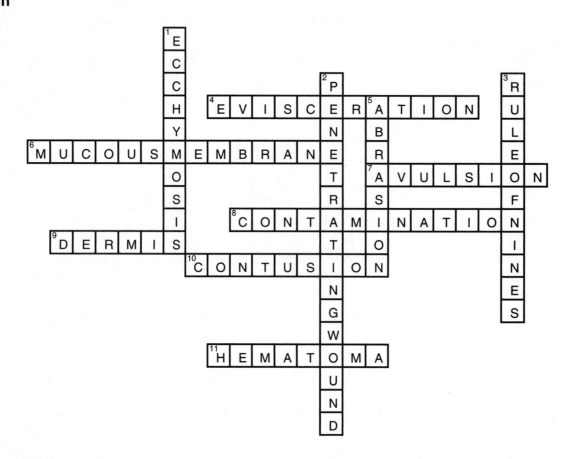

Calls to the Scene

1. -Partial thickness or second-degree

-BSI precautions.

-Immediately remove all clothing soaked in oil (cut, if necessary).

-Soak all areas in cool water or place wet, clean cloth on affected areas for 10 minutes.

-Call 9-1-1.

-Apply high-flow oxygen.

-Perform focused history and physical exam.

-Cover burned areas with sterile dressing loosely.

-Monitor vital signs.

2. -Hematoma to lower leg

-Laceration

-BSI precautions.

-Quickly assess ABCs.

-Treat hematoma with ICES.

-For laceration, treatment is pressure, sterile dressing, soft adherent bandage, splint, sling and swathe.

-Transport in position of comfort.

-Monitor vital signs en route.

-Complications: lower leg compartment syndrome; uncontrolled bleeding leading to hypovolemic shock, neurovascular injury to forearm

3. -Ensure personal safety.

-Check for loose wires, water on the floor, or other risks of electrical shock.

-Notify management (mountain operations).

-BSI precautions.

-Activate EMS and perform AVPU.

-Initiate CPR, if indicated.

-Check for serious bleeding.

-Assess for exit burn.

-Treat burns with dry, sterile dressings.

-Treat other identified injuries if time allows.

-Continue CPR until EMS arrives (prolonged CPR has a good outcome in electrical injuries)

Skill Drills

1. Skill Drill 19-1: Controlling Bleeding from a Soft-Tissue Injury (page 507)

1. Apply **direct pressure** with a **sterile** bandage.
2. Maintain pressure with a **roller** bandage.
3. If bleeding continues, apply a second **dressing** and **roller** bandage over the first and apply pressure to the corresponding arterial pressure point.
4. **Splint** the extremity.

2. Skill Drill 19-2: Sealing a Sucking Chest Wound (page 508)

1. Keep the patient **supine** and give **oxygen**.
2. Seal the wound with an **occlusive** dressing.
3. Follow **local protocol** regarding sealing or **leaving open** the dressing's fourth side

3. Skill Drill 19-3: Stabilizing an Impaled Object (page 509)

1. Do not attempt to **move** or **remove** the object.
2. Control **bleeding** and **stabilize** the object in place using **soft dressings**, **gauze**, and/or **tape**.
3. Add **bulky dressings** to stabilize and protect the impaled object during transport.

4. Skill Drill 19-4: Caring for Burns (page 515)

1. Follow BSI precautions to help prevent infection.

   Remove the patient from the burning area; extinguish or remove hot clothing and jewelry as needed.

   If the wound(s) is still burning or hot, immerse the hot area in cool, sterile water, or cover with a wet, cool dressing.
2. Give supplemental oxygen and continue to assess the airway.

   Estimate the severity of the burn, then cover the area with a dry, sterile dressing or clean sheet.

   Assess and treat the patient for any other injuries.

3. Prepare for transport.
   Treat for shock if needed.
4. Cover the patient with blankets to prevent loss of body heat.
   Transport promptly.

Chapter 20: Eye Injuries

Matching

1. D (page 525)	**6.** G (page 524)	
2. C (page 525)	**7.** A (page 524)	
3. B (page 525)	**8.** F (page 524)	
4. E (page 525)	**9.** I (page 524)	
5. J (page 524)	**10.** H (page 525)	

Multiple Choice

1. B (page 524)

2. D (page 524)

3. A (page 525)

4. A (page 525)

5. D (page 525)

6. C – Also record the severity and duration of signs and symptoms and any history of previous eye surgery. (page 526)

7. D (page 528)

8. D (page 530)

9. B (page 530)

10. D (page 530)

11. B (page 530)

12. C – Compression can interfere with the blood supply to the back of the eye and result in loss of vision from damage to the retina. (page 531)

13. D – Do not attempt to reposition an eyeball in its socket. Simply cover the eye, and stabilize it with a moist, sterile dressing. Have the patient lie supine during transport. (page 531)

14. A (page 531)

15. B (page 531)

16. A (page 532)

17. D – Signs of a possible head injury also include the eyes not moving together or pointing in different directions, and failure of the eyes to follow the movement of your finger as instructed. (page 532)

18. C (page 532)

Labeling

1. The Major Components of the Eye (page 524)

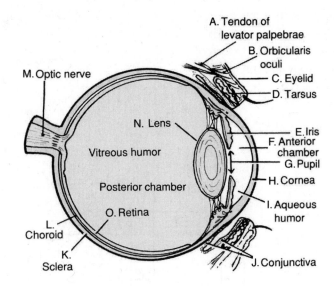

A. Tendon of levator palpebrae
B. Orbicularis oculi
C. Eyelid
D. Tarsus
M. Optic nerve
N. Lens
Vitreous humor
E. Iris
F. Anterior chamber
G. Pupil
H. Cornea
Posterior chamber
I. Aqueous humor
O. Retina
L. Choroid
K. Sclera
J. Conjunctiva

Vocabulary

1. Blowout fracture: Fracture of the orbit or of the bones that support the floor of the orbit. (page 532)
2. Hyphema: Bleeding into the anterior chamber of the eye. (page 531)
3. Conjunctivitis: Inflammation of the conjunctiva. (page 526)

Fill-in

1. lacrimal glands (page 524)
2. optic nerve (page 525)
3. camera, film (page 525)
4. chemical burn (page 528)
5. orbit (page 524)
6. abnormalities (page 525)
7. orbit (page 524)
8. Conjunctivitis (page 526)

True/False

1. F (page 527)
2. F (page 530)
3. T (page 530)
4. F (page 525)
5. F (page 532)

6. F (page 526)
7. F (page 526)
8. T (page 525)
9. F (page 526)

Short Answer

1. A condition in which the retina is separated from its attachments at the back of the eye. (page 525)

2. 1. Never exert pressure on the eye.

    2. If part of the eyeball is exposed, gently apply a moist, sterile dressing to prevent drying.

    3. Cover the eye with a protective shield or sterile dressing. (page 531)

3. 1. One pupil larger than the other

    2. Eyes not moving together or pointing in different directions

    3. Failure of the eyes to follow movement when instructed

    4. Bleeding under the conjunctiva

    5. Protrusion or bulging of the eye (page 532)

Word Fun

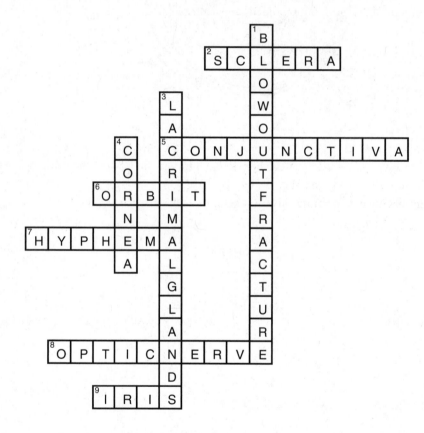

Calls to the Scene

1. -BSI precautions.

    -Stabilize object with bulky dressings.

    -Cover both eyes.

    -Place patient in position of comfort.

    -Reassure patient.

    -Arrange for rapid transport

2. -BSI precautions.

    -Position patient supine on stretcher.

    -Prepare an irrigation system.

    -Allow the fluid to run into the eyes.

    -Monitor patient and flush eyes continuously en route to medical attention.

    Arrange for rapid transport.

3. -BSI precautions.

-Position patient supine.

-Cover both eyes to minimize movement.

-Monitor patient and vital signs.

-Arrange for rapid transport.

Skill Drills

1. Skill Drill 20-1: Removing a Foreign Object from Under the Upper Eyelid (page 527)

1. Have the patient look **down**, grasp the **upper lashes**, and gently pull the lid away from the eye.
2. Place a **cotton-tipped applicator** on the upper lid, ½" from the lashes.
3. Pull the lid **forward** and **up**, folding it back over the applicator.
4. Gently remove the foreign object with a **moistened**, **sterile** applicator.

2. Skill Drill 20-2: Stabilizing a Foreign Object Impaled in the Eye (page 528)

1. To prepare a doughnut ring, wrap a 2" gauze roll around your fingers and thumb **seven or eight** times. Adjust the diameter by **spreading** your fingers.
2. Wrap the remainder of the roll…
3. …working around the ring.
4. Place the dressing over the **eye** to hold the impaled object in place, then **secure** it with a **gauze** dressing.

Chapter 21: Face and Throat Injuries

Matching

1. C (page 538)

2. B (page 538)

3. E (page 538)

4. F (page 538)

5. G (page 538)

6. D (page 540)

7. A (page 538)

Multiple Choice

1. D (page 538)

2. B (page 538)

3. C (page 538)

4. D (page 538)

5. A (page 538)

6. D (page 539)

7. C (page 540)

8. D (page 540)

9. A – Always place amputated or avulsed parts in a plastic bag and keep them cool. Placing the part directly on ice can cause frostbite. (page 542)

10. D (page 542)

11. B (page 542)

12. C (page 543)

13. A (page 542)

14. D – Also, assume a facial fracture in patients who have sustained a direct blow to the mouth or nose. A collision with a tree, lift tower, or windshield in a snowmobile or hit by a snowboard or falling rocks are examples of blunt impact that cause facial fractures. (page 544)

15. D (page 545)

16. A (page 545)

Labeling

1. Face/Skull (page 539)

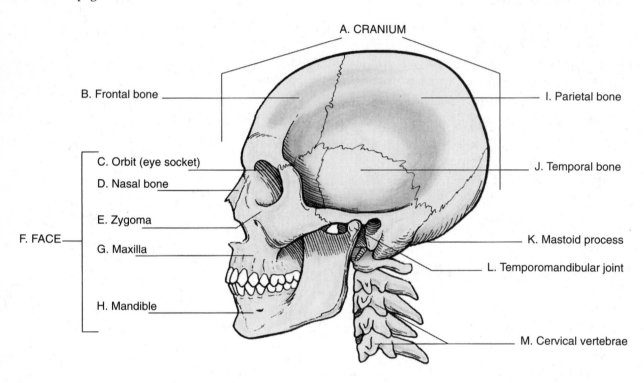

A. CRANIUM

B. Frontal bone

C. Orbit (eye socket)

D. Nasal bone

E. Zygoma

F. FACE

G. Maxilla

H. Mandible

I. Parietal bone

J. Temporal bone

K. Mastoid process

L. Temporomandibular joint

M. Cervical vertebrae

Vocabulary

1. Air embolism: The presence of air in the veins, which can lead to cardiac arrest if it enters the heart. (page 545)

2. Hematoma: The collection of blood in a space, tissue, or organ due to a break in the wall of a blood vessel. (page 540)

3. Sternocleidomastoid muscle: Muscles on either side of the neck that allow movement of the head. (page 540)

4. Subcutaneous emphysema: A characteristic crackling sensation on palpation, caused by the presence of air in soft tissues. (page 545)

5. Temporomandibular joint (TMJ): The joint that is formed where the mandible and the cranium meet, just in front of the ear. (page 538)

Fill-in

1. carotid arteries (page 540)

2. cervical (page 539)

3. temporal (page 539)

4. trachea (page 544)

5. cartilage (page 540)

6. men, women (page 539)

7. foramen magnum (page 538)

8. maxilla (page 538)

9. parietal (page 539)

10. trachea (page 540)

True/False

1. T   (page 540)
2. T   (page 541)
3. F   (page 541)
4. F   (page 543)
5. T   (page 545)
6. T   (page 540)
7. T   (page 543)

Short Answer

1. Direct manual pressure with a dry dressing. Use roller gauze around the circumference of the head to hold pressure dressing in place. (page 541)
2. Apply direct pressure above and below the injury. (page 545)

Word Fun

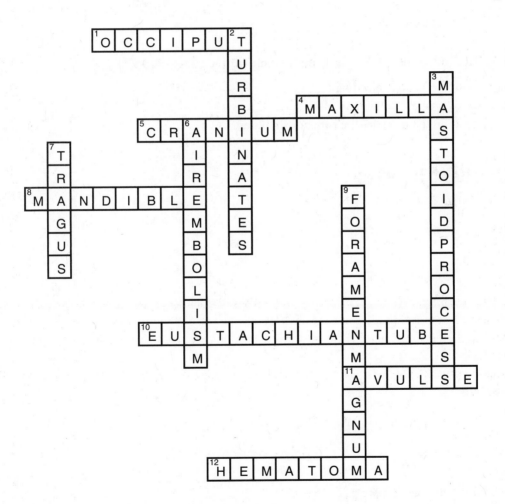

Calls to the Scene

1. -BSI precautions.

-Have patient lean forward while pinching the nostrils together.

-Assess the airway to assure patency.

2. -BSI precautions.

-Apply direct pressure, being careful not to compress both sides of the neck.

-Apply high-flow oxygen.

-Transport in a reclining position.

-Monitor vital signs.

3. -BSI precautions.

-Transport in position of comfort.

-Apply high-flow oxygen.

-Bandage ear when bleeding is controlled.

-Wrap avulsed part in moist, sterile dressing and place in plastic bag. Keep cool.

-Monitor vital signs.

Skill Drills

1. **Skill Drill 21-1: Controlling Bleeding from a Neck Injury (page 545)**

1. Apply **direct pressure** to control bleeding.
2. Use a **roller gauze** to secure a dressing in place.
3. Wrap the bandage around and under the patient's **shoulder**.

Chapter 22: Chest Injuries

Matching

1. B   (page 550)
2. D   (page 550)
3. C   (page 550)
4. A   (page 550)
5. E   (page 550)
6. H   (page 551)
7. I   (page 553)
8. J   (page 557)
9. F   (page 551)
10. G   (page 552)
11. M   (page 552)
12. K   (page 553)
13. L   (page 555)

Multiple Choice

1. B (page 550)
2. A (page 550)
3. C (page 550)
4. D (page 551)
5. D – (A), (B), and (C) are signs. (page 552)
6. D (page 552)
7. B – Flail segment (A) is a common cause of paradoxical motion (page 556)
8. C (page 553)
9. D (page 553)
10. C (pages 553–554)

11. D (page 554)

12. D (page 554)

13. D – It also includes tachycardia, low blood pressure, cyanosis, and decreased breath sounds on the injured side. (pages 554–555)

14. D (page 555)

15. D (page 555)

16. A (page 556)

17. C – Bruising of the lung (A) is called a pulmonary contusion. Broken ribs in two or more places (B) is called flail chest. (page 556)

18. D (page 556)

19. D – Signs and symptoms of pericardial tamponade also include jugular vein distention and a decrease in the difference between the systolic and diastolic blood pressure. (page 557)

20. B (page 557)

Labeling

1. Anterior Aspect of the Chest (page 551)

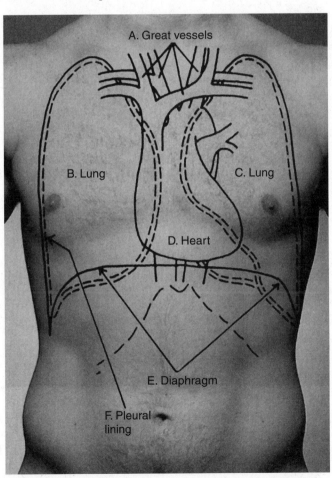

2. The Ribs (page 551)

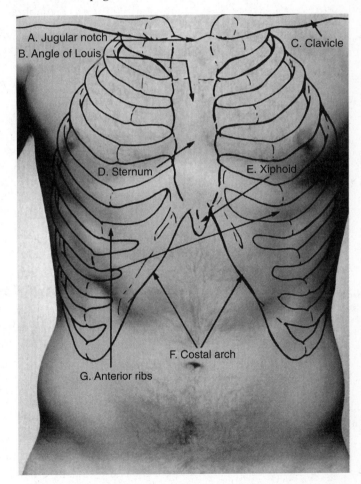

Vocabulary

1. Flail chest: A condition in which three or more ribs are fractured in two or more places, or in association with a fracture of the sternum, so that a segment of chest wall is effectively detached from the rest of the thoracic cage. (page 556)

2. Paradoxical motion: The motion of a portion of the chest wall that is detached in a flail chest; the motion—in during inhalation, out during exhalation—is exactly the opposite of normal motion during breathing. (page 556)

3. Pericardial tamponade: Compression of the heart due to a buildup of blood or other fluid in pericardial sac. (page 557)

4. Spontaneous pneumothorax: Pneumothorax that occurs when a weak area on the lung ruptures in the absence of major injury, allowing air to leak into the pleural space. (page 554)

5. Sucking chest wound: An opening or penetrating chest wall wound through which air passes during inspiration and expiration, creating a sucking sound. (page 553)

6. Tension pneumothorax: An accumulation of air or gas in the pleural cavity that progressively increases the pressure in the chest with potentially fatal results. (page 554)

Fill-in

1. back (page 550)
2. decreases (page 550)
3. sternum (page 550)
4. bronchi (page 550)
5. phrenic (page 550)
6. ribs (page 550)
7. diaphragm (page 550)
8. Pleura (page 553)
9. aorta (page 557)
10. contracts (page 550)

True/False

1. T (page 552)
2. F (page 552)
3. T (page 555)
4. F (page 555)
5. F (page 554)
6. F (page 557)
7. F (page 550)
8. T (page 550)
9. F (page 551)

Short Answer

1. -Pain at the site of injury

   -Pain localized at the site of injury that is aggravated by or increased with breathing

   -Dyspnea (difficulty breathing, shortness of breath)

   -Hemoptysis (coughing up blood)

   -Failure of one or both sides of the chest to expand normally with inspiration

   -Rapid, weak pulse and low blood pressure

   -Cyanosis around the lips or fingernails. (page 552)

2. 1. Seal the wound with a large airtight dressing that seals all four sides.

   2. Seal the wound with a dressing that seals three sides with the fourth side as a flutter valve.

   Your local protocol will dictate the way you are to care for this injury. (page 554)

3. Tape a bulky pad against the segment of the chest. (page 556)

4. Sudden severe compression of the chest, causing a rapid increase of pressure within the chest. Characteristic signs include distended neck veins, facial and neck cyanosis, and hemorrhage in the sclera of the eye. (page 556)

Word Fun

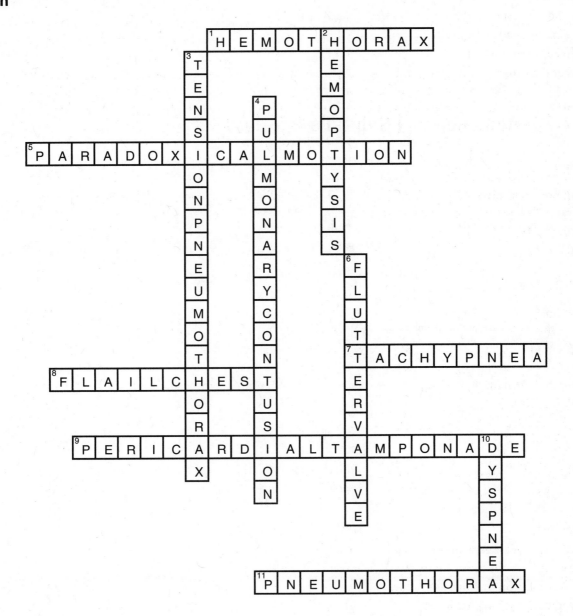

Calls to the Scene

1. -BSI precautions.

-Immediately begin assisting ventilations with a BVM attached to high-flow oxygen.

-Begin chest compressions.

-Arrange for rapid transport.

-Apply an AED as soon as possible.

-Continue CPR and continuously monitor the patient.

2. -BSI precautions.

-Apply high-flow oxygen.

-Monitor vital signs.

-Arrange for rapid transport.

-Continue to monitor patient for signs of distress.

3. -BSI precautions.

-Apply high-flow oxygen via nonrebreathing mask or BVM.

-Apply cervical collar and full-body immobilization.

-Arrange for rapid transport.

-Monitor vital signs.

Chapter 23: Abdomen and Genitalia Injuries

Matching

1. G   (page 562)

2. D   (page 562)

3. C   (pages 562, 572)

4. H   (page 568)

5. E   (page 568)

6. B   (page 566)

7. A   (page 569)

8. F   (page 562)

Multiple Choice

1. D (page 562)

2. D – The intestines are also hollow. (page 562)

3. C (page 562)

4. D (page 562)

5. B – The abdomen becomes distended and firm to touch (A), normal bowel sounds diminish or disappear (C). (page 562)

6. D (page 562)

7. A (page 563)

8. C (page 564)

9. B (page 563)

10. A (page 563)

11. D (page 563)

12. C (page 564)

13. B – (A) and (C) are types of open injuries (page 564)

14. A (page 564)

15. B – (A) is a symptom (page 564)

16. B (page 564)

17. B (page 564)

18. D (page 565)

19. D (page 566)

20. D (page 566)

21. D – Only a surgeon can accurately assess the damage. (page 566)

22. D – Never attempt to replace abdominal contents (A), always keep organs moist (B), and never use any type of adherent dressings (C). (page 566)

23. A – (B), (C), and (D) are all hollow organs (page 568)

24. C (page 568)

25. D (page 569)

26. D (page 569)

27. A (page 569)

28. B (page 570)

29. D (page 570)

Labeling

1. Hollow Organs (page 562)

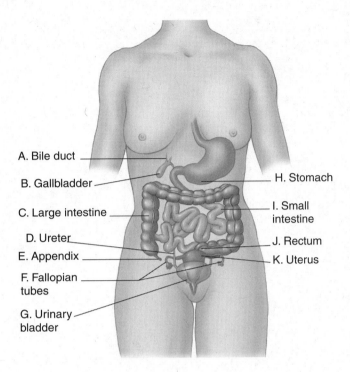

A. Bile duct

B. Gallbladder

C. Large intestine

D. Ureter

E. Appendix

F. Fallopian tubes

G. Urinary bladder

H. Stomach

I. Small intestine

J. Rectum

K. Uterus

2. Solid Organs (page 563)

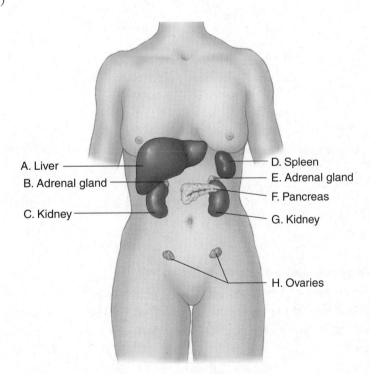

A. Liver

B. Adrenal gland

C. Kidney

D. Spleen

E. Adrenal gland

F. Pancreas

G. Kidney

H. Ovaries

Vocabulary

1. Closed abdominal injury: Any injury of the abdomen caused by a nonpenetrating instrument or force in which the skin remains intact; also called blunt abdominal injury. (page 563)
2. Open abdominal injury: Any injury of the abdomen caused by a penetrating or piercing instrument or force, in which the skin is lacerated or perforated and the cavity is opened to the atmosphere; also called penetrating injury. (pages 563–564)
3. Guarding: Contracting the stomach muscles to minimize the pain of abdominal movement; a sign of peritonitis. (page 565)

Fill-in

1. solid (page 563)
2. urinary (page 568)
3. retroperitoneal (page 568)
4. external signs (page 569)
5. peritonitis (page 562)
6. inflammatory response (page 563)
7. blunt injuries (page 565)

True/False

1. F   (page 562)
2. T   (page 564)
3. F   (page 564)
4. T   (page 562)
5. F   (page 566)
6. F   (page 569)

Short Answer

1. Stomach, intestines, ureters, bladder, gallbladder, and rectum (page 562)
2. Liver, spleen, pancreas, and kidneys (page 562)
3. Pain, shock signs, bruises, lacerations, bleeding, tenderness, guarding, and difficulty with movement because of pain (page 564)
4. -Inspect the patient's back and sides for exit wounds.

   -Apply a dry, sterile dressing to all open wounds.

   -If the penetrating object is still in place, apply a stabilizing bandage around it to control external bleeding and to minimize movement of the object. (page 566)
5. -Cover with moistened sterile dressing.

   -Secure dressing with bandage.

   -Secure bandage with tape. (pages 566–567)
6. -An abrasion, laceration, or contusion in the flank

   -A penetrating wound in the region of the lower rib cage (the flank) or the upper abdomen

   -Fractures on either side of the lower rib cage or of the lower thoracic or upper lumbar vertebrae (page 569)

Word Fun

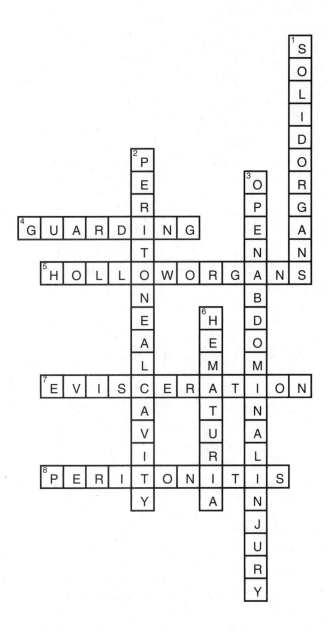

Calls to the Scene

1. -BSI precautions.
    -Assess the ABCs.
    -Apply high-flow oxygen.
    -Control any bleeding.
    -Stabilize the tree branch in place with bulky dressings – DO NOT REMOVE THE BRANCH.
    -Keep movement of patient to the bare minimum, so as not to create further injury. (Sliding the patient very carefully onto a backboard may help to minimize movement.)
    -Monitor vital signs.
    -Arrange for rapid transport.
    -Bandage minor lacerations if time allows.

2. -BSI precautions; be aware of possible vomitting.

   -Call for transport to definitive care.

   -Apply high-flow (15L/min) oxygen, but do not wait for O_2 to arrive before transport to base.

   -"Load and go" transport is essential

   -Watch for possible major shock complications

   -Monitor vital signs and airway continuously.

3. -BSI precautions.

   -Apply high-flow oxygen via nonrebreathing mask.

   -Cover the abdominal contents with moist, sterile gauze and an occlusive dressing.

   -Transport in the position of comfort (probably supine with knees bent).

   -Arrange for rapid transport.

   -Monitor vital signs and airway continuously.

Chapter 24: Principles of Musculoskeletal Injuries

Matching

1. G (page 576)
2. J (page 576)
3. D (page 576)
4. I (page 577)
5. F (page 577)
6. B (page 580)

7. K (page 582)
8. A (page 581)
9. C (page 577)
10. E (page 580)
11. H (page 587)

Multiple Choice

1. A (page 572)
2. B (page 576)
3. A – Minerals (B) and electrolytes (C) are stored in the bone marrow, which serves as a reservoir. (page 577)
4. B (page 577)
5. C (page 577)
6. B (page 578)
7. C – With a strain (B), no ligament or joint damage occurs. (page 578)
8. A (page 578)
9. D – The size of the zone of injury depends on the amount of kinetic energy the tissues absorb from forces acting in the body. (page 579)
10. A (page 579)
11. B (page 579)
12. C (page 580)
13. D (page 580)
14. B (page 580)
15. C (page 581)
16. D (page 581)
17. A (page 581)
18. C (page 582)
19. D (page 582)
20. A (page 581)
21. C (page 582)

22. B (page 582)

23. A (page 583)

24. C (page 583)

25. D (page 584)

26. D (page 590)

27. D (page 588)

28. C (page 589)

29. D (page 590)

30. B (page 596)

31. D – Hazards of improper splinting also include aggravation of the injury, and injury to tissue, nerves, blood vessels, or muscles as a result of excessive movement of the bone or joint. (page 604)

Labeling

1. The Human Skeleton (page 577)

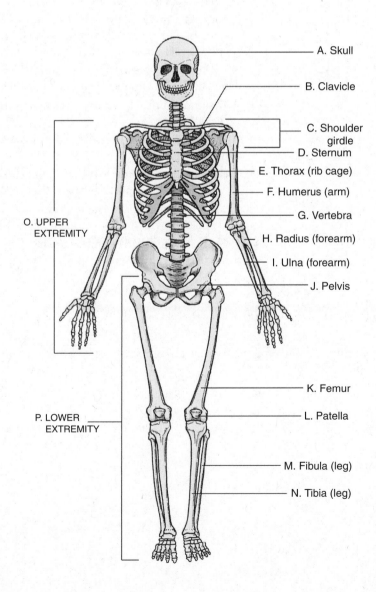

A. Skull
B. Clavicle
C. Shoulder girdle
D. Sternum
E. Thorax (rib cage)
F. Humerus (arm)
G. Vertebra
H. Radius (forearm)
I. Ulna (forearm)
J. Pelvis
K. Femur
L. Patella
M. Fibula (leg)
N. Tibia (leg)
O. UPPER EXTREMITY
P. LOWER EXTREMITY

Vocabulary

1. Traction: The act of exerting a pulling force on a structure. (page 609)

2. Dislocation: Disruption of a joint in which ligaments are damaged and the bone ends are completely displaced. (page 578)

3. Nondisplaced fracture: A simple crack in the bone that has not caused the bone to move from its normal anatomic position; also called a hairline fracture. (page 581)

4. Sling: A bandage or material that helps to support the weight of an injured upper extremity. (page 593)

5. Swathe: A bandage that passes around the chest to secure an injured arm to the chest. (page 593)

Fill-in

1. wasting (page 556)

2. red (page 557)

3. hinge (page 578)

4. mechanism of injury (page 579)

5. open fracture (page 580)

6. femur (page 587)

7. crepitus (page 583)

8. reduce (page 583)

9. neurovascular status (page 585)

10. **Quick splint:** Lower legs, some dislocations; possibly additional padding (page 590)

Cardboard splint: Lower legs, arms, some dislocations; padding, cravats (page 590)

Wire, ladder splint: Upper arms, forearms, hands, improvised splinting for legs, ankles, and feet; Padding, cravats, self-adhering roller bandages (page 592)

Malleable metal splint: Upper arms, forearms, hands, improvised splinting for rigid collar, splint of legs, ankles, and feet; padding, cravats, self-adhering roller bandages (page 592)

Air splint: Forearm, upper extremity, legs, lower extremity; no additional supplies required (page 593)

Vacuum splint: Upper or lower extremities; suction pump (page 593)

Sling and swathe: Clavicles, dislocations, upper extremity; cravats, possibly padding (page 593)

Hare traction splint: Midshaft femur fracture; all supplies provided with commercial package (page 599)

Sager or Kendrick traction splint: midshaft femur fracture; all supplies provided with commercial package (page 603)

Thomas (modified) splint: midshaft femur fracture; cravats, ankle hitch, or smaller rope for pulley system (page 597)

True/False

1. T   (page 588)

2. T   (page 588)

3. F   (page 596)

4. T   (page 596)

5. T   (page 588)

6. F   (page 589)

7. T   (page 587)

8. T   (page 585)

9. T   (page 587)

Short Answer

1. 1. Direct

2. Indirect

3. Twisting

4. High-energy (page 579)

2. Deformity

Tenderness (point)

Guarding

Swelling

Bruising

Crepitus

False motion

Exposed fragments

Pain

Locked joint (pages 582–583)

3. 1. Pulse

2. Capillary refill

3. Sensation

4. Motor function (page 587)

4. 1. Remove clothing from the area.

2. Note and record the patient's neurovascular status distal to the site of the injury.

3. Cover all wounds with a dry, sterile dressing before splinting.

4. Do not move the patient before splinting.

5. For a suspected fracture, immobilize the joints above and below the fracture.

6. For a joint injury, immobilize the bones above and below the injured joint.

7. Pad all rigid splints.

8. Maintain manual immobilization to minimize movement of the limb and to support the injury site.

9. Use a constant, gentle manual traction to align the limb.

10. If you encounter resistance to limb alignment, splint the limb in its deformed position.

11. Immobilize all suspected spinal injuries in a neutral in-line position on a backboard.

12. If the patient has signs of shock, align the limb in the normal anatomic position and provide transport.

13. When in doubt, splint. (pages 588–590)

5. 1. Stabilize the fracture.

2. Align the limb.

3. Avoid potential neurovascular compromise. (page 597)

Word Fun

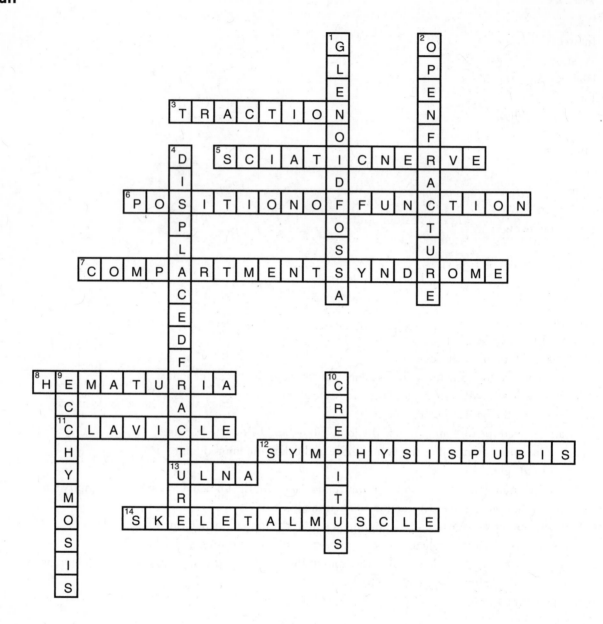

Calls to the Scene

1. -BSI precautions.

-Evaluate ABCs and pulse/motor/sensation in all extremities.

-Apply high-flow oxygen.

-Splint fractured scapula using a sling and swathe.

-Transport patient in position of comfort.

-Consider c-spine immobilization if patient fell, was thrown, or complains of any neck pain.

-Upgrade to rapid transport if patient shows any signs of altered mental status, respiratory distress/compromise, or circulatory compromise.

2. -BSI precautions.

-Splint the arm in position found, since circulation is intact.

-Use a board splint for support with a sling and swathe.

-Immobilize hand in the position of function.

-Apply oxygen as needed.

-Transport in the position of comfort.

-Arrange for normal transport.

-Monitor vital signs.

3. -BSI precautions.

-Verify scene safety.

-Be aware of documentation for risk management.

-Traction splint is contraindicated and should not be used.

-Splint leg with fixation splint in position found.

-Continue to reassess pulse, motion, and sensory function (CMS).

-Reassess transport decisions.

Skill Drills

1. Skill Drill 24-1: Assessing Pulse, Motor, and Sensory Functions (page 586)

1. Palpate the **radial** pulse in the upper extremity.
2. Palpate the **posterior tibial** pulse in the lower extremity. Remember to palpate the **dorsalis pedis** pulse as well.
3. Assess capillary refill by blanching a fingernail or **toenail**.
4. Assess sensation on the flesh near the **tip** of the **index** finger and thumb, and the **little finger** as well.
5. On the foot, first check sensation on the flesh near the **tip** of the **great toe**.
6. Also check foot sensation on the **lateral side**.
7. Evaluate motor function by asking the patient to **open** the hand. (Perform motor tests only if the hand or foot is not **injured**. **Stop** a test if it causes pain.)
8. Also ask the patient to **make a fist**.
9. To evaluate motor function in the foot, ask the patient to **extend (dorsiflex)** the foot.
10. Also have the patient **flex (plantar flex)** the foot and **wiggle** the toes.

2. Skill Drill 24-2: Caring for Musculoskeletal Injuries (page 589)

1. Cover open wounds with a **dry, sterile** dressing, and **apply pressure** to control bleeding. Assess **distal** CMS functions.
2. Apply a **quick** splint.
3. **Elevate** the extremity and **position** the patient for transport.
4. Assess distal **CMS** functions and **position** the patient for transport.

3. Skill Drill 24-3: Applying a Quick Splint (page 591)

1. Open the quick splint **flat** next to the patient's injured **extremity**.
2. Grasp the booted foot with one hand, using slight **longitudinal** traction, and place the other hand just below the **knee** or under the lower thigh to **support** the extremity.
3. The "**pant-leg pinch** lift" is another useful method for lifting and supporting the injured extremity.
4. Have a second rescuer **slide** the splint underneath the leg while you gently **lower** the injured extremity into the splint.
5. The second rescuer then **folds** up the sides of the splint like a **clamshell**, and secures the splint **straps** firmly.
6. Reassess **neurovascular** function.

4. Skill Drill 24-4: Applying a Sling and Swathe (page 594)

1. Bend the patient's elbow to just under a 90° angle and lay a **triangular** bandage on the chest wall under the injured arm. The injured forearm lays across the **chest**.

2. Tie the two ends together at the **side** of the neck. Bring the apex **forward** and pin it to the **front** of the sling, or tie a knot in the apex.

3. Wrap a **swathe** around the patient's chest, include the **upper arm** on the injured side, and tie it snugly under the **opposite** armpit.

4. To avoid pressure on an injured shoulder or fractured clavicle, bring the lower corner under the near **axilla**. Tie it to the opposite corner behind the patient's **back**.

5. Skill Drill 24-5: Forming and Applying a Blanket Roll Splint (page 595)

1. Fold a blanket **longitudinally** in thirds.

2. Lay **cravats** across the blanket. Tie knots in the two ends of one cravat(s) for **identification** purposes later.

3. Position the **rolled** blanket snugly and in the **abduction** angle of the dislocated shoulder.

4. Securely **tie** the cravats around the **neck** and **waist**.

5. Secure the injured arm with a **sling** and **swathe**.

6. Skill Drill 24-6: Initial Application of all Traction Splints (page 598)

1. One rescuer manually stabilizes the fracture site.

2. After the fracture has been stabilized, another rescuer(s) removes the ski or snowboard and assesses the CMS status of the extremity.

3. The first rescuer firmly grasps the injured leg below the knee and realigns the fracture by manual, longitudinal (axial) traction. The boot can be removed and CMS status assessed at this time as needed.

4. The second rescuer sizes and prepares the splint. The ankle hitch should be applied at this time and can be used to maintain manual traction.

5. The leg is placed in the splint, secured to the upper thigh, and mechanical traction is evenly substituted for manual traction.

6. Reassess the CMS status of the injured extremity after all straps have been applied.

7. Log roll the patient onto his or her uninjured side and place the patient on a long backboard. Secure the splint to the backboard to prevent movement.

8. Skill Drill 24-7: Applying a Sager Traction Splint (page 603)

1. Adjust the thigh strap so that it lies anteriorly when secured.

2. Estimate the proper length of the splint by placing it next to the uninjured limb.
   Fit the ankle pads to the ankle.

3. Place the splint at the inner thigh, apply the thigh strap at the upper thigh, and secure snugly.

4. Tighten the ankle harness just above the malleoli.
   Snug the cable ring against the bottom of the foot.

5. Extend the splint's inner shaft to apply traction of about 10% of body weight.

6. Secure the splint with elasticized cravats.

7. Check CMS functions.
   Secure the patient to a long backboard.

9. Skill Drill 24-8: Boot Removal (page 607)

1. Stabilize the **lower** leg and the **boot**.
2. While maintaining **manual** stabilization, spread the boot shell, pulling the **tongue** out or opening a rear entry boot as wide as possible. **Loosen** all devices and provide **instructions** to the assisting rescuer.
3. With the boot shell held open and the leg stabilized, apply **tension** to the boot. Firmly and smoothly **pull** and **rotate** the boot off the foot, while using your **shoulder** as counterpressure against the boot toe.
4. Monitor the patient for indications of excessive **pain** or **resistance**. Stop or modify the procedure as appropriate.
5. Assess distal **circulation** and **neurologic** function, swelling, **displacement**, or bruising (remove clothing).
6. Prepare to **splint** the lower extremity.

Chapter 25: Assessment and Care of Bone and Joint Injuries

Matching

1. A (page 624)
2. E (page 616)
3. B (page 634)
4. C (page 616)
5. D (page 617)
6. J (page 631)

7. H (page 625)
8. K (page 626)
9. G (page 627)
10. I (page 637)
11. F (page 634)

Multiple Choice

1. A (page 616)
2. D (page 617)
3. A (page 630)
4. C (page 630)
5. D (page 625)
6. C (page 631)
7. D (page 616)
8. C (page 637)
9. D (page 626)
10. C (page 628)

11. B (page 629)
12. C (page 631)
13. B (page 631)
14. A (page 635)
15. A (page 634)
16. D (page 624)
17. D (page 637)
18. C (page 627)
19. B (page 635)

Labeling

1. Anatomy of the Knee (page 629)

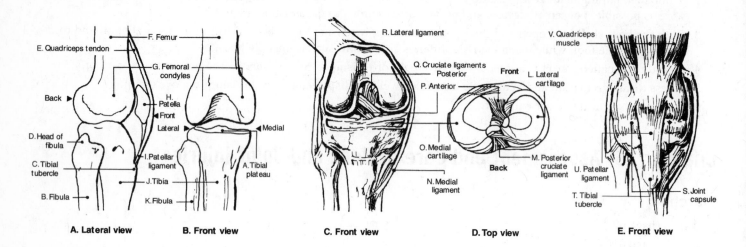

Vocabulary

1. Acromioclavicular (A/C) joint: A simple joint where the bony projections of the scapula and the clavicle meet at the top of the shoulder. (page 616)

2. Colles fracture: Fracture of the distal radius, a common upper extremity injury in snowboarders, aka "silver fork" deformity. (page 621)

3. Sciatic nerve: Major nerve in the lower extremity; a frequent complication of hip dislocation is injury to this nerve. (page 626)

4. Glenohumeral joint: The shoulder joint, the most commonly dislocated <u>large</u> joint in the body, where the head of the humerus meets the glenoid fossa of the scapula. (page 616)

5. Supracondylar fracture of the humerus: A fracture just above the elbow complicated by nerve and blood vessel injury. (page 619)

6. Retroperitoneal space: The space between the abdominal cavity and posterior abdominal wall. Contains the kidneys and pancreas. (page 624)

Fill-in

1. swelling (page 614)

2. scapula (page 615)

3. strong distal pulses, normal sensations (page 621)

4. direct compression (page 624)

5. Knee sprains (page 629)

6. upper femur (page 626)

True/False

1. T (page 616)

2. F (page 632)

3. F (page 627)

4. T (page 628)

5. F (page 635)

6. T (page 635)

7. T (page 618)

8. T (page 623)

9. F (page 628)

10. F (page 627)

Short Answer

1. Distal pulse to verify there is no change in CMS (page 623)
2. Blood in urine, severe abdominal pain, shock (page 624)
3. Stabilized and immobilized in near anatomical position (page 635)
4. Sprained shoulder or fractured upper arm. (page 614)
5. Fractured clavicle (page 614)
6. Anterior dislocation of the shoulder—patient holds arm slightly away from the chest and supports it with the opposite hand.

   Posterior dislocation of the shoulder—patient holds arm away from the body or over the head, unable to bring it near the chest. (page 616)

Word Fun

Calls to the Scene

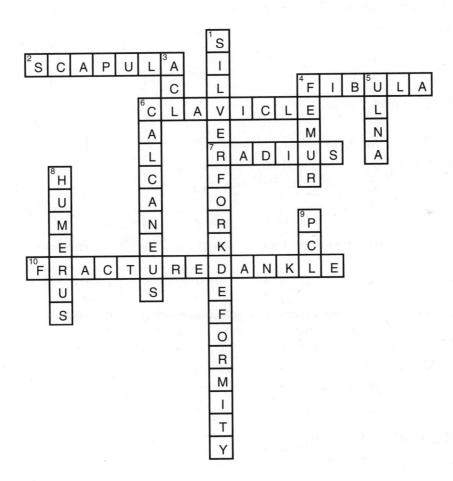

1. -BSI precautions.
   -Verify scene safety.
   -Follow assessment protocols.
   -Call for materials to improvise a splint to keep the patient's arm in the position found.
   -Assess CMS.
   -If the patient can be splinted in the sitting position, make sure she is supported during transport.
   -Reassess CMS.

2. -BSI precautions.

   -Assess distal pulse.

   -Perform thorough assessment. Make sure the patient did not hit his head or neck. While waiting for toboggan, obtain a SAMPLE history and rapid body survey.

   -Treat the open injury by realigning the deformity, if not associated with the joint.

   -Dress and bandage the open wound, being aware of potential problems of bone going back in, swelling, and infection.

   -Splint the lower extremity with a soft splint.

   -Reassess distal circulation.

   -Give oxygen, if necessary.

   -Transport to the aid room.

   -Reassess.

3. -BSI precautions.

   -Verify scene safety.

   -Stabilize ABCs, if necessary.

   -Perform trauma history and physical exam for responsive patient without significant MOI.

   -Care for chief complaint, assessing distal pulse, splint the leg in the position found.

   -Reassess distal pulse.

   -Record vitals.

   -Monitor patient.

   -Transport to aid room.

Skill Drills

1. Skill Drill 25-1: Splinting the Hand and Wrist (page 623)

1. Move the hand into the **position of function**. Place a soft **roller bandage** into the **palm**.
2. Apply a padded **board splint** on the palmar side with **fingertips** exposed.
3. Secure the splint with a **roller bandage**.
4. Stabilize a **thumb** ulnar collateral ligament sprain to the **hand** with a **roller gauze**.

2. Skill Drill 25-2: Realignment of Angulated, Rotated, Fractured Tibia/Fibula with Application of a Quick Splint (page 636)

1. Rescuer 1 grasps the boot heel of the injured leg with one hand, while the other hand is placed under the calf just below the knee.
2. When the splint is ready, rescuer 1 applies gentle longitudinal traction, and with both hands, lifts, straightens, and derotates the deformed tibia all in one continuous motion.
3. Rescuer 2 slides the splint under the leg from medial and below, then rescuer 1 lowers the leg into the splint.
4. Rescuer 2 closes the splint and secures the straps, while rescuer 1 removes his or her upper hand.
5. Rescuer 1 slides his or her hand out from around the heel, and then checks the CMS function in the foot.

Chapter 26: Head and Spine Injuries

Matching

1. D	(page 647)	**6.** C	(page 646)
2. E	(page 647)	**7.** B	(page 661)
3. H	(page 649)	**8.** I	(page 648)
4. G	(page 649)	**9.** J	(page 650)
5. A	(page 650)	**10.** F	(page 647)

Multiple Choice

1. D (page 647)
2. B (page 649)
3. C (page 647)
4. C (page 652)
5. A (page 647)
6. B (page 649)
7. D (page 648)
8. D (page 648)
9. C (page 649)
10. A (page 650)
11. D (page 651)
12. D (page 652)
13. B (page 650)
14. D – Assess pulse and motor and sensory function in all extremities (page 654)
15. B (page 653)
16. A (page 654)
17. A – Remember BSI. (page 659)
18. B (page 667)
19. D (page 659)
20. B (page 659)
21. D (page 660)
22. D – An intracerebral hemorrhage (B) is within the substance of the brain tissue itself. A subdural hematoma (C) is below the dura but outside the brain. (page 661)
23. B (page 661)
24. B (page 662)
25. D – Cyanosis (A) and hypoxia (B) are results of cerebral edema. Vomiting (C) results from increased intracranial pressure. (page 662)
26. C (page 661)
27. C (page 663)
28. D – An example of a congenital problem (B) that could cause unequal pupils is anisocoria. (page 663)
29. C (page 663)
30. B – BSI and scene safety always come first, but (B) is the best answer of the choices given. (page 664)
31. D (page 665)
32. C (page 668)
33. A (page 671)

Labeling

1. The Brain (page 647)

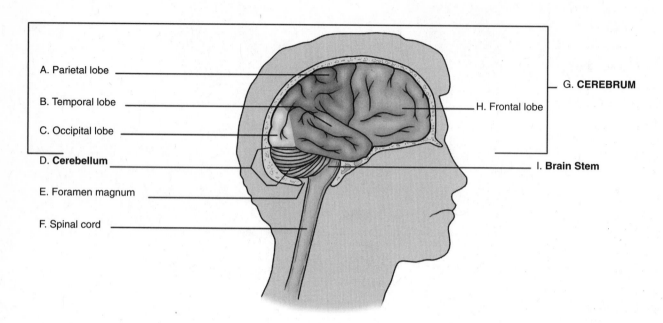

A. Parietal lobe

B. Temporal lobe

C. Occipital lobe

D. **Cerebellum**

E. Foramen magnum

F. Spinal cord

G. **CEREBRUM**

H. Frontal lobe

I. **Brain Stem**

2. The Connecting Nerves in the Spinal Cord (page 649)

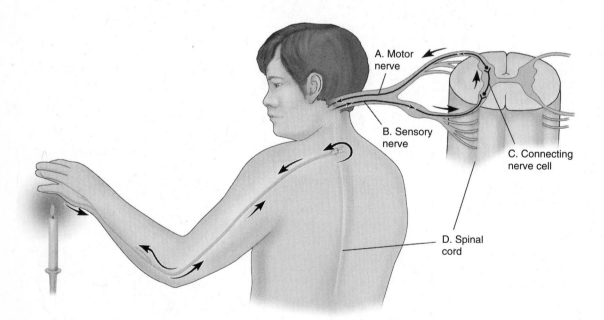

A. Motor nerve

B. Sensory nerve

C. Connecting nerve cell

D. Spinal cord

3. The Spinal Column (page 650)

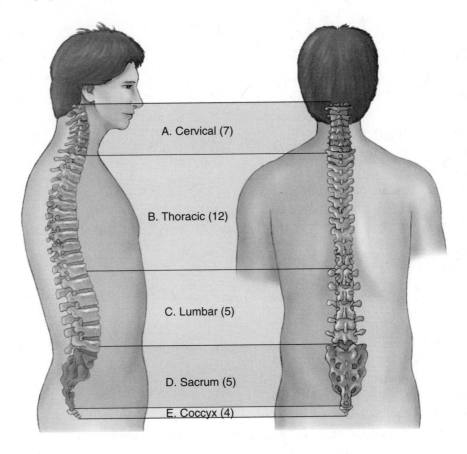

A. Cervical (7)

B. Thoracic (12)

C. Lumbar (5)

D. Sacrum (5)

E. Coccyx (4)

Vocabulary

1. Retrograde amnesia: The inability to remember events leading up to a brain injury. (page 660)

2. Anterograde (posttraumatic) amnesia: Inability to remember events after an injury. (page 660)

3. Closed brain injury: Injury usually associated with trauma in which the brain has been injured but the skin has not been broken and there is no obvious bleeding. (page 662)

4. Eyes-forward position: A position in which the head is gently lifted until the patient's eyes are looking straight ahead and the head and torso are in line. (page 665)

5. Open brain injury: Injury to the brain often caused by a penetrating object in which there may be bleeding and exposed brain tissue. (page 662)

Fill-in

1. motor (page 649)

2. meninges (pages 647–648)

3. central (page 646)

4. 31 (page 648)

5. cranial (page 648)

6. intervertebral disks (page 650)

7. cranium, face (page 649)

8. choroid plexus (page 647)

9. sympathetic (page 649)

10. parasympathetic (page 649)

True/False

1. T   (page 650)
2. F   (page 648)
3. F   (page 649)
4. T   (page 649)

5. F   (page 649)
6. F   (page 651)
7. F   (page 651)

Short Answer

1. 1. Does your neck or back hurt?

2. What happened?

3. Where does it hurt?

4. Can you move your hands and feet?

5. Can you feel me touching your fingers? Your toes? (page 651)

2. -Muscle spasms in the neck

-Increased pain

-Numbness, tingling, or weakness

-Compromised airway or ventilations (page 654)

3. 1. Concussion

2. Contusion

3. Intracranial bleeding (pages 659–660)

4. -Lacerations, contusions, or hematomas to the scalp

-Soft area or depression upon palpation

-Visible fractures or deformities of the skull

-Ecchymosis about the eyes or behind the ear over the mastoid process

-Clear or pink cerebrospinal fluid leakage from a scalp wound, the nose, or the ear

-Failure of the pupils to respond to light

-Unequal pupil size

-Loss of sensation and/or motor function

-A period of unconsciousness

-Amnesia

-Seizures

-Numbness or tingling in the extremities

-Irregular respirations

-Dizziness

-Visual complaints

-Combative or other abnormal behavior

-Nausea or vomiting (page 662)

5. 1. Establish an adequate airway.

2. Control bleeding.

3. Assess the patient's baseline level of consciousness. (page 664)

6. 1. Is the patient's airway clear?

2. Is the patient breathing adequately?

3. Can you maintain the airway and assist ventilations if the helmet remains in place?

4. How well does the helmet fit?

5. Can the patient move within the helmet?

6. Can the spine be immobilized in a neutral position with the helmet on?
(page 668)

Word Fun

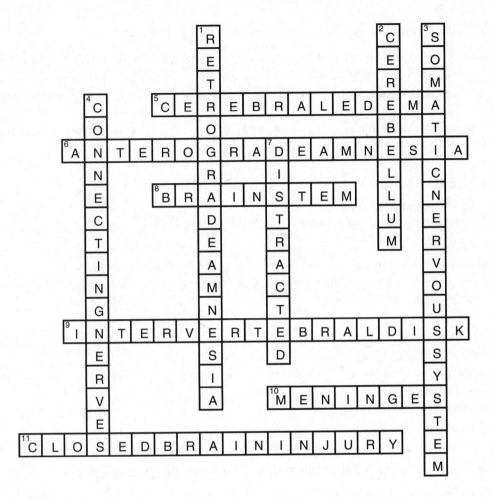

Calls to the Scene

1. -BSI precautions.
-Apply a cervical collar and hold manual stabilization.
-Secure patient to long backboard.
-Apply high-flow oxygen.
-Monitor vital signs and continue with assessment.
-Normal transport to base facility, arrange for ambulance transport to hospital

2. -BSI precautions.
-Cervical spine immobilization
-Maintain the airway/apply high-flow oxygen—suction as needed.
-Cover the open laceration with gauze, being careful to gently press over the area to avoid further damage.
-Put patient on long backboard and rapid transport.
-Monitor vital signs.

3. -BSI precautions.
-Manually guard cervical spine, stabilize ABCs.
-Pad appropriately to immobilize the patient for transport–rigid collar, long backboard.
-Use high-flow oxygen via nonrebreathing mask.
-Monitor vital signs and shock.
-Reevaluate neurological condition in extremities.
-Continue assessment.
-Rapid transport due to mechanism of injury with head uphill. Arrange for EMS transport to hospital.

Skill Drills

1. **Skill Drill 26-1: Performing Manual In-Line Stabilization** (page 653)

1. Kneel at the head of the patient and place your hands firmly around the **base** of the **skull** on either **side**.
2. Support the lower jaw with your **index** and **long** fingers, and the head with your **palms**.
3. Gently **align** the head into a **neutral, eyes-forward** position, aligned with the torso. Do not **move** the head or neck excessively.
4. Continue to **support** the head manually while your partner places a rigid **cervical collar** around the neck. Maintain **manual support** until you have the patient secured to a backboard.

2. **Skill Drill 26-2: Immobilizing a Patient to a Long Backboard** (pages 655–656)

1. Apply and maintain **cervical stabilization**.
   Assess **distal functions** in all extremities.
2. Apply a **cervical collar**.
3. Rescuers **kneel** on one side of the patient and place **hands** on the far side of the patient.
4. On command, rescuers **roll** the patient toward themselves, quickly examine the **back**, slide the backboard under the patient, and roll the patient onto the board.
5. **Center** the patient on the board.
6. Secure the **upper torso** first.
7. Secure the **pelvis**, and **legs**, and **feet**.
8. Begin to secure the patient's head using a commercial immobilization device, **blanket roll**, and/or **foam blocks**.
9. Place **tape** across the patient's forehead.
10. Check all **straps** and readjust as needed.
    Reassess **distal functions** in all extremities.

3. **Skill Drill 26-3: Immobilizing a Patient Found in a Standing Position** (page 658)

1. After **manually** stabilizing the head and neck, apply a **cervical collar**. Position the board **behind** the patient.
2. Position rescuers at **sides** and **behind** the patient.
   Side rescuers reach under patient's **arms** and grasp **handholds** at or slightly above **shoulder** level.
3. Prepare to lower the patient. Rescuers on the sides should be **facing** the rescuer at the head and **wait** for his or her **direction**.
4. On command, **lower** the backboard to the ground.

4. **Skill Drill 26-4: Application of a Cervical Collar** (page 666)

1. Apply **in-line** stabilization.
2. Measure the proper **collar size**.
3. Place the **chin support** first.
4. **Wrap** the collar around the neck and **secure** the collar.
5. Ensure proper **fit** and maintain **neutral, in-line** stabilization.

6. **Skill Drill 26-5: Removing a Helmet (page 670)**

1. Kneel down at the patient's head with another **rescuer** at one side.

   Open the face shield to assess **airway** and **breathing**. Remove **eyeglasses** or goggles if present.

2. Prevent head movement by placing your **hands** on either side of the helmet and fingers on the **lower jaw**. Have another rescuer **loosen** the strap.

3. Have another rescuer place one hand at the **angle** of the **lower jaw** and the other at the **junction** of the head and cervical spine.

4. Gently slip the helmet about **halfway** off, then stop.

5. Have another rescuer slide his or her hand from the **junction** of the patient's head and cervical spine to the **back** of the head to prevent it from snapping back.

6. Remove the helmet and **stabilize** the cervical spine.

   Apply a **cervical collar** and secure the patient to a **long backboard**.

   Pad as needed to prevent neck flexion or extension.

Section 6 Scene Techniques

Chapter 27: Rescue Techniques: Lifts and Loads

Matching

1. C   (page 698)
2. G   (page 702)
3. H   (page 707)
4. E   (page 703)
5. A   (page 703)

6. I   (page 702)
7. F   (page 695)
8. B   (page 707)
9. D   (page 704)

Multiple Choice

1. D (page 687)
2. D (page 694)
3. B (page 684)
4. D (page 686)
5. D (page 687)
6. D (page 689)
7. D (page 702)
8. A – The command of execution is done during each phase of moving. (page 689)
9. D (page 690)
10. D – When carrying a patient in a stair chair, you should also bend at the knees. (page 690)
11. D (page 690)
12. C – When you can move no farther, stop and move back another 15" to 20". (page 691)
13. D (page 684)
14. B (page 690)
15. D (page 692)
16. D (page 692)
17. C (page 692)
18. D (page 694)
19. D – An urgent move may also be necessary if the patient needs immediate intervention that requires a supine position, if the patient's condition requires immediate transport to the hospital, or if there is an extreme weather condition. (page 694)
20. D (page 689)
21. C (page 701)
22. D – To move a patient from the ground or the floor onto the cot, you may also log roll the patient onto a blanket, centering the patient on the blanket and rolling up the excess material on each side. Lift the patient by the blanket, and carry him or her to the nearby cot. (page 701)
23. B (page 703)
24. B (page 702)
25. A (page 703)
26. D (pages 703, 704)
27. D (page 708)
28. D (page 708)

Vocabulary

1. Jams and pretzels: Techniques for aligning and extricating a patient found in an awkward position or confined location. (page 681)
2. Log roll: A technique used to roll a patient 180° (usually from prone to supine) or to the side so that a backboard can be slipped underneath without bending or twisting the spine. (page 684)
3. Bridge lift: A lift performed by three or more rescuers. Each rescuer braces his or her head against the shoulder of an opposite rescuer, allowing lifting to occur with the arms instead of the back. (page 695)
4. Power lift: A lifting technique in which the rescuer's back is held upright, with legs bent, and the patient is lifted when the rescuer straightens the legs to raise the upper body and arms. (page 687)
5. Emergency move: A move in which the patient is dragged or pulled from a dangerous scene before initial assessment and care are provided. (page 692)

Fill-in

1. body mechanics (page 684)
2. upright (page 686)
3. power lift (page 692)
4. palm (page 688)
5. locked-in (page 690)
6. 250 (page 690)
7. sideways (page 691)
8. overhead (page 690)
9. less strain (page 692)
10. spine movement (page 692)
11. direct ground lift (page 695)
12. extremity lift (page 698)
13. backboard, stretcher, or blanket (page 701)

True/False

1. T (page 680)
2. T (page 707)
3. T (page 687)
4. F (page 690)
5. F (page 699)
6. T (page 692)
7. F (page 703)
8. F (page 702)
9. F (page 692)
10. F (page 689)

Short Answer

1. -Front cradle

   -Firefighter's drag

   -One-person walking assist

   -Firefighter's carry

   -Pack strap (page 694)

2. -The vehicle or scene is unsafe.

   -The patient cannot be properly assessed before being removed from the car.

   -The patient needs immediate intervention that requires a supine position.

   -The patient's condition requires immediate transport to the hospital.

   -The patient blocks the rescuer's access to another seriously injured patient.
   (page 692)

3. -Tighten back in normal upright position.

-Spread your legs apart about 15 inches.

-Grab device with palms up.

-Adjust orientation and position until weight is balanced.

-Reposition feet if necessary.

-Lift with arms extended downward by straightening your legs.

Note: Make sure back is locked. (page 687)

4. Always keep your back in a straight, upright position and lift without twisting. (page 687)

5. When placing a patient in a toboggan, the general rule is to position the injury uphill to decrease swelling, slow bleeding, and keep the patient's weight from jamming the injury against the toboggan. Patient comfort also is a strong guide when positioning. (page 705)

Word Fun

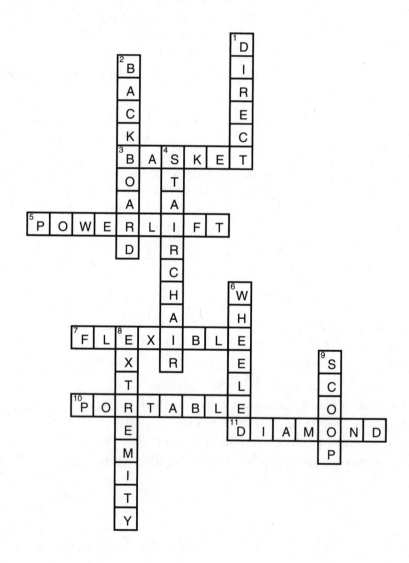

Calls to the Scene

1. -Immobilize the patient on a long backboard and apply high-flow oxygen.

   -Use four persons to carry the board back up the ledge.

   -Plan the route and brief your helpers before moving the patient.

   -Clarify whether you will move on "three" or count to three then move.

   -Coordinate the move until the patient is loaded into the ambulance.

2. -Move the patient's legs so they are clear of, or on one side of, the snowmobile.

   -Place your arms through the armpits and grasp either the patient's forearms or your own forearms.

   -Support the patient's head against your body.

   -While supporting the patient's weight, drag the patient from the snowmobile.

   -Place him supine on the ground and secure the airway.

   -Assist ventilations with 100% oxygen until further help arrives.

3. -After completing the rapid body survey, immediately roll the patient to the side, protecting the neck as well as possible.

   -Continue assessment, ensuring a secure airway.

   -Maintain ABCs until further help arrives.

Skill Drills

1. Skill Drill 27-1: Log Roll (page 685)

1. Manually stabilize the head and neck.
2. Position sufficient rescuers on the same side of the patient, kneeling as close to the patient's side as possible. Position hands on the far side, taking body mass into consideration. Keep your back straight and lean solely from the hips. Overlap hands if possible.
3. Roll the patient as a unit toward the rescuers on command from the leader (at the head), keeping the body in line and while monitoring vital signs. The patient's arm may be alongside the body or elevated, depending on local protocols.
4. Place the backboard, blanket, or stretcher alongside the patient and underneath as far as possible without excessive movement.
5. When using a backboard, bring the device as close as practical to the patient's back.
6. Roll the patient onto the device on command from the leader, keeping the body in line.

2. Skill Drill 27-2: Performing the Power Lift (page 688)

1. Lock your back into an **upright**, slightly inward curve. **Spread** and bend your legs. Grasp the backboard, palms up and just in front of you. **Balance** and **center** the weight between your arms.
2. Position your feet, **straddle** the object, and **distribute** weight.
3. **Straighten** your legs and lift, keeping your back locked in.

3. Skill Drill 27-3: The Bridge Lift (page 696)

1. Manually stabilize the head and neck.
2. With five rescuers, the first rescuer is at the head, rescuers 2 and 3 are at one side, and rescuers 4 and 5 are at the other side.
3. Position the rescuers and have them form a bridge over the patient, head-to-shoulder or shoulder-to-shoulder. All rescuers must use the same configuration.
4. Position hands underneath the patient to lift at points of body mass and ensure the rescuer's commitment and distribution across the bridge. Lift the patient just enough to place a backboard underneath.

4. Skill Drill 27-4: Direct Ground Lift (pages 697–698)

1. Line up on one side of the patient rescuer 1 at the patient's head, rescuer 2 at the patient's **waist**, and rescuer 3 at the patient's **knees**. All rescuers kneel on one knee, preferably the same knee.
2. The patient's arms should be placed on his or her **chest**, if possible.
3. Rescuer 1 then places the other arm under the patient's **shoulder**.
4. Rescuer 2 places both arms under the patient's **lower back** and **buttocks**.
5. Rescuer 3 places both arms under the patient's **legs**.
6. On command, the team lifts the patient up to **knee level** as each rescuer **rests** an arm on his or her knee.
7. As a team on **signal**, each rescuer **rolls** the patient in toward his or her chest. Again on **signal**, the team stands and carries the patient to the carrying or transportation device.
8. The steps are **reversed** to lower the patient onto the carrying or transportation device.

5. Skill Drill 27-6: Lifting a Patient into a Toboggan or Other Transportation Device (page 706)

1. Assess the factors:
   a. Position of the patient in the toboggan
   b. Nature and extent of the injury
   c. Patient responsive/unresponsive
   d. Patient mobility—ability to assist
   e. Number of people able to assist
   f. Terrain (steep or flat)
   g. Conditions (hard/soft; poor footing)
   h. Type of transportation device (with/without basket; height of edges)
2. Position the toboggan and all of the other equipment.
3. Ensure all rescuers are in appropriate position.
4. Perform the lift smoothly without compromising the injury.
5. Ensure that the patient clears the side of the device.

Chapter 28: Triage

Matching

1. C. Green (page 716)
2. B. Yellow (page 716)
3. D. Black (page 717)
4. A. Red (page 715)
5. C. Green (page 716)
6. B. Yellow (page 716)
7. A. Red (page 715)
8. C. Green (page 716)

Multiple Choice

1. B (page 702)
2. A (page 715)
3. C (page 716)
4. D (page 717)
5. A (page 715)
6. C (page 716)
7. C (page 716)
8. D (page 717)
9. B (page 719)

10. D (page 718)

11. A (page 716)

12. B (page 715)

13. D (page 716)

14. D (page 715)

15. B-You must triage when multiple patients are involved to ensure that as many patients as possible receive optimal care. (page 715)

16. A (page 716)

17. B (page 716)

18. D (page 716)

19. C (page 716)

20. A (page 716)

21. D (page 716)

22. A (page 716)

23. B (page 716)

24. D (page 716)

25. C (page 716)

Vocabulary

1. Mass-casualty incident: An emergency situation involving more than one patient, and which can place such demand on equipment or personnel that the system is stretched to its limit or beyond. (page 714)

2. Extrication: Removal of a patient from entrapment or a dangerous situation or position, such as removal from a wrecked vehicle, avalanche, or rockslide. (page 717)

3. Secondary triage: An in-depth reassessment of a patient's condition that allows for a change in triage category. (page 719)

4. Triage: The process of sorting patients based on the severity of injury and medical need, to establish treatment and transportation priorities. (page 715)

5. Golden Hour: The average amount of time before a patient with multiple injuries starts to deteriorate rapidly; for every half hour after the first hour, the patient's chances of survival are cut in half. (page 720)

Fill-in

Initial Assessment	Triage Assessment (START)
1. Form general impression of the patients; Assess Mental Status	1. Get up and walk! Make clear announcement to all injured who can walk to proceed to a designated area (Green patients). Move through remaining patients assessing each casualty with triage tag. Provide minimal treatment (15 to 30 seconds/patient)
2. A-Assess the Airway – If necessary, open airway.	2. Respirations – open airway, tag
3. B-Assess Breathing – Provide rescue breathing, oxygen	3. Perfusion – radial pulse, stop excessive bleeding
4. C-Assess Circulation – Take pulse, control external bleeding, evaluate skin color, temperature, and condition	4. Mental status (do simultaneously with steps 2 and 3) - Tag

(page 719)

True/False

1. F (red tag) (page 716)
2. T (page 717)
3. T (page 720)
4. F (circulatory and respiratory systems have highest priority) (page 719)
5. T (page 716)
6. T (page 719)
7. T (page 720)
8. T (page 717)

Short Answer

1. Survival is probable with immediate care and stabilization without constant attention. (page 715)
2. -Get up and walk!
   (Patients sort themselves out. Those who walk are tagged GREEN.)
   -Respiration
   (Check for respiratory compromise. Open airway if closed.
   No respirations = tag BLACK;
   Respirations more than 30 breaths/min = tag RED;
   Respirations less than 30 breaths/min = proceed to perfusion)
   -Perfusion (Radial pulse check)
   -Mental status (Compromise of mental status)(pages 717–719)
3. Patients are transported to a treatment area where an in-depth reassessment takes place and allows for the patient's triage category to be changed. (page 719)
4. -Disruptive or hysterical patient, or patient with hysterical relative
   -Children
   -Patient is/becomes hypothermic (page 720)

Word Fun

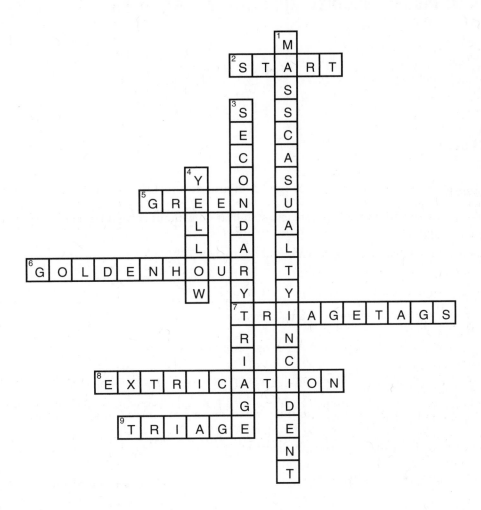

Calls to the Scene

1. #1 in first toboggan on a backboard; #3 in second toboggan on a backboard; until toboggans return, remaining patroller should treat #2 and #4 and reassure #5.

2. 1. BSI precautions include gloves at a minimum. Consider different gloves for each patient.

2. This will be a patient-by-patient decision based on assessment and availability. The highest identified need receives oxygen soonest upon availability.

3. Scene size-up, resource requests for personnel and equipment, triage assessment of patients, patient care as time permits after triage. Maintain command and assign personnel to most serious injuries as they arrive on the scene. You provide initial care to the three with life-threatening conditions after completing triage. Conduct initial airway maintenance immediately.

4. Confusion, chaos, public reaction, media, local public safety agencies arriving, lack of immediate resources, you are by yourself for five minutes (stress).

5. As personnel arrive, assign one individual to coordinate the movement of patients to an intermediate location or directly transfer to EMS as available. Consider staging of ambulances and any helicopters.

6. Initially use triage tags. Later complete detailed documentation. Obtain same from EMS. Detailed incident report, witness statements, and others as directed by area management.

3. -The 4-year-old should be triaged as first priority (red).

-The 27-year-old should be triaged as third priority (green).

-The 42-year-old should be tagged as fourth priority (black).

Chapter 29: Mass-Casualty Incident Management

Matching

1. F   (page 727)
2. A   (page 731)
3. E   (page 731)
4. C   (page 730)
5. D   (page 730)
6. B   (page 729)

Multiple Choice

1. D (page 728)
2. D – Extended operations also have finance and administrative sectors as part of their typical incident command structure. (page 728)
3. A (page 729)
4. D (page 730)
5. C (page 730)
6. D (page 731)
7. B (page 729)
8. D – Bus crashes are also an example of a mass-casualty incident. (page 726)

Vocabulary

1. Command post: The designated field command center where the incident commander and support personnel are located. (page 728)
2. Casualty collection area: A designated location where victims of a mass-casualty incident may be taken for triage and initial medical care prior to transport to a hospital. (page 731)
3. Triage officer: The individual in charge of the incident command triage section, who directs the sorting of patients into triage categories in a mass-casualty incident. (page 729)
4. Incident commander: The individual who has overall command of the scene in the field. (page 728)

Fill-in

1. incident command system (page 727)
2. command post (page 728)
3. safety officer (page 728)
4. disaster (page 731)
5. Triage (page 729)

True/False

1. T (page 727)
2. F (page 727)
3. F (page 726)
4. T (page 728)

Short Answer

1. -Incident commander, command post, and incident command system
   -On-site communications system
   -Adequate supply of long backboards, straps, or ties
   -Extrication/retrieval team
   -Triage office and designated triage area
   -Staffed patient collection area
   -Supply location adjacent to the treatment area
   -Staffed patient treatment area
   -Transportation officer and transport area
   -Staging area to hold resources until they are needed
   -Fire and law enforcement personnel
   -A secure perimeter
   (page 728)

2. Extrication area is where patients are disentangled and removed from a hazardous environment, allowing them to be moved to the triage area. (page 729)

3. In a disaster, a rescuer is to respond when requested and to report to the incident command system for assigned roles. (page 731)

Word Fun

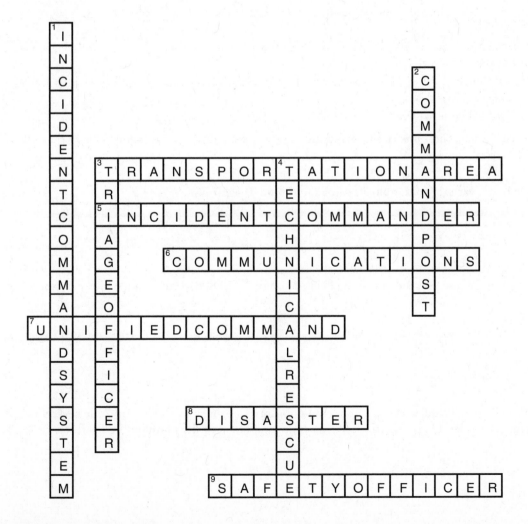

Calls to the Scene

1. -Direction and control of operations (incident commander identified, command post identified)

   -Security of the site (safety officer)

   -Coordination of search for potential missing/injured people at the avalanche site (skiers, riders, pedestrians in parking lot, people in cars)

   -Location for evacuation, triage, and emergency medical care (medical group coordinator)

   -Communications with local EMS and any other rescue services (transport)

   -Communication, via public relations department/individual at the area

Chapter 30: Pediatric Outdoor Emergency Care

Matching

1. F   (page 741)
2. B   (page 742)
3. A   (page 743)
4. E   (page 740)
5. D   (page 740)
6. C   (page 738)
7. K   (pages 745, 752)
8. L   (page 746)
9. M   (page 752)
10. N   (page 746)
11. I   (page 755)
12. P   (page 746)
13. O   (page 758)
14. J   (page 751)
15. H   (page 755)
16. G   (page 751)
17. R   (page 765)
18. S   (page 761)
19. Q   (pages 740, 762)

Multiple Choice

1. D (page 739)
2. C – Infants have very little use of their chest muscles to make their chest expand during inspiration, so they depend on the diaphragm. (page 739)
3. B (page 740)
4. C – Physical stimuli include light, warmth, cold, hunger, sound, and taste. (page 740)
5. D (page 751)
6. C (page 739)
7. A (page 739)
8. D (page 745)
9. D – Signs of complete airway obstruction also include an ineffective cough (no sound) and/or loss of consciousness. (page 746)
10. C – Cyanosis (C) is a late sign if seen at all. (page 751)
11. A (page 754)
12. B (page 755)
13. C – Never use alcohol or cold water to cool a patient. (page 756)
14. B (page 760)
15. A – In children, shock is rarely due to a cardiac event. Other common causes of shock in children include severe infection, traumatic injury with blood loss, severe allergic reaction, and blood or fluid around the heart. (page 758)
16. B (page 758)
17. B (page 759)
18. D (page 739)

19. C – Elevate (A) only injured extremities if needed. Only assist ventilations (B) if needed. Remove helmets (D) as the situation or local protocols dictate. (page 760)
20. C –Airway is top priority in ANY patient. (pages 749, 760)
21. C (page 760)
22. A (page 763)
23. B (page 753)
24. C (page 767)

Vocabulary

1. Work-of-breathing (WOB): Often seen as faster breathing, retractions along the chest wall, or the way the child sits and positions himself or herself. (page 743)
2. Altered level of consciousness: A mental state in which infants and children may be unresponsive, combative, or confused, may thrash about, or may drift into and out of an alert state. (page 756)
3. Epiglottitis: An infection of the soft tissue in the area above the vocal chords. (page 752)
4. Shaken baby syndrome: Bleeding within the head and damage to the cervical spine of an infant who has been intentionally and forcibly shaken; a form of child abuse. (page 766)

Fill-in

1. Pale skin (page 743)
2. adolescents (page 743)
3. status epilepticus (page 754)
4. Skin condition (page 745)
5. seizure (page 754)
6. ribs (page 761)
7. head (page 760)
8. head injury (page 760)
9. shock (page 758)
10. Growth plates (page 762)

True/False

1. T (page 740)
2. T (page 742)
3. F (page 743)
4. T (page 764)
5. F (page 760)
6. T (page 741)
7. F (page 749)
8. F (page 755)
9. F (page 755)
10. F (page 738)
11. T (page 758)
12. F (page 760)
13. T (page 758)
14. T (page 761)

Short Answer

1. These children are beginning to act more like adults and can think in concrete terms, respond sensibly to direct questions, and help take care of themselves. Talk to the child, not just the parent when obtaining a history. Give the child choices and explain any procedures. Give them simple explanations and carry on a conversation to distract them. Reward the child after a procedure. (page 740)

2. Minor: Partial-thickness burns involving less than 10% of the body surface.

    Moderate: Partial-thickness burns involving 10% to 20% of the body surface

    Critical: Any full-thickness burn; any partial-thickness burn involving more than 20% of the body surface; any burn involving the hands, feet, airway, or genitalia

    (page 763)

3. -Alcohol

    -Epilepsy, endocrine, or electrolyte abnormalities

    -Insulin or low blood glucose levels

    -Opiates or other drugs

    -Uremia

    -Trauma or temperature

    -Infection

    -Psychogenic or poison

    -Shock, stroke, or shunt obstruction (page 756)

4. -Nasal flaring

    -Grunting

    -Wheezing, stridor, or other abnormal airway sounds

    -Use of accessory muscles

    -Retractions

    -Tripod position (page 751)

Word Fun

Calls to the Scene

1. - BSI precautions.
   - Talk to the child directly.
   - Explain that you need to check for a pedal pulse before touching the child
   - Once equipment is prepared, show it to the child and explain how it will work.
   - Explain that moving the injured leg will be painful and ask the mother to help by allowing the child to squeeze her hand, etc.
   - Manipulate the leg as little as possible, but be expedient.
   - Transport in the position of comfort, allowing the child to dictate movement within reason.
   - Arrange for EMS transport.
2. - BSI precautions.
   - Position the child with the airway in a neutral sniffing position.
   - Insert a nasopharyngeal airway.
   - Assist ventilations with a BVM and 100% oxygen.
   - Arrange for rapid transport.
   - Continue assessment.
   - Obtain SAMPLE history.
3. - BSI precautions.
   -Suction the airway if needed.
   -Immediately begin assisting ventilations with a BVM and 100% oxygen.
   -Determine if c-spine control is needed.
   -Arrange for rapid transport.
   -Continue assessment.
   -Continue to monitor the airway and be alert for vomiting.
   -Monitor vital signs and keep patient warm to prevent hypothermia.

Chapter 31: Outdoor Adaptive Athletes

Matching

1. C   (page 777)
2. G   (page 775)
3. I   (page 774)
4. J   (page 779)
5. B   (page 777)

6. H   (page 778)
7. E   (page 777)
8. D   (page 778)
9. F   (page 777)
10. A   (page 774)

Multiple Choice

1. D (page 774)
2. C (page 775)
3. D (page 775)
4. D (page 775)
5. D (page 775)
6. A (page 776)
7. D (page 776)
8. C (page 777)
9. D (page 777)
10. D (page 777)

11. A (page 778)

12. D (page 778)

13. D (pages 778–779)

14. A (page 779)

15. D (page 779)

16. C (page 780)

17. B (page 780)

18. A (page 780)

19. D (page 781)

20. D (page 781)

Vocabulary

1. Impairment: Any loss or abnormality of psychological, physiologic, or anatomic structure or function. (page 774)

2. Disability: Any restriction in or lack of ability to perform an activity in the manner or within the range considered normal for a human being. (page 774)

3. Mental retardation: Refers to below-average intellectual capacity from birth or childhood associated with difficulties in learning and socialization. (page 775)

4. Cognitive disability: Is from damage or deterioration on any portion of the brain that affects the ability to process information, coordinate and control the body, and/or move in space. (page 776)

5. Amputation: Can be traumatic or surgical, or an individual can be born without one or more limbs. (page 777)

6. Spina bifida: A congenital malformation of the spinal cord (usually the bony spine in the same area) resulting in an anomaly. (page 779)

Fill-in

1. nordic, alpine (page 775)

2. mental, physical (page 775)

3. supervising adult, information (page 776)

4. Down syndrome (page 775)

5. assessment (page 777)

6. muscular dystrophy (page 779)

7. spina bifida, spinal cord injury (page 779)

8. spinal column (page 779)

9. stroke, brain trauma (page 780)

10. braces, appliances (page 781)

True/False

1. T (page 774)

2. F (page 775)

3. F (page 776)

4. F (page 777)

5. T (page 777)

6. T (page 780)

7. F (page 780)

8. F (page 781)

9. T (page 783)

Short Answer

1. Learning disabilities, cognitive disabilities, mental retardation, psychological disorders. (page 775)

2. Paraplegia, quadriplegia. (page 780)

3. A surgically created port on the abdominal wall to facilitate excrement of urine or feces. (page 781)

Word Fun

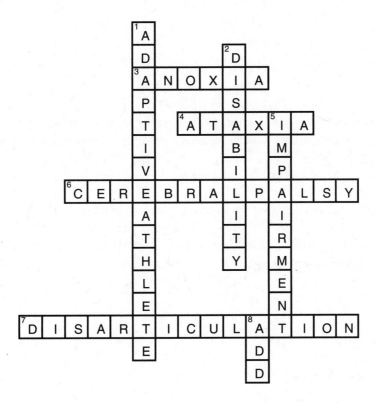

Calls to the Scene

1. -BSI precautions.

-Scene size-up and initial assessment, stabilizing ABCs. Initiate rapid transport.

-Remove patient from monosled.

-Perform rapid history and physical exam, concentrating on chief complaints as described by the patient.

-Stabilize the patient for rapid transport off the slope.

2. -BSI precautions.

-Perform initial assessment, stabilizing ABCs. Follow local procedures for deaf and hearing problems. For example, find an individual who can communicate to this patient or have an assistant write things on a pad as you ask questions.

-Follow procedures to ask permission to assist and to do a focused history and physical exam.

-Care for the patient's injuries.

-Evaluate and initiate transport as appropriate.